Treatment of Child Abuse

Treatment of Child Abuse

*Common Ground for Mental Health,
Medical, and Legal Practitioners*

EDITED BY

Robert M. Reece, M.D.

The Johns Hopkins University Press

BALTIMORE AND LONDON

Note to the Reader: This book discusses the treatment of child abuse *in general.* It is not intended to provide medical or legal advice regarding specific cases.

Drugs: The authors and publisher have made reasonable efforts to determine that the selection of drugs discussed in this text conforms to the practices of the general medical community. The medications described do not necessarily have specific approval by the U.S. Food and Drug Administration for use in the diseases for which they are recommended. In view of ongoing research, changes in governmental regulations, and the constant flow of information relating to drug therapy and drug reactions, the reader is urged to check the package insert of each drug for any change in indications and dosage and for warnings and precautions. This is particularly important when the recommended agent is a new and/or infrequently used drug.

© 2000 The Johns Hopkins University Press
All rights reserved. Published 2000
Printed in the United States of America on acid-free paper

9 8 7 6 5 4 3 2 1

The Johns Hopkins University Press
2715 North Charles Street
Baltimore, Maryland 21218-4363
www.press.jhu.edu

Library of Congress Cataloging-in-Publication Data will be found at the end of this book.
A catalog record for this book is available from the British Library.

ISBN 0-8018-6320-1

Contents

PART III / NEGLECT

PART IV / MUNCHAUSEN BY PROXY

PART V / MULTIPLE TRAUMATIZATION

PART VI / DISPOSITION ISSUES

Contents

PART VII / CHILD MALTREATMENT AND SOCIETY

Contributors

Randell C. Alexander, M.D., Ph.D.
Associate Professor of Pediatrics
Director, Center for Child Abuse
Morehouse University School of
   Medicine
Atlanta

Catherine C. Ayoub, R.N., M.N., Ed.D.
Assistant Professor of Psychiatry
Harvard University
Massachusetts General Hospital
Boston

Carol D. Berkowitz, M.D.
Professor of Clinical Pediatrics
Acting Chair, Harbor–UCLA Medical
   Center
University of California at Los Angeles
   School of Medicine

Maureen M. Black, Ph.D.
Professor of Pediatrics
Director, Growth and Nutrition Clinic
University of Maryland School of
   Medicine
Baltimore

Barbara W. Boat, Ph.D.
Associate Professor of Clinical
   Psychiatry and Pediatrics
The Childhood Trust
University of Cincinnati College of
   Medicine

Frank P. Cervone, J.D.
Executive Director
Support Center for Child Advocates
Philadelphia

Mark Chaffin, Ph.D.
Center on Child Abuse and Neglect
University of Oklahoma Health Sciences
   Center
Oklahoma City

Cindy W. Christian, M.D.
Assistant Professor of Pediatrics
University of Pennsylvania School of
   Medicine
Director, Child Abuse Services
The Children's Hospital of Philadelphia

Robin M. Deutsch, Ph.D.
Instructor, Harvard Medical School
Director of Training, Law, and
   Psychiatry Service
Massachusetts General Hospital
Boston

Lesley Devoe, M.S.W., L.C.S.W.
Adjunct Professor and Therapist
University of Maine, Orono
Graduate School of Social Work
Rockland, Maine

David B. Doolittle, Psy.D.
Clinical Instructor in Psychology
Clinical Associate, Law and Psychiatry
   Service
Harvard Medical School
Massachusetts General Hospital
Boston

Kerry M. Drach, Psy.D.
Child Abuse Program at the Spurwink
   Clinic
Portland, Maine

Howard Dubowitz, M.D.
Professor of Pediatrics
Director, Child Protection Program
University of Maryland School of
    Medicine
Baltimore

Megan L. Elam, J.D.
Deputy District Attorney
Cumberland County District Attorney's
    Office
Portland, Maine

Martin A. Finkel, D.O.
Associate Professor of Pediatrics
Medical Director, Center for Children's
    Support
University of Medicine and Dentistry of
    New Jersey
School of Osteopathic Medicine
Stratford, New Jersey

Richard J. Gelles, Ph.D.
Joanne and Raymond Welsh Chair of
    Child Welfare and Family Violence
Professor of Social Welfare
Research Director, Center for the Study
    of Youth Policy
University of Pennsylvania
Philadelphia

Stephanie Hamerman, M.D.
Medical Director, Child and Adolescent
    Outpatient Psychiatry
Assistant Professor of Psychiatry
New Jersey Medical School
University of Medicine and Dentistry of
    New Jersey
Brunswick, New Jersey

Rochelle F. Hanson, Ph.D.
Assistant Professor of Psychology
Medical University of South Carolina
Charleston

Robert Kinscherff, J.D., Ph.D.
Children and the Law Program
Law and Psychiatry Service
Massachusetts General Hospital
Boston

David J. Kolko, Ph.D.
Associate Professor of Child Psychiatry
    and Psychology
Director, Special Services Unit
University of Pittsburgh Medical Center
Western Psychiatric Institute and Clinic
Pittsburgh

Stephen Ludwig, M.D.
Professor of Pediatrics
Associate Physician-in-Chief
Children's Hospital of Philadelphia
University of Pennsylvania School of
    Medicine

Mary B. Meinig, M.S.W.
Office of the Family and Children's
    Ombudsman
State of Washington
Tukwila, Washington

John E. B. Myers, J.D.
Professor of Law
University of the Pacific
McGeorge School of Law
Sacramento, California

Erna Olafson, Ph.D., Psy.D.
Assistant Professor of Clinical Psychiatry
    and Pediatrics
The Childhood Trust
University of Cincinnati College of
    Medicine

Cris Ratiner, Ph.D.
Staff Psychologist
The Human Relations Service
Wellesley, Massachusetts

Robert M. Reece, M.D.
Clinical Professor of Pediatrics
Tufts University School of Medicine
Director, Institute for Professional
    Education
Massachusetts Society for the Prevention
    of Cruelty to Children
Boston

Lawrence R. Ricci, M.D.
Clinical Associate Professor of Pediatrics
University of Vermont College of
    Medicine
Clinical Associate Professor of Pediatrics
University of New England College of
    Osteopathic Medicine
Director, Spurwink Child Abuse
    Program
Portland, Maine

Thomas A. Roesler, M.D.
Director, Hasbro Pediatric Partial
    Hospital Program
Brown University School of Medicine
Providence, Rhode Island

Suzanne Rosenberg, M.D.
Instructor, Harvard University
Attending Pediatric Psychiatrist
Spaulding Rehabilitation Hospital
Boston

Daniel P. Ryan, M.D.
Assistant Professor of Surgery
Harvard Medical School
Massachusetts General Hospital
Boston

Anita M. St. Onge, J.D.
Research Associate
Edmund S. Muskie School of Public
    Service
Portland, Maine

Benjamin E. Saunders, Ph.D.
Associate Professor of Psychology
Director, Family and Child Program
National Crime Victims Research and
    Treatment Center
Medical University of South Carolina
Charleston

Toni Seidl, R.N., M.S.W.
Senior Health Consultant
Support Center for Child Advocates
Children's Hospital of Philadelphia

Robert L. Sheridan, M.D.
Associate Professor of Surgery
Harvard Medical School
Assistant Chief of Staff
Shriners Burn Institute
Boston

Cynthia Cupit Swenson, Ph.D.
Assistant Professor of Psychology
Medical University of South Carolina
Charleston

Robert H. Wharton, M.D.
Chief, Developmental and Behavioral
    Pediatrics
Assistant Professor of Pediatrics
Massachusetts General Hospital
Spaulding Rehabilitation Hospital
Boston

Cathy Spatz Widom, Ph.D.
Professor of Criminal Justice and
    Psychology
School of Criminal Justice
The University at Albany

Preface

Since the 1960s there has been a prodigious outpouring of literature on the subject of child maltreatment from the disciplines of mental health, medicine, and the law. Through the decades, several definitions of child abuse have evolved, with different disciplines favoring different emphases and each state establishing its own legal and legislative parameters. For our purposes here, an overarching definition from the federal Child Abuse Prevention and Treatment Act (1974) provides a useful framework. Child abuse, the act states broadly, is "the physical and mental injury, sexual abuse, negligent treatment or maltreatment of a child under the age of 18 by a person who is responsible for the child's welfare under circumstances which indicate that the child's health and welfare is harmed or threatened thereby."[2]

During the early period of this discourse, the major emphasis was on means of establishing the diagnosis. This involved the development and testing of various techniques in interviewing children about possible abuse. It involved closer examination and reevaluation of what was normal and what was abnormal in childhood behavior and development. For medical personnel, it meant taking a closer look at what characteristics of injury distinguished abuse from nonintentional injuries and from conditions of a medical etiology. An additional dimension was introduced when professionals whose traditional ethical obligation was the well-being of their client or patient were given the new task of formulating sensitive information to fit the needs of the legal process.

The growing and continuing attention to diagnosing child abuse and its designation as a legally reportable offense in all fifty states has resulted in an increasingly solid statistical base from which child abuse can be examined, although—as you will read in the following pages—much work is still needed to accurately quantify and analyze information about this sometimes elusive but all too pervasive occurrence. According to the National Clearinghouse on Child Abuse and Neglect Information, in 1996 there were more than two million reports alleging maltreatment of more than three million children, a rate of 44 per 1,000 children in the population. Child protective services substantiated abuse or neglect in nearly one million of those children—an 18 percent increase since 1990.[4]

Who is reporting? You are. More than half the reports came from professionals, and almost two-thirds of those that were eventually substantiated came from professionals—medical, social services, education, or law enforcement sources.

Who is being abused? Fifteen children of every 10,000 in the population, according to the National Clearinghouse (1996 statistics). They are almost half and half boys and girls—47 percent male, 53 percent female. Approximately one-quarter of them are under the age of 4, more than half under the age of 7. Approximately 15 percent of them are eventually removed from their homes. In 1996, at least 1,077 children officially died from maltreatment, most of them under the age of 4. The true incidence of fatality from child maltreatment is unknown.

And who is doing the abusing? More than 75 percent of the perpetrators are parents, another 11 percent other relatives of the victimized child. Males are more likely to sexually abuse, women more likely to neglect.

Beyond the statistics, those of us who work with abused and neglected children are witness to the suffering, degradation, and damaged lives that are the painful and tragic human side of child maltreatment. As we have become more competent at diagnosis, investigators have broadened their scope to examine the short- and long-term consequences of childhood victimization. Outcome studies are seen more regularly in the peer-reviewed literature in recent years, particularly with regard to sexually abused victims but increasingly also focusing on outcomes in physically and emotionally abused and neglected children.

The subject of this book is what occurs during the intervening period between diagnosis and outcome. There is a growing realization that treatment of the devastating effects of child maltreatment simply does not occur for the majority of victims. This may be due to any of a number of reasons—a lack of understanding of what is needed, the unavailability of trained professionals, or the increasingly limited access of these victims to health and social services.

Information about how to care for victims of the various forms of child maltreatment over the long term is sparse. When found at all, it is usually narrowly focused, attending to only one category of abuse. There has been no single reference source for the clinician who needs to know which modality of treatment might be most appropriate for a given child trying to cope with the aftermath of physical, emotional, or sexual abuse. The clinician also may not have the luxury of locally available specialists to whom referrals can be made. Although a book alone cannot equip the mental health or medical practitioner to help with all the problems of abused patients, much of the long-term treatment is, of necessity, delivered near home. This book seeks to provide guidelines for such treatment. Consultation with others in the provision of treatment is a well-established model in other fields of practice, and it can and should be employed by the primary care clinician in this complex field, as well.

As the reader of these pages will see, even those whose professional lives are dedicated to establishing treatment norms do not always agree about philosophy of and approach to treatment.

Especially because the treatment of child abuse is uncharted territory, it is helpful for the caregiver to keep the goals of treatment in mind. Although these goals obviously differ from child to child, some general principles can apply. The general goals of treatment for child abuse are, as nearly as possible, to restore or create in the child and family a state of good physical and mental health.

How to Use This Book

The book is divided into parts that address four categories of abuse, which are described below and in the text. Within each part, the chapters are arranged to provide the current thinking about the different forms of child abuse treatment, both in the immediate postdiagnostic period and for the longer term. In general, the initial postdiagnostic period can be thought of as the first few weeks following diagnosis. Also included are chapters that address so-called treatment-resistant families, treatment of offenders, forensic implications, and the current state of research in treatment.

A brief introduction here of each of the forms of abuse considered in this volume will give the practitioner an overview of the problem and perhaps some idea of how a particular case may be classified and treated.

Sexual abuse.　The American Academy of Pediatrics defines childhood sexual abuse as "the engaging of a child in sexual activities that the child cannot comprehend, for which the child is developmentally unprepared and cannot give informed consent, and/or that violate the social and legal taboos of society." Sexual abuse describes a range of behaviors from sexual touching or fondling to forced masturbation to digital or object penetration to sexual intercourse. Exposing a child to exhibitionism or other forms of sexual behavior are also considered forms of sexual abuse, as is inappropriate talk about sex. Using a child in the production of pornography is another form of childhood sexual abuse.

The incidence of childhood sexual abuse is difficult to determine, but recent statistics suggest that about 1 percent of all children will experience some form of sexual abuse each year.[1] Twelve percent of the approximately one million cases of substantiated child abuse annually in this country involve sexual abuse.

Physical abuse.　According to the National Center on Child Abuse and Neglect, physical abuse is child abuse that "results in physical injury, including fractures, burns, bruises, welts, cuts, and/or internal injury. Physical abuse often occurs in the name of discipline or punishment and ranges from a slap of the hand to use of an object."[3]

As you will see in chapters 6 through 10, the results of physical abuse encompass a spectrum of injuries, from minor bruises to broken bones to serious head injury to severe multisystem trauma and death. Twenty-four percent of child abuse victims suffer physical abuse. Of these children, 160,000 are thought to suffer from serious or life-threatening injuries.

Neglect.　More children are neglected than suffer from all the other types of child maltreatment combined. Neglect can be physical or psychological/emotional or both. Often defined as an act of omission rather than commission, neglect accounts for more than half the *substantiated* reports of child maltreatment in this country—more than 500,000 children a year. Nearly half of all deaths related to child maltreatment are attributed to neglect.

Neglect means that a child's essential needs are not met—from the basics of food, clothing, shelter, education, and medical care to the positive emotional interaction that is necessary for a child to develop and maintain a sense of security and psychological safety. The results can be fatal, and many survivors of neglect suffer lifelong physical and emotional effects.

Munchausen by proxy.　A relatively uncommon disorder that is receiving increasing attention, Munchausen by proxy (MBP) is the name given to a subset of factitious disorders in which a caretaker—almost always a mother or mother surrogate—simulates or produces illness in a child to enhance her role as caretaker. It is hard to know how widespread this disorder is, because secrecy is at its very core. It is probably more common than suspected. What is known about MBP is the damage it causes—some sort of morbidity results for nearly all the children who are victims of MBP, and some studies have found the mortality rate to be as high as 22 percent.

We hope that professionals caring for children and their families will find this book useful and that children and their families will be the ultimate beneficiaries.

R E F E R E N C E S

1. American Academy of Pediatrics, Committee on Child Abuse and Neglect Policy Statement. Guidelines for the evaluation of sexual abuse of children (RE 9202). *Pediatrics* 1991;87:254–260. Also at http://www.aap.org/policy/03773.html.

2. Child Abuse Prevention and Treatment Act of 1974, Public Law 92-247, U.S. Statutes at Large, 88, 4–8.

3. National Center on Child Abuse and Neglect. Washington, DC. 1988.

4. National Clearinghouse on Child Abuse and Neglect Information. *Reports from the States to the National Child Abuse and Neglect Data System* (NCANDS). http://child.cornell.edu. 1994.

Acknowledgments

The "team approach" has become so hackneyed a concept that I am somewhat reluctant to use it when thanking the many who have helped shape this book, but this was truly an expedition into uncharted territory, and a team was necessary for doing it. From the inception of the idea of the book nearly five years ago to the dispatching of the final copy to the Johns Hopkins University Press, I have been blessed by help from a team at the Press.

First I would like to thank Jackie Wehmueller, who had the initial idea of compiling a book such as this. She has been unfailingly pleasant, patient, and committed to the project, despite delays and changes in the complexion of the book. She is an ideal editor with whom to work. Ronnie Henderson, the developmental editor, took the chapter manuscripts and sculpted them into a graceful, unified whole. The book owes much of its elegance to her work, and I thank her for that. Thanks also to Anne Whitmore, our copyeditor at the Press, the last person to touch the text with her talent. Anne's attention to the meaning of each and every sentence has rendered the book accessible and understandable to all who may read it. Her precision and attention to detail have minimized errors of content and citation.

My part in this project, representing many hours and much energy, I dedicate to my wife, Betsy, and to our children.

Finally, my heartfelt thanks go to the authors. Not only do these dedicated people provide care to the victims of child abuse, but they conduct research, contribute to the generation of new knowledge in the field, and help in the dissemination of that knowledge. Their reward for this effort is the satisfaction of contributing to the betterment of the lives of children they will never know.

PART I

Sexual Abuse

Chapter 1

Initial Medical Management of the Sexually Abused Child

Martin A. Finkel, D.O.

Victims of childhood and adolescent sexual abuse and their families have complex medical needs. Clinicians involved with initial medical management of the sexually abused child must address a number of concerns—the significance of the physical lesions associated with sexual abuse, the child's personal body image, continued follow-up to detect sexually transmitted diseases, evaluation of genitourinary and gastrointestinal injury, the possibility of pregnancy, and the framing of the medical diagnosis. This diagnosis, which should be as specific as possible, will be involved in subsequent medical, social, and legal considerations. The role of the medical clinician continues to expand into the postdiagnostic period, as more becomes known about the treatment needs of victims.

GENERAL CONSIDERATIONS

Society's recognition of the sexual victimization of children has resulted in a partnership among physicians, child protection workers, and law enforcement. Physicians have an important role in the recognition and validation of allegations of child sexual abuse. Sexual abuse constitutes approximately 10 percent of referrals to child protective services. Prevalence studies suggest that one in four girls and one in five boys will experience some form of inappropriate sexual contact before turning 18. Every physician will need to learn about the dynamics of sexual victimization and behavioral indicators of abuse and be able to conduct a thorough examination to diagnose and treat residua of sexual abuse.

Sexual victimization of children is very different from physical maltreatment in two important dynamics. The first is that most perpetrators do not intend to actually harm their victims; because of this, few children present with significant and diagnostic injuries. The second dynamic is that few children disclose their experience immediately following the sexually inappropriate action, and this results in some diagnostic challenges in identifying residua and collecting forensic evidence. The most available evidence in child sexual abuse is the child's statement about the experience. Therefore, physicians must understand the dynamics of sexual victimization and be able to obtain a medical history from the child in a manner that is nonleading, facilitating, and empathetic. An appropriately obtained medical history will assist the physician in assessing the residual effects, both physical and psychological, as well directing a treatment plan.

Once disclosure of sexual abuse has been made, physical examination completed, and laboratory results received, decisions about treatment can be made. (The importance of documentation and its legal implications, an important component of the therapeutic goal of recovery, are discussed in chapter 23.)

For the treating health professional the most relevant issues are

- the child's concern about her or his body image,
- the interpretation of the lesions residual to the sexual abuse,
- the medical follow-up for sexually transmitted diseases,
- conditions in the genitourinary and gastrointestinal systems associated with the abuse, and
- the formulation of a final medical diagnosis.

BODY IMAGE CONCERNS

The literature suggests that an abusive experience may change the way sexually abused children view themselves.[5] An important initial focus of therapy is to discuss with abused children their anxiety about what may be wrong with their body as a result of the abuse. The stigmatization and shame experienced by most victims contribute to a feeling of being "damaged goods."[18] There is also an association between eating disorders, body image, and sexual victimization.[36]

Concerns about body intactness may stem from a child's incorrect perception about the degree of physical invasion that was experienced. Children may say that objects have been placed all the way inside of them although a medical examination does not support this. It is important to understand this common discrepancy and to articulate the reason for this discrepancy in the medical record, when this misperception is present. This discrepancy should not be surprising; children should not be expected to have an adult understanding of sexual activities. Limited research documents that children's abilities to understand the difference between "in" and "on" vary at different developmental ages.[16]

That events were not physically invasive, however, does not mean they were not psychologically invasive. The medical clinician should assume that any sexually inappropriate contact has the potential for significant psychological sequelae. A comprehensive assessment of the impact of the victimization is most often made by a mental health professional, but medical personnel are in an ideal position to observe and record distress or alterations of mood during the child's examination.

Children should be given an opportunity to express any worries or concerns about their body while the medical history is being taken. This may be the first time they have an opportunity to voice concerns and reveal distortions of thinking about bodily integrity. Knowing these concerns prior to proceeding with the examination is essential and is an important component of diagnosing and treating the residual trauma of the sexual victimization.

Such concerns may sometimes take unusual forms:

- An 8-year-old girl asked if it was true that you could get breast cancer if someone put his mouth on your breast.
- A 9-year-old girl worried for months that sperm was still inside her after the perpetrator had ejaculated onto her genitalia.

- A 6-year-old girl was convinced that she was pregnant because when she sat on the potty and looked in the mirror her tummy puffed out.
- A 13-year-old thought that people could tell by the way she walked that "she had done those disgusting things."
- A 10-year-old boy was worried that he was going to get the "dying disease"— AIDS.

Each of these worries was successfully addressed by identifying the specific concerns and discussing them during a general physical examination. Even children who express no concerns about their body during the encounter with the physician may breathe a sigh of relief when the physician tells them after the examination that they are fine. Some children may require continued reassurance for a long period of time.

Nonoffending parents also need the reassurance that their child is not physically altered. After the examination, the physician must decide what information to share with the victim and nonoffending parent. The extent of the information will depend on the child's age, emotional stability, and expressed concerns. It is important to remember that an overly paternalistic attitude in withholding information to "protect the child" may inadvertently represent to children a further betrayal of trust. In most cases, it is sufficient to tell children that any injuries have now healed, that they are fine, and that no one could ever tell they had been injured. Older children may need reassurance that their experience will not directly interfere with their ability to have children when they are adults. Male victims may worry that their experience will make them become homosexual, and a discussion should address these fears.

INTERPRETATION OF RESIDUAL LESIONS

Two of the most significant challenges for the examining physician are differentiating between accidental and nonaccidental patterns of injury and interpreting the significance of healed changes in anogenital anatomy without knowledge of the premorbid state. The retrospective interpretation of healed posttraumatic findings can be difficult. There are several reasons for this, among them:

- Acute injuries to the genitalia are infrequent. For most children, sexually inappropriate activities are with a person they know, who does not intend to harm them physically.
- When injuries do occur they are generally superficial and heal without posttraumatic residua.

Most children do not disclose abuse until they feel safe, sometimes long after the last contact. Consequently, at the time of disclosure, they may have no acute signs of trauma. Only a small percentage of children sustain significant injuries that heal with distinct and diagnostic posttraumatic findings. When acute injuries are significant enough to heal with the formation of granulation tissue, the chronic healed posttraumatic lesion may appear different than anticipated.

Acute injuries should be reexamined to verify complete healing and to document the resolution of the injury. The frequency of reexamination will depend on the extent of the injury. Superficial injuries generally heal within 96 hours if not complicated by an infection. Consequently, one follow-up examination is usually sufficient to document the somewhat predictable healing of acute superficial injuries. More extensive injuries heal with the development of scar tissue, and so examinations over a longer period (up to a year) may be required. There are three stages of healing—fibrin clot formation, proliferation of neo-vascularized granulation tissue, and eventual wound retraction—and each provides a distinctly different appearance to the injury and should be observed and documented.

Longitudinal studies reflect the difficulty of predicting the appearance of the healed posttraumatic findings based on the appearance of the acute injury.[14,30] Although some injuries will heal with predictable posttraumatic findings, many will heal with unanticipated residua, such as distortions of genital structures due to scar tissue or surprisingly minimal residua that would not appear to be reflective of the extent of the initial injury. Larger clinical studies are necessary to understand the subtle alterations of anogenital anatomy that reflect healed trauma.

Another variable in interpreting residua is the age of the child. If a girl was injured when prepubertal, the effect of puberty and estrogen's effect on the vestibular tissues complicate the recognition of scar tissue. Estrogen changes the thin mucosa of the prepubertal hymen and vestibular structures to a thickened, redundant, elastic appearance, from a pink to white coloration similar to scar tissue. In puberty, only the most obvious changes in the hymenal membrane can be said to be a result of sexual contact if no knowledge of the premorbid state exists. Longitudinal studies demonstrating developmental changes of genital structures will help clinicians differentiate the residua from sexual trauma and changes in the appearance of the hymen as a result of normal development.

In spite of the increasingly common use of child-sensitive examination techniques, for some children the examination can be an emotionally difficult experience. To minimize the need for reexamination, every attempt should be made to assure that the initial examination is thorough and conducted appropriately. When follow-up examinations are necessary, they should be conducted by the same examiner whenever possible.

FOLLOW-UP EXAMINATIONS FOR SEXUALLY TRANSMITTED DISEASES

Guidelines for treatment and follow-up care for sexually transmitted diseases (STDs) have been established by the Centers for Disease Control and Prevention. Follow-up care is required when an STD has been diagnosed.

When a sexually transmitted disease has been diagnosed and treated in a child, therapeutic efficacy must be assessed. Serologic retesting 12 weeks following sexual contact will provide time for antibodies to have developed for syphilis, human immunodeficiency virus (HIV), and hepatitis B.[21,25,35] The decision to retest periodically will depend upon risk factors known to be present in the abuser. Whenever an STD has been identified in a child, be sure to confirm the specific test utilized and its specificity for the infection.[3,33] Use confirmatory tests to minimize the potential for false positives or misinterpretations.[24,37]

The follow-up schedule is less clear for the child who has had a history of genital-to-genital or genital-to-anal contact, or contact with potentially infected genital secretions, but who shows no signs and symptoms of an STD in the initial exam. Human papillomavirus (HPV) is a particular problem; it may not become apparent clinically for months to years following contact and has the potential for malignant transformation, raising many questions regarding long-term management.[20] Guidelines for management and follow-up examinations when HPV is present in young children are yet to be developed.

HIV presents another challenge. Screening for HIV should be integrated into diagnostic and follow-up protocols.[7,15,19,23] Gellert and colleagues[22] surveyed professionals in health and social services to begin to identify the number of children who contracted HIV as a direct result of sexual abuse. In the survey, of the 41 children identified nationwide as seropositive for HIV, 28 had sexual abuse as the only risk factor. Knowledge of the alleged perpetrator's serostatus and behavioral risk profile simplifies clinical decision making regarding testing; if either of these aspects is positive or the child has symptoms of HIV or another STD, then follow-up testing of the child victim must be done at six-month intervals for two years, until seronegativity can be assured. Whenever possible, the alleged perpetrator should be tested. Knowledge of the perpetrator's serologic status for HIV, syphilis, and hepatitis B, as well as the presence of HPV, has the potential to reduce the retesting of the child victim.

Whenever contact with infected genital secretions has occurred, screening for hepatitis B should be done. The prevalence of hepatitis B as a result of sexual abuse is unknown.

Although fomites have been considered a mode of transmission of STDs in children, since the studies by Shore[34] and Elmrost[11] in the 1970s, no scientific papers have been published about this subject. Position statements by the American Academy of Pediatrics,[2] the American Academy of Dermatology,[1] and the Centers for Disease Control and Prevention[6] have recommended that sexually inappropriate contact be considered the mode of transmission when a sexually transmitted disease is present in a child, until proven otherwise, except when vertical transmission or transmission through blood products is a possibility. When children present with a sexually transmitted disease whose mode of transmission is not apparent, it is not appropriate to simply assume that the mode of transmission is through fomites. The failure to identify the mode of transmission may be due to limitations of our investigatory skills. Until scientific support exists for the nonsexual transmission of microbes, we must assume that direct transmission occurs from infected person to noninfected person.

When testing for sexually transmitted diseases has been completed and if children are old enough to understand the implications of the results, they should be assured that they will be informed of all test results and retested as appropriate. A follow-up phone call as soon as the results of outstanding tests are available is comforting to children and parents and also provides the clinician another opportunity to address any additional concerns.

GENITOURINARY COMPLICATIONS

Obtaining information about symptom-specific complaints associated with inappropriate sexual contact is important in addressing medical needs and follow-up care, but it is equally important in confirming alleged contact. Symptom-specific complaints may be elicited when obtaining a history from the child. Whenever possible, the history of the alleged events should be obtained from the child alone, without the presence of an adult caretaker.

One way to obtain a history of symptom-specific complaints is to ask children if any of the things that happened to them hurt. This question is obvious, both in regard to the information it may elicit as well as establishing the fact that the examining physician is seeing the child to diagnose and treat residual effects of the alleged abuse. If the child responds by answering yes, then it is appropriate to ask what happened that hurt. A child might state that the alleged perpetrator placed his finger in her coochie. If so, continue by asking the child to explain whether it hurt while she was being touched or afterwards. If she responds that it hurt afterwards, ask her to explain in what way it hurt.

Genitourinary complications that must be evaluated include infection, voiding dysfunction, urethral prolapse, labial agglutination, pregnancy prophylaxis or termination, and the presence of foreign bodies.

Infection and Voiding Dysfunction

Trauma to the urethral meatus that occurs in the context of intercourse is known in the adult literature as honeymoon cystitis and can be associated with urinary tract infections.[28] Trauma to the urethra appears to increase the potential for bacteria to ascend into the bladder. The development of an infection depends in part on the colonization of the urethra and urodynamic characteristics of the patient. Similarly, trauma to the urethral meatus, which may occur during genital fondling, vulvar coitus, or intercourse, may result in temporally related voiding symptoms and urinary tract infections. The prevalence of this syndrome of urinary tract infections and subsequent voiding dysfunction (dysuria, urgency, frequency, incontinence) has not been thoroughly studied in sexually abused children.[10]

In a pilot study to assess the frequency of the complaint of dysuria as the result of genital fondling, Finkel[17] found that 23 percent of 105 children responded that it hurt to urinate following genital fondling. A full genitourinary review of systems could eliminate or explain all other causative factors. Thus, in the absence of alternative explanation, complaints of dysuria temporally related to a specific event establish that the child experienced trauma to the periurethral area with a degree of medical certainty. When a child presents in close temporal proximity to the alleged sexual contact, a urinalysis may demonstrate microscopic hematuria. A urine culture will also assist in establishing the possibility of infection. Although most children report resolution of their symptomatology, some may go on to develop voiding dysfunction.[10]

Urethral Prolapse

Urethral prolapse is also seen in association with trauma related to sexual abuse of girls. Urethral prolapse can present in a rather dramatic way and may be interpreted as acute genital trauma.[27] Although there is an association between sexual abuse and prolapse, this condition may also present itself spontaneously or in association with a urinary tract infection.[29] An appropriately obtained history can generally assist in determining whether sexual abuse is a contributing factor. Urethral prolapse is most commonly seen in African American patients and can generally be managed medically.[38] When urethral prolapse is sufficient to obscure the vestibule, follow-up examinations may be necessary to observe the hymenal membrane fully.

Labial Agglutination

Agglutination of the medial aspects of the labia minora may be seen as the healed effect of inflammation. Its association with sexual abuse has been well documented, but agglutination is a commonly acquired condition, seen also in nonabused girls.[4] When agglutination is present in alleged victims of sexual abuse, care must be taken to establish a temporal relationship between the agglutination and the alleged abuse; otherwise this finding is considered nonspecific.

Some girls will present with agglutination sufficient to obscure the visualization of the hymenal membrane and the structures of the vaginal vestibule. With this degree of agglutination, treatment is required to reveal the structures posterior to the agglutination and determine the presence of hymenal injuries. Topical estrogen cream generally will produce successful dehiscence of the labia, although thick agglutinations may require treatment over several weeks. If the agglutination has resulted in a pinpoint opening in the labia minora, there is the potential for hydronephrosis secondary to an outlet obstruction, and an ultrasound should be obtained immediately. If there is no evidence of back-pressure, then medical management is indicated regardless of the apparent degree of obstruction.

Exogenous estrogen will dehisce the agglutination but will result in a leukorrhea and change the appearance of the genital tissues. Therefore, it may be necessary to examine the child not only shortly following the dehiscence but also after the estrogen effect wears off. Published reports associating agglutination and substantiated sexual abuse are insufficient to conclude an abusive etiology for labial agglutination.

Pregnancy Prophylaxis or Termination

If the victim of sexual abuse is an adolescent female and the assault involved intercourse, the possibility of pregnancy must be addressed. Because only a small percentage of adolescent victims of sexual abuse will experience their contact as a result of forcible rape, few adolescents will present immediately following the experience. Of those who are raped, many will not disclose the rape immediately, due to either threats by the perpetrator or embarrassment and feelings of shame. Therefore, the opportunity for postcoital contraception is uncommon. When adolescents present within 48 hours of an assault, the postcoital use of high-dose estrogens should be offered and its efficacy and complications explained.[12]

Whenever an adolescent victim is being evaluated for allegations of sexual abuse and is not presenting as an acute assault, it is important to obtain a pregnancy test. The adolescent can generally provide information regarding the extent of sexual contact and whether the perpetrator used any pregnancy prophylaxis. If the victim is pregnant, then options regarding continuation or termination of the pregnancy must be discussed. This counseling must be carried out with objectivity and sensitivity in order to reduce the emotional sequelae of this untoward event and help the adolescent make the most appropriate decision.

Adolescents who experience intercourse as a result of sexual abuse and are not pregnant remain at risk for developing sexually reactive behaviors, placing them at risk for future assault, pregnancy, and sexually transmitted diseases.[26] To avoid these potential complications, adolescents must be directed to appropriate mental health services. (See chapter 3 for further discussion of these behaviors and how they can be treated.)

Whenever an adolescent presents with a pregnancy, the clinician should consider sexual abuse as a possibility and tactfully explore this with the patient. A pregnancy may be the first opportunity to disclose sexual abuse, or it may raise concerns that a pregnancy that appeared to result from consensual intercourse with an age-mate actually is the result of acting-out behaviors that can be traced to an abusive experience.

Foreign bodies

Foreign bodies in the vagina may be observed in sexually abused children, as well as in those presenting with a history of persistent vaginal discharge but no history of sexual abuse.[32] The most commonly found foreign body in the vagina of prepubertal children is the wood spicules of toilet paper. Unusual foreign bodies will raise greater concern about the possibility of sexual abuse as a contributing factor. When toilet paper is present, removal without anesthesia, facilitated by the use of video colposcopy, has proven to be an appropriate alternative to an examination under anesthesia. Some children will present with a vaginal discharge and bleeding, triggering the suspicion of sexual abuse. Removal of the foreign body and a follow-up examination once the friable inflamed mucosa heals is necessary to determine whether trauma-specific injuries are present.

GASTROINTESTINAL COMPLICATIONS

Gastrointestinal complications include anal trauma and encopresis.

Anal Trauma

Children who experience anal abuse may be able to provide a history of symptom-specific complaints temporally related to the alleged sexual contact. Because the anorectal canal is not naturally lubricated, penetration into the canal without the use of a lubricant will generally result in subsequent pain associated with bowel movements. Because of the external anal sphincter's ability to dilate to large diameters for defecation, the residual tissue damage due to anal penetration can be variable. In a study of consenting adults engaged in sodomy, only 3 percent noted bleeding following anal intercourse.[13] Although this population is different in many regards from sexually abused children, this study reflects an incidence of residual damage that appears consistent with the infrequent history of bleeding in older children experiencing anal intercourse. As in the case of vaginal penetration, a problem exists regarding a potential discrepancy between the child's perception of penetration and the actual event. Significant controversy exists regarding the interpretation of anal findings following sexual abuse. Caution should be used until a more substantive clinical research base exists.[8,9]

Encopresis

Some children who experience trauma to the anus may develop encopresis, with or without fecal retention. The exact incidence of this complication is not known. When a child presents with a history of anal trauma, it is important to obtain a stooling history encompassing not only the period prior to the alleged abuse but also subsequent to it, to identify whether preexisting conditions were operative and if treatment and follow-up are indicated. When a child presents with encopresis, it is appropriate to address sexual abuse as one of the differential considerations.

FORMULATION OF THE FINAL REPORT

A medical record that clearly states the physician's diagnostic assessment and the basis for it should be written in a clear, objective, and noneditorial style. The report should have a consistent format that assures inclusion of all information used to reach the diagnosis and recommended treatment plan. A report that is factual and educates its reader is invaluable to child protective services, law enforcement officers, courts, defense attorneys, and other medical practitioners. Reports that are illegible, lacking in detail, and/or biased serve little purpose and are a disservice to the child. A complete medical report will play an important role should the case proceed to either civil or criminal actions and may reduce the need for court testimony. (See chapter 23 for a further discussion of the importance of a report for forensic purposes.)

When articulating a diagnosis, it is insufficient simply to conclude that evidence from the physical examination is consistent with the history and neither confirms nor denies the allegations. Conclusions such as these are easily challenged. Examination findings may be categorized as follows:

- medical findings that can be stated to confirm the allegations with medical certainty,
- nonspecific findings temporally related to specific events that can be corroborated by history or other investigative details and thus support an association between the findings and the alleged contact,
- findings that are nonspecific and thus are seen in both abused and nonabused children, and
- findings that have no relevance to the allegations.

When there are no physical findings but clear historical details reflective of sexual contact, the clinician must explain the factors that account for such a possibility. If there are no residua to an alleged contact, then state the reasons this may be the case. If a child provides a history that reflects his perception of penetration and the physical examination does not confirm it, potential reasons for this discrepancy need to be explained.

Supplemental reports will be necessary to summarize the outcome of follow-up examinations, test results, and additional recommendations emanating from multidisciplinary review. Routine components too often overlooked by physicians are a referral for a mental health assessment of the impact of the abuse, and treatment recommendations. The recommendation may influence child protective services' decision to provide mental health services. Increasingly, child protective services are limiting their involvement to "protection," and once the child appears no longer to be at risk, agencies are closing cases. Consequently, the responsibility for providing therapeutic services is shifted to the child's family. Obviously there are mental health sequelae of abuse that require skilled therapeutic intervention. In addition, nonoffending parents need guidance in addressing the sexually stylized behaviors that the child might exhibit. These behaviors increase the risk for future victimization. Injuries and sexually transmitted diseases can be treated and resolved in relatively short order, but unrecognized and untreated psychological impact has the potential for serious long-term sequelae. Although physicians will not be providing mental health therapy for these children, they do have an important role in the postdiagnostic period in advocating these services and monitoring their progress.

CONCLUSION

With the complex needs of child and adolescent victims and their families, early and meticulous medical management is a challenging but necessary process. The role of the clinician continues to expand into the postdiagnostic period as we become more knowledgeable about the needs of the victims and more sophisticated in our response. There remains ample opportunity to build on the scientific footings of the field and provide further insight into the diagnostic quandaries that remain.

REFERENCES

1. American Academy of Dermatology Task Force on Pediatric Dermatology. Genital warts and sexual abuse of children. *J Am Acad Dermatol* 1989;11:529.

2. American Academy of Pediatrics Committee on Early Childhood, Adoption, and Dependent Care. Gonorrhea in prepubertal children. *Pediatrics* 1983;71:553.

3. Bays J, Chadwick D. The serologic test for syphilis in sexually abused children and adolescents. *Adolesc Pediatr Gynecol* 1991;4:148–151.

4. Berkowitz CD, Elvik SL, and Logan MK. Labial fusion in prepubescent girls: A marker for sexual abuse? *Am J Obstet Gynecol* 1987;156:16–20.

5. Byram V, Wagner H, and Waller G. Sexual abuse and body image distortion. *Child Abuse Negl* 1995;19:507–510.

6. Centers for Disease Control. Sexually transmitted diseases treatment guidelines-1993. *Morb Mortal Wkly Rep* 42 1993;(RR-14):9.

7. Centers for Disease Control. Technical guidance on HIV counseling. 1993;42(RR-2):8–17.

8. Clayden GS. Anal appearance and child sexual abuse. *Lancet* 1987;1:620.

9. Clayden GS. Reflex anal dilatation associated with severe chronic constipation. *Arch Dis Child* 1988;63:832.

10. Ellsworth PI, Mergurerian PA, and Copening ME. Sexual abuse: Another causative factor in dysfunctional voiding. *J Urol* 1995;153:773–776.

11. Elmrost T, Larsson P. Survival of gonococci outside the body. *Br Med J* 1972;2:403.

12. Emans SJ, Goldstein DJ. Contraception. In: *Pediatric and Adolescent Gynecology.* Boston. Little, Brown. 1990:492–493.

13. Feigen GM. Proctologic disorders in sex deviates. *Calif Med* 1954;81:79–83.

14. Finkel MA. Anogenital trauma in sexually abused children. *Pediatrics* 1989;84:317.

15. Finkel MA. Guidelines for HIV testing of sexually abused children. *APSAC Advisor* 1990;3:8.

16. Finkel MA. Medical findings in child sexual abuse. In *Child abuse: Medical diagnosis and management.* RM Reece, ed. Philadelphia: Lea and Febiger. 1994.

17. Finkel MA, Debasi L. *Postfondling dysuria in sexually abused children: A pilot study.* Foundation of University Medicine and Dentistry of New Jersey, Summer Student Research Program. 1992.

18. Finkelhor D, Browne A. Impact of child sexual abuse: A review of the research. *Psychol Bull* 1986;99:66–77.

19. Fost N. Ethical considerations in testing victims of sexual abuse for HIV infection. *Child Abuse Negl* 1990;14:5–7.

20. Frasier LD. Human papilloma virus infections in children. *Pediatr Ann* 1994;23:354–360.

21. Gellert GA, Durfee MJ, and Berkowitz CD. Developing guidelines for HIV antibody testing among victims of child sexual abuse. *Child Abuse Negl* 1990;14:9–17.

22. Gellert GA, Durfee MJ, and Berkowitz CD. Situational and sociodemographic characteristics of children infected with HIV from pediatric sexual abuse. *Pediatrics* 1993;91:39–44.

23. Gutman LT, Herman-Giddens PA, and McKinney RE. Pediatric acquired immunodeficiency syndrome, barriers to recognizing the role of child sexual abuse. *Am J Dis Child* 1993;147:775–779.

24. Hammerschlag MR, Rettig PJ, and Shields ME. False-positive results with the use of chlamydial antigen detection tests in the evaluation of suspected sexual abuse in children. *Pediatr Infect Dis J* 1988;7:11.

25. Hanson RM. Sexually transmitted diseases and the sexually abused child. *Current opinion in Pediatrics* 1993;5:41–49.

26. Harter S, Alexander PC, and Neimyer RA. Long-term effects of incestuous child abuse in college women: Social adjustment, social cognition, and family characteristics. *J Consult Clin Psychol* 1988;58:5–8.

27. Johnson CF. Prolapse of the urethra: Confusion of clinical and anatomic characteristics with sexual abuse. *Pediatrics* 1991;87:722–724.

28. Kunin CM. Sexual intercourse and urinary infections. *N Engl J Med* 1978;298:336–337.

29. Lowe FC, Hill GS, Jeffs RD et al. Urethral prolapse in children: Insights into etiology and management. *J Urol* 1986;135:100.

30. McCann J, Voris J. Genital injuries resulting from sexual abuse: A longitudinal study. *Pediatrics* 1992;89:307.

31. Myers JEB. The role of the physician in preserving verbal evidence of child abuse. *J Pediatr* 1986;109:409.

32. Paradise JE, Willis ED. Probability of vaginal foreign body in girls with genital complaints. *Am J Dis Child* 1985;139:472–476.

33. Schwarcz SK, Whittington WL. Sexual assault and sexually transmitted diseases: Detection and management in adults and children. *Rev Infect Dis* 1990(suppl.);6:S682–90.

34. Shore WB, Winkelstein JA. Non-venereal transmission of gonococcal infections in children. *J Pediatr* 1971;79:661.

35. Sirotnak AP. Testing sexually abused children for sexually transmitted diseases: Who to test, when to test and why. *Pediatr Ann* 1994;23:370–374.

36. Waller G, Hamilton K, and Rose N. Sexual abuse and body image distortion in the eating disorders. *Br J Clin Psychol* 1993;32:350–352.

37. Whittington WL, Rice RJ, and Biddle JW. Incorrect identification of Neisseria gonorrhoeae from infants and children. *Pediatr Infect Dis J* 1988;7:3–10.

38. Zager RP. Urethral prolapse in young girls. *Am J Dis Child* 1957;94:196–199.

Chapter 2

Long-term Management of the Sexually Abused Child: Considerations and Challenges

Erna Olafson, Ph.D., Psy.D., and Barbara W. Boat, Ph.D.

The painful consequences of child sexual abuse can persist throughout a victim's life. Although children are adaptable, they are not truly resilient, and severe and prolonged abuse can irreversibly alter the developing nervous system; this underscores the need for early intervention and consideration of developmental issues in treatment. Since sexual abuse is not a disorder or syndrome but something experienced by a child, there is no single type of treatment that can be recommended. However, sexually abused children often exhibit common behaviors, including traumatic sexualization, stigmatization, and—in the most severe cases—dissociation. There are gender differences both in response to abuse and in response to therapy. One of the first principles of therapy is that trauma cannot be effectively treated if it is ongoing, so the child's current safety must be addressed. Individual and group therapies both have a role in treatment, and cognitive behavioral therapy is a modality that has been shown to be effective with many children. The longer and more intense the abuse, the longer duration of therapy needed. It is also essential to involve nonoffending parents in treatment so they can cope with their own distress and help their children cope. The therapist needs an open-door policy to provide the ongoing care required by these often difficult patients.

GENERAL CONSIDERATIONS

Near the conclusion of Ingmar Bergman's film *Fanny and Alexander,* the child Alexander is safely back at a festive celebration with his extended family after his escape from a sadistically abusive stepfather who has now died in a fire. At bedtime, as Alexander walks down an empty hallway, the ghost of his stepfather brutally knocks him to the floor, stands over him, and tells him, "You can't escape me." Because of his own childhood experiences, Bergman knew that the pain and terror of child abuse can persist and intrude into times of safety and peace. In this insight, Bergman is supported by researchers such as Bruce

Perry and others, who are showing us the ways in which severe and prolonged child abuse irreversibly alters the developing human nervous system.[66,67] As Judith Herman writes in *Trauma and Recovery,* "Repeated trauma in adult life erodes the structure of the personality already formed, but repeated trauma in childhood forms and deforms the personality."[46]

What treatment approaches hold the greatest promise to enhance long-term coping? The few research studies on treatment of child sexual abuse that have appeared in this emerging field indicate that early identification and treatment can mitigate the negative effects of child sexual abuse, although the long-term studies that would assess the effects of treatment into adulthood remain to be done. Abuse-focused treatment for children dates back only to the 1980s, and there is much still to be learned.

CHILD SEXUAL ABUSE: NOT A UNITARY CONCEPT

In a recent literature review about treatment research of sexually abused children, Finkelhor and Berliner remind us that sexual abuse is an experience, not a disorder or syndrome, and that it seems to be associated with a very wide range of symptom patterns.[29]

Two theoretical models to describe the effects of child sexual abuse have been developed. Finkelhor and Browne identify four traumagenic dynamics of child sexual abuse:

- trauma sexualization
- stigmatization
- betrayal
- powerlessness[30]

Briere's Trauma Symptom Checklist for Children (TSCC) has six subscales:

- anxiety
- depression
- posttraumatic stress
- sexual concerns
- dissociation
- anger[11]

However, despite more than a decade of effort, researchers have been unable to identify a unified sexually abused child's disorder, similar to the battered child syndrome, that can be applied as a predictive cluster of symptoms to differentiate sexually abused children from their nonabused peers.[20] A recent review of 45 studies by Kendall-Tackett, Williams, and Finkelhor[58] found that, although sexually abused children had more symptoms than nonabused children, there appeared to be an absence of any specific syndrome in children who had been sexually abused and no single traumatizing process. In addition, approximately one-third of these sexually abused children had no symptoms, at least as assessed in these cross-sectional studies. The authors argue that longitudinal studies (such as the one currently under way by Trickett and Putnam[87]) may reveal more about the course of a sexually abused child's symptomatology and recovery over time; they also recommend that future studies of child sexual abuse outcomes be more precisely differentiated by age and gender.

In the Kendall-Tackett literature review, sexually abused children showed more posttraumatic stress disorder and sexualized behavior, but not, interestingly, higher rates of other symptoms, when compared to other children in mental health treatment. The authors caution that the clinical control group may contain abused children whose abuse has not been discovered. Symptoms found to be more common among sexually abused children than among comparison groups of children not in treatment included poor self-esteem, behavior problems, aggression, anxiety, depression, and withdrawal. These symptoms are also found, of course, in children undergoing mental health treatment who do not have sexual abuse histories. Other studies have also found increased somatic symptoms, attention deficit hyperactivity disorder, sleep disturbances, suicidality, self-mutilation, substance abuse, and dissociative symptoms among sexually abused children when compared to nonabused cohorts.[5,6,85,86]

The Kendall-Tackett literature review also found that the degree of symptoms in sexually abused children was affected by whether or not the child had been abusively penetrated, the duration and frequency of the abuse, the presence or absence of force or violence as part of the assault, and the degree of closeness of the perpetrator to the child (e.g., whether the perpetrator was a father figure). Maternal support was found to be a protective factor in determining the degree of symptomatology.

The Many Forms of Sexual Abuse

One problem in the search for a unified sexually abused child's disorder for which unified treatment measures could be developed is that the term *sexual abuse* encompasses a wide variety of acts in varied contexts and with differing emotional valences, in contrast, for example, to the *battering* of a child or woman, which covers a narrower range of behaviors and emotional tones. Contact sexual abuse can range from one-time genital fondling of a child in a crowded subway or bus, to seductive and sexually stimulating fondling in an atmosphere of coaxing and apparent paternal tenderness, to intrusive and prolonged sexual touching disguised by a mother or father as genital hygiene, to sexual assaults by multiple perpetrators, to anal or vaginal rape in an atmosphere of terror, pain, and sadism. These are just some of the acts gathered under the rubric *sexual abuse*. It may be that the symptoms of sexual abuse vary greatly because the sexual acts perpetrated on children and their contexts, meanings, and emotional contents vary greatly.[62] In addition, sexual abuse is often accompanied by physical abuse, psychological abuse, and neglect, making it difficult to isolate the effects of one type of abuse from another.

Traumatic Sexualization

Traumatic sexualization has been identified as one of four traumagenic dynamics of child sexual abuse.[30] This dynamic can entail distorted ideas about sexuality and disturbances in sexual behavior in young victims. Instruments to assess the level of sexual disturbances in children include Briere's recently validated Trauma Symptom Checklist for Children, a self-report measure for children aged 8 to 15, and Friedrich's Child Sexual Behavior Inventory, a parent report measure appropriate for female caregivers of male and female children aged 2 to 12 years. Both the TSCC and the CSBI are now commercially available from Psychological Assessment Resources.[11,37,38] These instruments, targeted to assess the impact of interpersonal victimization in children, appear to be superior to more general instruments such as the Achenbach Child Behavior Inventory[1] in assessing traumagenic dynamics in children, although the Achenbach is still widely used in treatment outcome studies.[29]

In children, sexualized behaviors include frequent, overt masturbation, inappropriate sexual overtures toward other children and adults, and compulsive sexualized talk, play, and fantasy. Sexually abused preschoolers may grab at adult genitals or try to stroke them as a form of play or affection, without awareness that these behaviors are inappropriate. Children of all ages may engage in compulsive, repetitive, joyless self-stimulation or sexual enactments on dolls or pets.[7]

When victims of childhood sexual assault reach adolescence or young adulthood, sexual dysfunctions may emerge for the first time. Many adolescent sex offenders have been molestation victims; their treatment issues are addressed in other chapters in this book (see chapters 21 and 22). Avoidance of sexual contact, flashbacks during sexual intercourse, vulnerability to revictimization, and increased rates of high-risk sexual behavior have all been reported in studies of sexual abuse victims when compared with people who were not abused. A recent study of young women who became pregnant as adolescents found that 62 percent of them had been sexually victimized by child sexual molestation or rape before their first pregnancy. Reported age at first voluntary intercourse was 14.5 for the abused girls.[9,10] The mean age of first intercourse for nonabused female adolescents is 16.2.[48] Abused adolescent girls were less likely to use contraceptives and more likely to have repeated pregnancies, to become pregnant by different men, and to become single parents with less paternal involvement in child rearing, than were nonabused sexually active adolescent girls.[9,10]

These data, as well as other data showing that child sexual abuse victims have higher rates of revictimization, including subsequent experiences of sexual assault, rape, and physical violence, pose particular challenges to pediatricians and others whose tasks include long-term clinical management of sexual abuse victims. There has been little research about why some victims—but not all victims—are vulnerable to revictimization, or about how to help them learn to protect themselves. Research on younger victims and on those older victims who become sexual offenders is more extensive.

Stigmatization

Because of the sexual component, sexual victimization differs from other forms of stress and trauma in another crucial aspect, one that is not covered in standard diagnostic manuals: stigmatization. A stigma originally was a distinguishing mark burned or cut into the flesh, as of a slave or criminal. The word comes from the Greek. A stigma is a mark of disgrace, reproach, or shame, and it detracts from the character or reputation of a person or group. Like an ancient Greek slave or criminal branded with a stigma, many sexual abuse victims feel branded in the flesh by what has been done to them.

How does a clinician deal with a 14-year-old promiscuous girl who, when describing her sexually stimulating molestation by her stepfather, states, "Let's face it, I was a slut when I was 5." This stigmatizing conviction can be strengthened in those cases of sexual abuse where the victim experienced sexual arousal or the perpetrator blamed the victim as "irresistible." An adolescent who "knows" she was a slut when she was five may carry this negative self-image into compulsive, high-risk, and self-destructive sexual acting out with multiple partners. Thus, a treating clinician will help her confront her cognitive distortions, including the reality of childrens' ability to be sexually aroused, her powerlessness at age 5, and a child's need to take some control and blame in these situations. Sometimes contrasting the handprint of a 5-year-old with that of an adult male helps make the point of size and power difference. Also, the reinforcing properties of promiscuity and the excuse to be promiscuous need to be addressed. Stigmatization is not, however, a universal outcome among victims; one study of younger victims found that most did not internalize blame for sexual abuse.[52,64]

SAFETY FIRST; THEN HEALING CAN BEGIN

Trauma cannot be effectively treated if it is ongoing. There are two circumstances under which we cannot provide intervention: if we do not know or suspect that sexual victimization has occurred and if sexual victimization is continuing. Thus, it is imperative to ask. Interventions will be of little use unless the child is safe and feels safe. Unfortunately, routine questions that could invite disclosures of ongoing abuse in the home, at school, or during other activities are still not included in many standard pediatric examinations or mental health intakes.

Earlier estimates have shown that 95 percent of sexual abuse experienced by girls was never reported to the authorities and that a majority of these girls never told anyone.[77] Many of those who disclosed child sexual abuse during a recent nationwide telephone survey told the surveyors that the interviewer was the first person to whom this abuse had ever been disclosed.[33] A question such as, "Has anyone touched you in a way that you did not like?" may elicit responses such as, "Jason pushed me in lunch line"; but such responses can be pursued to ask about other touches that may have been intrusive, such as hitting, kicking, pinching, as well as touching of private parts. Schoolyard bullying, although not the focus of this chapter, can be very damaging to children, and some bullying involves abusive genital touching. In addition, high rates of peer sexual harassment are reported in schools among children of all ages.[8,31,32,76]

Abuse Histories as a Routine Part of Medical and Mental Health Assessments

Clinical histories of children must include questions about physical, emotional, and sexual abuse. In mental health settings, children who show sexualized behaviors or posttraumatic stress symptoms may be signaling us about past or current sexual abuse and should clearly be questioned in a nonleading manner.

For those who treat a child known to have a history of abuse, it is advisable to assess the child's physical and emotional safety periodically. Pediatricians, family practitioners, or therapists should gather information at least every six months about the child's current environment, including changes in family members or others with access to the child, school performance, assessment of sexualized behaviors and questions, and any concerns about the sexual abuse that linger, have surfaced for the first time, or have resurfaced. The goal is to implement proactive protection for the child against the lasting consequences of ongoing abuse by attempting to ascertain if the child continues to be at risk. The skill of the professional to attend to the possibility of ongoing abuse can make the difference in reporting—or not reporting—to mandated agencies. If abuse continues or recurs and practitioners do not find this out and report it, there is little chance of protecting the child and providing opportunity for healing.

Clinicians and the Courts

Many clinicians have had the frustrating experience of seeing the courts return a child to caretakers whom the clinician believes to be dangerous or abusive. Faller has shown in her sample of separated parents that even after sexual abuse had been clinically substantiated, over one-third of children continued to have unsupervised contact with their alleged parental abuser.[27] In some of these cases, judges refused even to hear the clinical evidence of sexual abuse, and one judge threw the clinical reports to the courtroom floor unread.

When a professional has intervened to protect a child and then believes that social services and the courts have not responded adequately, only limited alternatives are available. The professional can keep careful records about what the child continues to say, avoid leading questions, document the child's observed and reported symptoms, and report as mandated to protective services if there are indications that abuse continues or has recurred. In many states, treating clinicians are not asked to give expert opinions in court, but a professional's willingness to appear as a fact witness in court may help protect a child. Familiarity with laws and legal precedents on such matters must be part of a practitioner's knowledge base. See chapter 23 for further discussion of forensic implications.

TREATMENT SPECIFICS: CHILDREN

Treatment outcome research has established some guidelines and principles which are summarized here and discussed in greater detail below.

- Cognitive behavioral treatment approaches have been shown to be effective both with severely traumatized children and with victimized but not traumatized children.
- Sexually victimized young children may respond to time-limited behavioral interventions limited to ten or twelve sessions. However, victimized children with trauma symptoms require longer times in treatment.
- There is not agreement about the efficacy of individual versus group therapy for sexually abused children. It is generally believed (but not yet shown in research studies) that adolescents may respond better in group therapy than in individual treatment when dealing with issues such as secrecy, shame, stigmatization, and interpersonal deficits.
- Boys and girls generally respond differently to sexual abuse and to treatment interventions, especially for that majority of male victims who are sexually molested by men.[16,34,35,66]
- Although studies show that sexual acting out in older children is more resistant to treatment than anxiety and depression, preschoolers in one study were found to respond within two sessions when parents were instructed in behavioral interventions to control this behavior. This result underscores the necessity for early identification and treatment so that dysfunctional sexual behaviors do not become embedded and habitual as victimized children mature. It also underscores the importance of developmental factors when considering the effects and treatment of sexual abuse.[4,66]
- Outcome studies for adolescent victims who are not perpetrators are scarce, and research in this area is urgently needed.

- The same trauma can be amplified in some individuals and not in others, although we do not understand this process.[36] Similarly, some children respond to treatment and some do not, although the variables that predict treatment responsiveness are not well known. It has been suggested that the defenses of denial and avoidance may slow recovery.[61]
- It is essential to involve nonoffending parents in treatment and to teach them child behavioral management strategies to apply at home. The younger the child, the more important parental involvement appears to be.

COGNITIVE BEHAVIORAL THERAPY FOR SEXUALLY ABUSED CHILDREN AND THEIR NONOFFENDING PARENTS

Cognitive behavioral therapy (CBT) is a promising treatment modality and is being investigated by a number of clinicians and researchers. CBT seeks to change negative patterns of thought and behavior by teaching the relationships among thoughts, feelings, and actions and applying practical behavioral solutions to specific problems. A very useful new book by Deblinger and Heflin gives detailed instructions for the application of CBT to children aged 3 to 13 and their nonoffending parents.[23] Lipovsky offers cognitive and behavioral guidelines for treatment of child survivors of sexual assault who have posttraumatic stress disorder.[62] Cohen and Mannarino provide a cognitive behavioral model for preschoolers and their nonoffending parents and have demonstrated its effectiveness in an outcome study.[17] Further outcome studies are under way on this treatment approach.

In their treatment manual, Deblinger and Heflin[23] argue that cognitive behavioral interventions are particularly suited to addressing the problems of sexually abused children and their families for a number of reasons. The wide range of interventions in this treatment approach matches the wide range of symptoms victims experience. The approach is flexible and can be individually tailored while remaining grounded in a theoretical model. Although CBT is generally a short-term approach, the education and coping skills it teaches parents and children can be applied through different life cycle stages. The authors cite the authority of Paniagua to argue that because the cognitive behavioral approach is active, practical, directive, and structured, it appears to be preferred by minority groups, including African Americans, Native Americans, Hispanics, and Asians.[65]

The rationale and strategies of cognitive behavioral interventions are made explicit to clients, and goals and intervention strategies are designed collaboratively by therapists and clients. In this way, children and their nonoffending parents may again experience a measure of control and self-respect in their lives, if, as is often the case, the abusive experiences and their investigative and legal sequelae have caused them to feel helpless and disempowered. Many children and their parents enter treatment overwhelmed both by their own strong emotional reactions to the abuse and by the novel experience that strangers—social workers, lawyers, judges, detectives—seem to have taken control of their private lives. Finally, preliminary empirical evidence demonstrates the greater effectiveness of therapy that is abuse-focused and cognitive behavioral when compared with nondirective, supportive psychotherapy for child victims and their families.[18]

The treatment focus of the Deblinger and Heflin model, intended for children aged 3 to 13 and their nonoffending parents, is tripartite:

- to alleviate posttraumatic, generalized anxiety, oppositional, and depressive symptoms in the child;
- to correct misconceptions or distortions the child has about the abuse; and
- to ameliorate behavior problems developed by the child as a consequence of the abuse.

The cornerstone of the CBT treatment approach is *gradual exposure and cognitive and affective processing*. Sessions with parent and child are initially separate and last as long as necessary for symptoms to decrease and coping skills to develop. Individual sessions are followed by joint sessions between parent and child. Coping skills include cognitive restructuring to modify catastrophic and other dysfunctional thoughts about the abuse, and breathing and relaxation training. Deblinger and colleagues have found that the prolonged exposure techniques proven effective with adults who suffer from posttraumatic stress disorder (PTSD) were not appropriate for children; instead, they combined elements of systematic desensitization and prolonged exposure in an approach they call *gradual exposure,* which they also use in therapy with parents. They also teach behavior management techniques to parents in order to address acting out or avoidant behaviors in their children between sessions or when therapy has terminated. Education of parent and child about healthy sexuality, personal safety skills, and child sexual abuse occurs throughout treatment, which can range from 12 to 40 sessions, depending on how complex and severe a situation is.

Deblinger and Heflin's manual is rich with practical guidelines and clinical cautions about the application of abuse-focused cognitive behavioral therapy for the sexually abused child. In their generally positive review of the publication, Chaffin and Champion[15] caution that proper application of this "deceptively simple and straightforward" protocol to an individual case or problem requires training, experience, and careful thought. They also note that the approach may not be applicable to the full range of children and non-offending parents affected by sexual abuse. The collateral parent component requires a parent who is able and willing to implement it. Finally, Chaffin and Champion warn that this approach may not be appropriate or should be applied cautiously to abused children who have psychotic or dissociative symptoms.

In a treatment outcome study of abuse-focused CBT with preschool child sexual abuse victims and their nonoffending mothers, Stauffer and Deblinger[84] found improvements in symptom levels for mothers and children. Some children, however, did not improve and one became more symptomatic. Mean scores on standard instruments such as the Child Behavior Checklist reached the normal range by the conclusion of 11 sessions. Children's sexualized behaviors diminished, parenting skills increased, and reported levels of distress declined. No improvements occurred during the baseline period, suggesting that improvements were not due to the passage of time alone. Stauffer and Deblinger caution that the study is limited by the absence of a control group and of long-term follow-up to determine whether clinical improvements endured for longer than the three-month follow-up.

Another study looked at 100 sexually abused children with posttraumatic symptoms and their nonoffending parents, using random assignment to one of three treatment conditions (parent only, child only, parent-child) and a community control condition.[24] Children were aged 7 to 13 and received short-term cognitive behavioral treatment. Not surprisingly, child PTSD symptoms decreased when the child was directly treated, and parenting skills reportedly improved when parents were treated. Some of the children's symptoms (depression, aggression, and sexual acting out), however, reportedly improved not with direct treatment to children but rather when their parents were treated. Although the results are preliminary and longer-term follow-up assessments continue, this study strongly suggests that optimal treatment includes both the sexually abused child and the nonoffending parent.

In one of the few outcome studies to randomly assign sexually abused preschoolers and their nonoffending parents to treatment modalities (cognitive behavioral therapy versus nondirective supportive therapy), Cohen and Mannarino[18] found that children who received abuse-focused cognitive behavioral therapy showed significant improvement in symptomatology during 12 individual treatment sessions, relative to the control group of children who received nondirective, supportive, individual therapy. They conclude that therapy that requires children to address their sexual abuse experience directly is more effective in reducing symptoms than nondirective therapies. Their research also shows that sexually inappropriate behaviors by preschoolers respond well to behavioral interventions and do not respond to play therapy. Problematic sexual behaviors were eliminated in two cognitive behavioral individual treatment sessions for parents and children, whereas six of the children receiving supportive therapy had to be removed from this category because of the persistence of sexually inappropriate touching of others. Finally, the Cohen and Mannarino study strongly supports the inclusion of nonoffending parents, to teach them behavioral management strategies to apply at home and allow them to process their reactions to their child's sexual abuse in the context of their own personal histories.

Cohen and Mannarino have recently completed a similar study of cognitive behavioral therapy with sexually abused children aged 7 to 14 and their primary caregivers. They are now collaborating with Deblinger in a large treatment-outcome study (Cohen and Mannarino, personal communication, 1997). Treatment professionals should look for publication from these researchers as the outcome studies are completed and analyzed.

The use of CBT for children who have suffered multiple abuse is discussed in chapter 20.

THE TRAUMATIZED CHILD SEXUAL ABUSE VICTIM

All sexually abused children are victimized, but not all are traumatized. Children with severe posttraumatic or dissociative symptoms have more intense treatment needs and need treatment for longer duration than sexually victimized children who exhibit less severe and pervasive symptoms. Lanktree and Briere[60] find that children's symptoms continue to improve throughout 12 months of treatment. Friedrich[36] warns against complacency about the efficacy of brief therapies and reminds us that we do not know how long it might take to treat severe abuse that occurred in a chaotic household. Outcome research generally does not include these families, because they either never enter treatment, drop out, or are lost to follow-up.

For children traumatized or severely neglected in infancy and early childhood, some of the neurodevelopmental effects may be irreversible. Children may be adaptable, but they are not truly resilient. As Perry has found in a number of excellent studies,[66,67] there appear to be critical and sensitive periods in the development of the central nervous system during which disruptions of experience-dependent neurochemical signals may lead to major abnormalities or deficits. He and his coauthors write:

> The simple and unavoidable result of this sequential neurodevelopment is that the organizing, sensitive brain of an infant or young child is more malleable to experience than the mature brain. While experience may alter the behavior of an adult,

experience literally provides the organizing framework for an infant and child. Because the brain is most plastic (receptive to environmental input) in early childhood, the child is most vulnerable to variance of experience during this time.[66]

We can, however, in many cases help traumatized children adapt to their distress, offering medications for severe anxiety and/or impulsiveness, cognitive and behavioral interventions for symptoms, and therapy and education for caregivers so that the work of recovery can continue at home as well in the therapy setting.

In cases of severe, prolonged abuse, where the child's identity consolidation has been compromised, therapy should be carefully titrated in order to avoid more intensity of emotional processing than the child can tolerate. Even for adults with traumatic symptoms, concerns have been raised that exposure therapies such as systematic desensitization and flooding may retraumatize some victims.[25,83] Friedrich[34] recommends "keeping the child within the 'therapeutic window,' or that moderate distress area between denial and intrusion."

Fragmented, dissociating, chaotic children who suffer from chronic autonomic nervous system arousal, accelerated heartbeats, startle reactions, and hypervigilant, distrustful, approach-avoidance to adults will require safe, predictable, structured therapeutic (and living) settings in order to begin to heal. Even the administration of the Rorschach can frighten and destabilize such children. Many of them are keeping nearly intolerable memories of terror, humiliation, and pain at bay only with enormous effort.

For these children, unstructured and nondirective play therapy may be destabilizing. We recall Mindy, aged 4, who had made a clear allegation of repeated sexual molestation by her violent and frightening stepfather. In the course of subsequent nondirective play therapy, Mindy became increasingly agitated, tried repeatedly to reach up her therapist's skirt, grabbed at her crotch and breasts, tried to hurt her, and began to chant and sing in sessions that Big Bird, Oscar, and her "Nana" had hurt her pee pee. As therapy continued, Mindy's symptoms worsened. Within weeks after transfer to a therapist who instituted standard cognitive behavioral therapy and training for the nonoffending parent, Mindy's sexual acting out and bizarre allegations stopped, and she gradually became less symptomatic. Bizarre allegations by children have been the focus of two recent papers.[22,26]

When abuse has been prolonged and severe, it may be that splitting off, denial, or avoidance is adaptive for some period of time, especially when victims are very young. As these children achieve greater internal structure, they can begin gradually to process their memories and attendant emotions. They should always have some control of the process. Feeling pushed or pushed around in a therapy session, by an adult who tells them that this is for their own good (just as their molesters may have done), can impede healing for these severely traumatized children. The child will experience the well-meaning but overly intrusive therapist as just another adult who ignores her or his protests and pain. Lipovsky[62] reports a case in which a therapist pressed a 10-year-old girl who had been severely abused by her father to talk about what had happened to her. The child, who became upset, told the therapist, "I'm not going to do anything that I don't want to, even if you tell me it's for my own good."

The American Academy of Child and Adolescent Psychiatry has published practice parameters for the assessment and treatment of children and adolescents with posttraumatic stress disorder, along with a good, current bibliography about childhood PTSD ("Practice Parameters for the Assessment and Treatment of Children and Adolescents with Posttraumatic Stress Disorder," *J Am Acad Child Adolesc Psychiatry* 1998 [Suppl.]; 37:4S-26S).

The Dissociative Child

Dissociation is defined as a psychophysiological process that alters a person's thoughts, feelings, or actions, so that for a period of time certain information is not integrated normally or logically with other information.[90] Certain forms of dissociation, such as daydreaming, fantasizing, or relating to an imaginary playmate, are normal in children. Normative dissociative behavior tends to peak at 9 to 10 years of age and then decrease with age.[69,70,71]

It is generally agreed that pathologically dissociative behaviors are associated with early childhood traumatic experiences. The child uses dissociation as an adaptive coping mechanism to protect against the potentially overwhelming nature of trauma. When repeated trauma such as recurrent sexual or physical abuse occurs, the child learns to dissociate as soon as a stressful situation threatens. When dissociation affects the continuity of memory or disturbs integration of self, a dissociative disorder results.

A National Institute of Mental Health survey of 100 cases of dissociative identity disorder found that 97 percent of these patients reported significant childhood trauma, with incest being the most commonly reported trauma (68%).[72]

Until recently, a low index of suspicion among child clinicians and the absence of substantial clinical profiles of childhood dissociative disorders has made it difficult to differentiate these cases from more commonly diagnosed childhood conditions.[51,69] The validity of the diagnosis has been strengthened by two recent studies.[50,68] The only current standardized measure for quantifying dissociative behaviors in children is the Child Dissociative Checklist.[73] Normative data on the Adolescent Dissociative Experiences Scale[2] has now been published.[3]

In considering long-term management of a dissociative child, a risk factor for the child is a parent or caretaker who has a dissociative disorder, or may be a substance abuser or have an antisocial personality, sexual paraphilias, or a manic, paranoid, or impulsive disorder. In a recent pilot study by Silberg and Waters,[80] parental consistency and length of treatment were the best predictors of favorable outcome for dissociative children. In addition, pediatric and school management of the dissociative child are important considerations.[89]

Dissociative children are polysymptomatic and frequently have somatic complaints. Pediatricians need to be aware that a dissociative disorder can share common symptom presentation with attention-deficit/hyperactivity disorder (ADHD), eating disorders, and seizure disorders/conversion disorders.[44] Treatment challenges include management of possible legal issues related to a perceived history of abuse, sleep complaints, confusing psychophysiological changes and many issues related to conduct, school performance, and family relationships. To manage the dissociative sexually abused child, it is critical to share information among all professionals who have contact with the child. Schools are often underutilized resources in treatment planning and implementation. Waterbury[89] offers a number of ideas for school-based interventions, techniques, and game plans that treatment professionals can share with school personnel as they plan a joint treatment strategy.

The symptom of dissociative coping as a response to overwhelming stress has been found to require more time to resolve than other symptoms sexually abused children experience.[29,60] Silberg and Waters[80] recommend that treatment involve cognitive techniques to help the child learn how to cope with the aftereffects of trauma, directive approaches to deal with the traumatic content, sensitivity to the family context, and emphasis on the child's need for mastery of developmentally appropriate tasks.

In his comprehensive recent book on dissociation in children and adolescents, Frank Putnam warns that traumatized, dissociative children "wear down the patience" of therapists and others, and suggests that "more than anything else, patience and persistence are necessary to make progress" with these youngsters.[71] A key treatment process issue that Putnam highlights involves management of the often severe behavioral problems these children display and their erratic ability to respond to treatment interventions and to learn from experience. Putnam writes, "This profound inability to incorporate learning into reliably accessible behavioral responses is a result of traumatized children's state dependency of learning and memory, as well as of their metacognitive integrative deficits.[71] Putnam reminds us that little is known about the efficacy of treatment for dissociative children, and he recommends long-term follow-up to monitor developmental changes and the delayed emergence of symptoms ("sleeper effect") observed in many of these children.

Group versus Individual Therapy

Lanktree,[59] who has treated and assessed outcomes for sexually abused young children, emphasizes the importance of rapport-building and safety for such children before they can explore their memories and feelings associated with the trauma. In the Stuart House Model of treatment, which Lanktree applies, rapport building is essential. Lanktree argues that a trusting, one-to-one relationship with an individual therapist is necessary before children can feel safe engaging in group therapy. She writes that "a stable sense of self and inner resources may be required before in-depth work on traumatic events and feelings can be initiated."

However, the intensity of one-to-one interaction in a small treatment room with a relatively unfamiliar adult may be more than some sexually victimized children can tolerate. Parents may also fear leaving a child alone with a therapist. In such cases, the diffusion of intensity that group therapy and cotherapy foster may feel safer for distrustful children and suspicious parents. Friedrich[34] has written that group therapy can offer opportunities for therapeutic movement not available in individual or family therapy, and he shows that it is the most widely used treatment modality for all ages of victims. He maintains that group treatment counteracts the incestuous family's secrecy and denial, offers resocialization experiences in a setting of empathy and support, and allows the therapist to view aspects of patients not visible in individual treatment.

Like Lanktree, however, Friedrich cautions that for some children, group therapy may be too intense and that they may need prior individual therapy. Friedrich urges that outcome studies comparing individual versus group treatment for victimized children of all ages be undertaken to resolve the treatment modality question. Noting that the question of group versus individual therapy remains unresolved, Friedrich writes: "The message is that if a victimized child presents with anger, treat the anger. Modality may not matter. This may also be the case with PTSD and a range of other symptoms."[36]

Gender Differences in Symptoms and Treatment

Research shows that in childhood more boys than girls display externalizing disorders such as ADHD, oppositionality, conduct disorders, and delinquency; and more girls than boys appear to have internalizing disorders such as depression and dissociation.[16] Perry and colleagues[66] speculate that the fight or flight response to threat more common among males and the freezing/dissociation response to threat more common among females may have had evolutionary survival value. Kaschak[54] argues that the radically different socialization experiences of males and females, evident in studies of the responses of parents and others to a child from the first hours of infancy throughout childhood, may shape gendered responses to danger.

Both externalizing and internalizing responses in children and adolescents generally receive inadequate treatment. The social service and court systems often respond to the desperate acting out of the male victim by labeling him as a delinquent or criminal and responding punitively, whereas the quieter female victim is too often simply missed. As Perry and colleagues write:[66]

> The vast majority of young children from backgrounds of abuse and neglect and other trauma who present to the mental health system with symptoms of aggression, inattentiveness, and noncompliance are male. . . . One wonders what happens to all the young girls who have been similarly traumatized. Children present to the mental health system because some adults in their world have been upset by their symptoms (which have almost always been caused by other adults). A compliant, dissociative, depressed young girl will generally not be brought to the attention of the mental health system, while her combative, verbally abusive and behaviorally-impulsive hyperaroused sibling (coming from the exact same abuse setting) will be. The potential homicide threatens, the potential suicide inconveniences.

Girls respond better to most current mental health treatment modalities than boys do, for reasons that we do not understand.[16,45] Research to develop and test treatment modalities for male child victims of abuse is needed. We must also identify and learn how to treat the compliant, depressed, or dissociating female child victims who do not upset adults enough to be brought to treatment and who are too often left to their isolation and quiet hopelessness.

ABUSED ADOLESCENTS WHO ARE NOT OFFENDERS

The true incidence of adolescent abuse may far exceed the documented statistics. In a study of 3,998 nonclinical and nonreported teenaged students, 20 percent reported some form of physical or sexual abuse.[47] Although victimization is viewed by some as a violation of the dependency status of a child,[32] it is also a fact that sexual maturation makes children, especially females, more vulnerable to sexually motivated crimes.[28] One survey found that 32 percent of forcible rapes occur when the victims are aged 11 to 17.[74] Gil[42] writes that because adolescents are viewed as being at lower risk than younger children, public perceptions may affect the reporting and protecting of them. Adolescents are perceived as having increased ability to fight, escape, or fend off abuse, as deserving the punishments they receive, as being able to sustain abuse without damage, and as more likely to be potential victimizers than potential victims. Furthermore, common reactions by adolescents to abuse—for example, running away, stealing, failing or skipping school, fighting, setting fires, and abusing drugs—often lead to involvement with the juvenile justice system, where there may be little attention paid to the safety and mental health needs of these abused children. This is especially true when desperate youngsters resort to illegal means of self-care such as prostitution, drug dealing, criminal activities, and gang participation.[42]

In her recent book on treatment of abused adolescents, Gil recommends that abuse-focused therapy (processing the abuse directly in a structured way) is indicated when there are the following:

- acute or chronic PTSD symptoms;
- behaviors such as self-injury, sexual acting out, or revictimization;
- attitudes such as vigorous denial of any impact of sexual abuse experiences or in-discriminate, affect-free disclosures of victimization.

She uses narrative therapy as an intervention to help adolescents rescript their personal stories and develop an orientation toward personal safety. Gil recommends that clinicians explore the meanings that adolescents have attributed to their abuse experiences and determine whether the abuse background has a link to current behaviors. The Hussy and Singer Adolescent Sexual Concerns Questionnaire[53] assists adolescents in defining physical and behavioral symptoms and worrisome thoughts, and the Guide to Family Observation and Assessment[81] is a useful conceptual framework for assessing families in a systematic and ongoing way.

With adolescents, the choice of individual, group, or family therapy needs to be made sensitively and individually. Severe anxiety can be elicited in some abused adolescents who are alone in a room with an authority figure who is focusing attention on them and asking them questions about private and often embarrassing matters. For other teens, the group experience may lead to overstimulation, noncompliance, or withdrawal. Although family therapy is effective for some adolescents, for others a family-focused approach can compromise their sense of identity, safety, and personal power.[21]

Long-term management of the sexually abused adolescent will be affected by whether the abuse is current or cumulative. Because of the difficult and often deeply embedded behaviors associated with it, ongoing cumulative abuse is especially likely to be resistant to clinical intervention. Adolescents need advocates who will help ensure a safe environment that supports and encourages growth and development. This means that a cardinal principle in long-term management of the sexually abused adolescent must be to protect the child from further abuse and to do everything possible to ensure safety. Adolescents live in a system where interventions are often sporadic and appear cursory at best. Information on treatment outcomes is sorely lacking, and we must rely largely on clinical observations to guide treatment approaches. No one minimizes the fact that working with abused adolescents and their families is an enormous challenge.

TREATMENT SPECIFICS: PARENTS

Parents of children abused out of the home, as well as nonoffending parents of incest victims, have immediate and longer-term treatment needs, both for their own recovery and for that of their children. Paternal or maternal support following disclosure has been found to be significant in predicting postabuse adjustment for children.[34,84] Traumagenic responses in parents, such as feelings of guilt, anger, and betrayal, are common. Several studies have shown that nonoffending parents continue to have very high levels of psychosocial distress as long as two years after discovery of the abuse.[55] We have seen parents of sexually abused children who, on testing, met criteria for posttraumatic stress disorder. Stauffer and Deblinger write, "Given the importance of parental support to the child victim's postabuse adjustment, sexually abused children may best be served by assisting nonoffending parents in coping with their own distress, while also teaching them how to help their children cope with the negative experience of CSA [child sexual abuse]."[84]

Important considerations for parental therapy include the following:

- Parents with unresolved abuse histories of their own have special treatment needs and may need to be referred for intensive individual work.
- Although recent research has laid the myth of the "collusive" incest to rest,[43,82] some parents are unsupportive, accusatory, and blaming of their victimized children, and research has shown that such attitudes can exacerbate symptoms[84] as well as jeopardize the child's ongoing safety. If this psychological maltreatment continues, it may become necessary to remove a child from such a home.
- Parents who see their children as irrevocably damaged or ruined by the sexual assault can be helped to soften this belief so that they do not transmit this toxic message to their children. We have seen this "damaged goods" message most strikingly when boys are homosexually assaulted. We worked with one mother of a child molested by a male teacher who described her son in the past tense, as if he had died.
- Avoidant, suppressing, and denying mothers have been shown to be responsive to group treatment and to become more emotionally available, so that their children may share their thoughts, worries, and feelings with them.[84]
- Friedrich[34,35,39] offers a flexible, sensible, compassionate approach and includes useful suggestions for inclusion of parents in treatment. Clinicians should, however, be cautious about his suggestion that hypnotherapy can be useful in aiding recall of abuse experiences.
- Teaching behavior management techniques to parents to apply at home with their children has been shown to be effective, especially with younger children.[18]

OUTCOME ASSESSMENT INSTRUMENTS

Friedrich recommends simplified assessment instruments to measure treatment outcomes: Briere's Trauma Symptom Checklist for Children,[11] his own Child Sexual Behavior Inventory,[37,38] the Child Behavior Checklist,[1] and Goal Attainment Scaling.[49] In addition, the Weekly Behavior Report,[19] a parent-report measure developed by Cohen and Mannarino for use with sexually abused preschool children, shows promise. In *Trauma Assessments: A Clinician's Guide,* Eve Carlson recommends administration of trauma assessment measures at the outset of treatment and readministration of brief symptom measures every four to eight weeks to monitor treatment progress. Carlson states that there is evidence that clinician and client impressions about treatment effectiveness in the absence of outcome measures can be mistaken. Carlson's book contains a very thorough description of current trauma assessment instruments for children, adolescents, and adults, including a number of good measures for posttraumatic stress disorder and dissociation.[12,88]

CHALLENGES FOR LONG-TERM MANAGEMENT OF THE SEXUALLY ABUSED CHILD

The Asymptomatic Child and the Open Door Policy

Because child sexual abuse is an experience, not a disorder, there is no single pattern of responses to it and not every child responds with overt distress. Perhaps the most challenging children are those known to have been sexually abused who appear to be without symptoms. Are these children well-functioning and resilient, or are they suppressing internal distress? Does one treat a child who shows no symptoms? It is widely believed among clinicians that sexually abused children who show no symptoms may develop them later at crucial periods such as puberty, entry into sexual relationships, and child bearing. A "sleeper effect" has been found in which children who appeared to have the fewest symptoms when initially evaluated were the most symptomatic upon later evaluation.[63] Another study found greater deterioration in the shorter term among children who showed the fewest initial symptoms. Are we hurting children when we coax those who are avoidant or may truly not be distressed to engage in exposure therapies or group therapies to process a known history of sexual victimization? On the other hand, are we neglecting children clinically if we allow them to continue to deny, avoid, and suppress their pain? We cannot answer these questions, and in the absence of general guidelines, each case should be assessed and treated individually.

In the absence of research for managing such children, an open door policy of treatment may be the recommended course. Certainly, education about sexual boundaries, education for parents and children about sexual abuse and its possible sequelae, and the offer to remain available should problems arise can be a basic intervention strategy. As a caution, however, we recall assessing 12-year-old Amelia, who had been sexually abused by a teacher and who presented herself to us as pleasant, polite, excelling in school, and behaviorally appropriate. Her parents maintained that Amelia had completely recovered from the experience and that they were a family who did not fuss when things went wrong. Despite the fact that projective testing at age 12 showed signs of dissociation, suppressed rage, disturbed thinking, and a negative self-image, her parents decided that Amelia did not need treatment. By the age of 15, Amelia was abusing drugs, cutting on her arms, and failing at school. She and her parents sought treatment at this time. Although Amelia appears to be doing well now, in case future life cycle transitions disturb her equilibrium, she and her parents have been told that the door to treatment remains open.

The Child Who Appears to Be Traumatically Sexualized but Discloses No Abuse

This situation must be handled by parents and clinicians with great care. A few therapists have lost malpractice lawsuits and even their licenses to practice by subjecting such children to repeated and sometimes very leading questions. Research indicates that some preschoolers who are repeatedly interrogated may recount experiences that have not taken place.[14] When all reasonable steps, such as extended evaluations, have been taken to ascertain what is happening and to protect the child, and the professional still cannot determine what is going on, is treatment possible? Deblinger and Heflin[23] recommend in such cases that behavioral therapy for parents and children can be instituted to address target symptoms, but they caution that verbal and cognitive focus on abuse must not be applied in such cases. These children should not be in group therapy for sexual abuse. As with the asymptomatic child, an open door policy is recommended.

Severely Symptomatic Children in Chaotic Homes

Management issues for severely abused children who live in fragmented and chaotic homes are extremely difficult. The most severely abused children may be from families so compromised that they are unable to sustain participation in therapy, so most outcome studies may not include them.[36] In spite of the dominance of family preservation theory in much child protection work today, Gelles[40,41] now argues that there exist families who differ not only in degree but also in kind from the more mildly or moderately abusive ones. In order to save children's lives and protect their welfare, we need to learn to identify these treatment-resistant families early and place their children in safe homes.

In addition, reductions in social service budgets and the limitations of managed medical care have made treatment much less available for severely troubled families who could be capable of responding to intervention. It is the children who suffer. The ethical codes of many of our professions suggest that some of our time be devoted to providing care for no fees. In the absence of legislative and budgetary changes on the governmental and corporate level, this may be the best we have to offer such families.

CAUTIONS: THE LIMITATIONS OF ABUSE-FOCUSED TREATMENT OUTCOME STUDIES

In recent overview of 29 outcome studies by Finkelhor and Berliner,[29] all but one study showed significant improvements on at least some measures. However, only five of the studies showed convincingly that the observed recovery of these children was related to treatment rather than to the mere passage of time or other factors. Two well-designed studies showed that structured, abuse-specific, cognitive behavioral therapy for parents and children was superior to supportive psychotherapy.[18,24]

A summary of outcome research for children edited by Joann Grayson[45] in the *Virginia Child Protection Newsletter* strongly suggests that treatment is effective and that many child victims require more than crisis intervention or short-term counseling services. Referring to research by Lanktree and Briere,[60] Grayson argues that short-term interventions, such as the maximum of ten visits under managed care, are not sufficient to alter some known sequelae of child sexual abuse, such as dissociation, posttraumatic stress symptoms, aggression, and sexualized behaviors. Because children are so often sexually abused by trusted caretakers, their sense that adults may betray and exploit them makes it difficult for many of them to trust a therapist. Six months of treatment may be needed to gain the trust of a maltreated child, and one to two years of treatment may be necessary.[30] Symptoms that are often seen in abused children, such as anxiety, depression, hyperactivity, sleep disturbances, damaged self-esteem, and interpersonal problems, are also seen and treated in nonabused children. Because abuse-focused treatment is still new and treatment outcome studies relatively few, clinicians may also wish to consult outcome studies for treatment of those symptoms from which both abused and nonabused children may suffer.[13,56,57,75]

CONCLUSION

Because this field is so new, and outcome studies with random assignment to treatment groups have appeared only in the last year or two, we need to be aware of the limitations of our knowledge.[79] There are no longitudinal studies tracing treatment outcomes over time and through life cycles yet. We have found no comparative studies of treatment effectiveness with nonoffending adolescents, that large population of vulnerable victims who are statistically more likely than the nonabused to be revictimized and exploited. We also need to learn more about attachment issues when an offender or a nonprotective parent is otherwise loved by the child. In an eloquent passage from her most recent book, Anna Salter[78] describes such attachment figures as "load-bearing walls," part of the client's sense of who she or he is, to be approached with care in therapy because of the risk of threatening client stability and balance. Finally, as Friedrich writes about his own clinical work, "Treatment-manual-based therapy is a useful framework, and I have used several in the past. However, I adhere to the manual only when I am part of a study. This is not just oppositionality on my part. Good therapy for victimized children must be grounded in theory but flexible in approach. Two children with the same diagnosis may still each require a different approach."[36]

REFERENCES

1. Achenbach TM, Edelbrock C. *Manual for the Child Behavior Checklist and the Revised Child Behavior Profile.* Burlington: University of Vermont, Department of Psychiatry. 1983.

2. Armstrong JG, Carlson EB, Putnam FW, et al. Reliability and validity of an adolescent dissociative experiences scale. (Data in preparation.)

3. Armstrong JG, Putnam FW, Carlson EB, Libero DZ, and Smith SA. Development and validation of a measure of adolescent dissociation: The Adolescent Dissociative Experiences Scale. *J Nerv Ment Dis* 1997;185(8):491–497.

4. Azar ST, Siegel BR. Behavioral treatment of child abuse: A developmental perspective. *Behav Modif* 1990;14:279–300.

5. Beitchman JH. A review of the short-term effects of child sexual abuse. *Child Abuse Negl* 1991;15:537–556.

6. Beitchman JH, Zucker KJ, Hood JE, et al. A review of the long-term effects of child sexual abuse. *Child Abuse Negl* 1992;16:101–118.

7. Boat BW. The relationship between violence to children and violence to animals: An ignored link? *J Interpers Viol* 1995;10:229–235.

8. Boney-McCoy S, Finkelhor D. Psychosocial sequelae of violent victimization in a national youth sample. *J Consult Clin Psychol* 1995;63:726–736.

9. Boyer D. Adolescent pregnancy: The role of sexual abuse. *National Resource Center on Child Sexual Abuse News* 1995;4:1–3.

10. Boyer D, Fine D. Sexual abuse as a factor in adolescent pregnancy and child maltreatment. *Family Planning Perspectives* 1992;24:4–19.

11. Briere J. Trauma Symptom Checklist for Children (TSCC). Odessa, FL: Psychological Assessment Resources. 1996.

12. Carlson EB. *Trauma assessments: A clinician's guide.* New York: Guilford Press. 1997.

13. Cautela JR, Groden J. *Relaxation: A comprehensive manual for adults, children and children with special needs.* Champaign, IL: Research Press. 1978.

14. Ceci JJ, Loftus EF, Leichtman M, et al. The role of source misattributions in the creation of false beliefs among preschoolers. *Int J Clin Exp Hypn* 1994;62:304–320.

15. Chaffin M, Champion K. Treating sexually abused children and their nonoffending parents: A cognitive behavioral approach. *Child Maltreatment* 1997;2:81–83.

16. Chandy JM, Blum RW, Resnick MD. Gender-specific outcomes for sexually abused adolescents. *Child Abuse Negl* 1996;20:1219–1231.

17. Cohen JA, Mannarino AP. A treatment model for sexually abused preschoolers. *J Interpers Viol* 1993;8:115–131.

18. Cohen JA, Mannarino AP. A treatment outcome study of sexually abused preschool children: Initial findings. *J Am Acad Child Adolesc Psychiatry* 1996;35:42–50.

19. Cohen JA, Mannarino AP. The weekly behavior report: A parent-report instrument for sexually abused preschoolers. *Child Maltreat* 1996;1:353–360.

20. Corwin DL. Early diagnosis of child sexual abuse: Diminishing the lasting effects. In Wyatt GE, Powell GL (eds.), *Lasting effects of child sexual abuse,* 251–269. Newbury Park, CA: Sage. 1988.

21. Culley DC, Flanagan CH. Assessment of sexual problems in childhood and adolescence. In Rekers GA (ed.), *Handbook of child and adolescent sexual problems,* 14–30. New York: Lexington Books. 1995.

22. Dalenberg CJ: Evaluation and treatment: Fantastic elements in child disclosure of abuse. *APSAC Advisor* 1996(summer);9:1–9.

23. Deblinger ED, Heflin AH. *Treating sexually abused children and their nonoffending parents: A cognitive behavioral approach.* Thousand Oaks, CA: Sage. 1996.

24. Deblinger ED, Lippmann J, Steer R. Sexually abused children suffering posttraumatic stress symptoms: Initial treatment outcome findings. *Child Maltreat* 1996;1:310–321.

25. Dutton MA. Assessment and treatment of post-traumatic stress disorder among battered women. In Foy DW (ed.) *Treating PTSD: Cognitive-behavioral strategies,* 69–94. New York: Guilford Press. 1992.

26. Everson MD. Understanding bizarre, improbable and fantastic elements in children's accounts of abuse. *Child Maltreat* 1997;2:134–149.

27. Faller KC. Allegations of sexual abuse in divorce. *J Child Sexual Abuse* 1995;4:1–25.

28. Finkelhor D. The victimization of children: A developmental perspective. *Am J Orthopsychiatry* 1995;65:177–193.

29. Finkelhor D, Berliner L. Research on the treatment of sexually abused children: A review and recommendations. *J Am Acad Child Adolesc Psychiatry* 1995;34:1408–1423.

30. Finkelhor D, Browne A. The traumatic impact of child sexual abuse: A conceptualization. *Am J Orthopsychiatry* 1985;55:530–541.

31. Finkelhor D, Dziuba-Leatherman J. Children as victims of violence: A national survey. *Pediatrics* 1994;94:413–420.

32. Finkelhor D, Dziuba-Leatherman J. The victimization of children. *Am Psychol* 1994;49:173–183.

33. Finkelhor D, Hotaling G, Lewis IA, et al. Sexual abuse in a national survey of adult men and women: Prevalence, characteristics, and risk factors. *Child Abuse Negl* 1990;14:19–28.

34. Friedrich WN. *Psychotherapy of sexually abused children and their families,* p. 66. New York: Norton. 1990.

35. Friedrich WN. *Psychotherapy with sexually abused boys: An integrated approach.* Thousand Oaks, CA: Sage. 1995.

36. Friedrich WN. Clinical considerations of empirical treatment studies of abused children. *Child Maltreat* 1996;1:343–347.

37. Friedrich WN. *CSBI Child Behavior Inventory: Professional manual.* Odessa, FL: Psychological Assessment Resources. 1997.

38. Friedrich WN, Grambsch P, Damon L, et al. Child sexual behavior inventory: Normative and clinical comparisons. *Psychological Assessment* 1992;4:303–311.

39. Friedrich WN, Luecke WJ, Beilke RL, et al. Psychotherapy outcome of sexually abused boys. *J Interpers Viol* 1992;7:396–409.

40. Gelles RJ. *The book of David.* New York: Basic Books. 1996.

41. Gelles RJ. Physical violence, child abuse, and child homicide: A continuum of violence, or distinct behaviors? *Human Nature* 1991;2:59–72.

42. Gil E. *Treating abused adolescents.* New York: Guilford Press. 1996.

43. Gomes-Schwartz B, Horowitz JM, Cardarelli AP. *Child sexual abuse: The initial effects.* Newbury Park, CA: Sage. 1990.

44. Graham DB. The pediatric management of the dissociative child. In Silberg JL (ed.), *The dissociative child: Diagnosis, treatment and management,* 297–314. Lutherville, MD: Sidran Press. 1996.

45. Grayson J. Treatment outcome part III: Intervention for the child. *Virginia Child Protection Newsletter* 1996;48:1–3,12–13.

46. Herman JL. *Trauma and recovery,* p. 96. New York: Basic Books. 1992.

47. Hibbard RA, Ingersoll GM, Orr DP. Behavioral risk, emotional risk, and child abuse among adolescents in a nonclinical setting. *Pediatrics* 1990;86:896–907.

48. Hofferth SL, Kahn IR, Baldwin W. Premarital sexual activity among U.S. teenage women over the past three decades. *Family Planning Perspectives* 1987;19:46.

49. Hogue TE. Goal attainment scaling: A measure of clinical impact and risk assessment. *Issues in Criminological and Legal Psychology* 1994;21:96–102.

50. Hornstein NL, Putnam FW. Clinical phenomenology of child and adolescent dissociative disorders. *J Am Acad Child Adolesc Psychiatry* 1992;31:1077–1085.

51. Hornstein NL, Tyson S. Inpatient treatment of children with multiple personality/dissociative disorders and their families. *Psychiatric Clinics of North America* 1991;14:631–638.

52. Hunter J, Goodwin D, Wilson R. Attributions of blame in child sexual abuse victims: An analysis of age and gender differences. *J Child Sexual Abuse* 1992;1:75–89.

53. Hussey D, Singer MI. Sexual and physical abuse: The Adolescent Sexual Concern Questionnaire. In Singer MI, Singer LT, and Anglin TM (eds.) *Handbook for screening adolescents at psychosocial risk,* 131–163. New York: Lexington Books. 1993.

54. Kaschak E. *Engendered lives: A new psychology of women's experience.* New York: Basic Books. 1992.

55. Kelley SJ. Parental stress response to sexual abuse and ritualistic abuse of children in day care centers. *Nursing Research* 1990;39:25–29.

56. Kendall PC. *Child and adolescent therapy: Cognitive behavioral procedures.* New York: Guilford. 1991.

57. Kendall PC. Treating anxiety disorders in children: Results of a randomized clinical trial. *J Consult Clin Psychol* 1994;62:100–110.

58. Kendall-Tackett KA, Williams LM, Finkelhor D. Impact of sexual abuse on children: A review and synthesis of recent empirical studies. *Psychol Bull* 1993;113:164–180.

59. Lanktree CB. Treating child victims of sexual abuse. In Briere J (ed.), *Assessing and treating victims of violence,* 55–66. San Francisco, CA: Jossey Bass. 1994.

60. Lanktree CB, Briere J. Outcome of therapy for sexually abused children: A repeated measures study. *Child Abuse Negl* 1995;19:1145–1155.

61. Larzelere RE, Sinclair JJ, Collins LE, et al. Practical methods for evaluating treatment for child sex abuse. Presented at the Second National Colloquium of the American Professional Society on the Abuse of Children, Cambridge, MA. 1994.

62. Lipovsky JA. Assessment and treatment of post-traumatic stress disorder in child survivors of sexual assault. In Foy DW (ed.), *Treating PTSD: Cognitive-behavioral strategies,* 127–159. New York: Guilford Press. 1992.

63. Mannarino A, Cohen J, Smith J, and Moore-McTily S. Six- and twelve-month follow-up of sexually abused girls. *J Interpers Viol* 1991;6:494–511.

64. McMillen C, Zuravin S. Attributions of blame and responsibility for child sexual abuse and adult adjustment. *J Interpers Viol* 1997;12:30–48.

65. Paniagua F. *Assessing and treating culturally diverse clients: A practical guide.* Thousand Oaks, CA: Sage. 1994.

66. Perry BD, Pollard RA, Blakley TL, et al. Childhood trauma, the neurobiology of adaptation, and "use-dependent" development of the brain: How "states" become "traits." *Infant Mental Health Journal* 1996;16:271–291.

67. Perry BD, Putnam FW, Wherry JN. Psychophysiological effects of childhood trauma and their influence on development. Presented at International Society for Traumatic Stress Studies, Chicago. 1994.

68. Peterson G, Putnam FW. Preliminary results of the field trial of proposed criteria for dissociative disorders of childhood. *Dissociation* 1994;7:212–220.

69. Putnam FW. Dissociative disorders in children and adolescents: A developmental perspective. *Psychiatric Clinics of North America* 1991;14:519–531.

70. Putnam FW. Dissociative disorder in children: Behavioral profiles and problems. *Child Abuse Negl* 1993;17:39–45.

71. Putnam FW. *Dissociation in children and adolescents: A developmental perspective,* 283. New York: Guilford Press. 1997.

72. Putnam FW, Guroff JJ, Silberman EK, et al. The clinical phenomenology of multiple personality disorder: A review of 100 recent cases. *J Clin Psychiatry* 1986;47:285–293.

73. Putnam FW, Helmers K, Trickett PK. Development, reliability and validity of a child dissociation scale. *Child Abuse Negl* 1993;17:731–741.

74. *Rape in America: A report to the nation.* Arlington, VA: National Victim Center. 1992.

75. Reinecke MA, Daltilio FM, Freeman A. *Cognitive therapy with children and adolescents.* New York: Guilford. 1996.

76. Richters JE, Martinez P. The NIMH community violence project: Part I: Children as victims of and witnesses to violence. *Psychiatry* 1993;56:7–21.

77. Russell DEH. *The secret trauma: Incest in the lives of girls and women.* New York: Basic Books. 1986.

78. Salter AC. *Transforming trauma: A guide to understanding and treating adult survivors of child sexual abuse.* Thousand Oaks, CA: Sage. 1995.

79. Saunders BE, Williams LM. Introduction. *Child Maltreat* 1996;1:293.

80. Silberg JL, Waters FS. Factors associated with positive therapeutic outcome. In Silberg JL (ed.), *The dissociative child: Diagnosis, treatment and management,* 103–112. Lutherville, MD: Sidran Press. 1996.

81. Singer MI, Singer LT, Anglin TM (eds.). *Handbook for screening adolescents at psychosocial risk.* New York: Lexington Books. 1993.

82. Sirles A, Franke P. Factors influencing mothers' reactions to intrafamilial sexual abuse. *Child Abuse Negl* 1989;13:131–139.

83. Solomon SD, Gerrity ET, Muff AM. Efficacy of treatment for posttraumatic stress disorder. *JAMA* 1992;268:633–638.

84. Stauffer LB, Deblinger E. Cognitive behavioral groups for nonoffending mothers and their young sexually abused children: A preliminary treatment outcome study. *Child Maltreat* 1996; 1:65–76.

85. Stein J, Golding J, Siegel J, et al. Long-term psychological sequelae of child sexual abuse: The Los Angeles Epidemiologic Catchment Area Study. In Wyatt GE, Powell GJ, (eds.), *Lasting effects of child sexual abuse,* 135–154. Newbury Park, CA: Sage. 1988.

86. Strick FL, Wilcoxon SA. A comparison of dissociative experiences in adult female outpatients with and without histories of early incestuous abuse. *Dissociation* 1991;4:193–199.

87. Trickett P, Putnam F. Impact of child sexual abuse on females: Toward a developmental psychobiological integration. *Psychol Sci* 1993;4:81–87.

88. van der Kolk BA, McFarlane AC, and van der Hart O. A general approach to treatment of

posttraumatic stress disorder. In van der Kolk BA, McFarlane AD, and Weisaeth L (eds.), *Traumatic stress: The effects of overwhelming experience on mind, body, and society,* 417–440. New York: Guilford Press. 1996.

89. Waterbury M. School interventions for dissociative children. In Silberg JL (ed.), *The dissociative child: Diagnosis, treatment and management,* 316–329. Lutherville, MD: Sidran Press. 1996.

90. West LJ. Dissociative reaction. In Freeman AM, Kaplan HI (eds.), *Comprehensive textbook of psychiatry,* 885–899. Baltimore: Williams and Wilkins. 1967.

Chapter 3

Immediate Issues Affecting Long-term Family Resolution in Cases of Parent-Child Sexual Abuse

Benjamin E. Saunders, Ph.D., and Mary B. Meinig, M.S.W.

When sexual abuse occurs in a family, medical, social service, mental health, and legal systems will converge. Their presence is time-limited, but the continuing needs of the family and long-term family functioning must be considered in the services it receives and the issues that are addressed. These issues include separation/removal, continuing manipulation of the family by the parent offender, conflicting feelings of family members (child victim, nonoffending parent, nonabused siblings), and shared familial cognitive distortions. Successful family therapy will consider all the problems incest families will face over time, help develop ways of anticipating and managing these problems, affirm the positive parts of existing relationships, and seek to achieve some form of long-term family resolution in the best interest of child victims, allowing them both physical safety and the benefits of a positive parent-child relationship, when possible.

GENERAL CONSIDERATIONS

The notion that families are important and powerful social systems that affect the behavior of individuals throughout the life span is hardly a new idea.[5,6,21] However, although some authors have considered the salience of family systems in treatment of sexual abuse[2,14,15,20,24,28] treatment issues focused on these relationships have received surprisingly little attention in the abuse literature compared to the individual treatment of victims and offenders. This chapter discusses important—but often neglected—family relationship issues in cases of parent-child sexual abuse that should be taken into account to achieve an effective, long-term family resolution (not necessarily reunification) that will benefit child victims. Although some recommendations for intervention are made, the objective of the chapter is not to present a formal protocol of treatment procedures. Rather, its purpose is to encourage child abuse professionals to consider the complex, multifaceted and long-term developmental nature of the relationships within incest families that likely will persist well after the crisis of discovery and period of professional intervention are over.

SOCIETAL VALUE CONFLICTS

Responding to cases of parent-child sexual abuse presents enormous challenges to deeply held societal values. As a culture we have strong proscriptions against violence in general, and adult-child sexual violence in particular. Sexual assault of children is a crime, and public sentiment mandates prosecution and ever-increasing sentences for sexual offenders.[16] However, we as a society also have strong values about the sanctity and independence of families and the importance of parent-child relationships in the development of children. Cases of parent-child sexual abuse bring these strongly held values into conflict that can result in a confused, fragmented, and potentially harmful community response.[3,12,25] Some forms of child violence, such as corporal punishment, are allowed and even encouraged, while others, such as child rape, trigger severe social control mechanisms. Society continually questions itself—at what point does parental violence towards children overwhelm the value of familial independence and justify societal intervention? On what basis should society mandate the temporary separation or permanent dissolution of families because of parental violence toward children? Standards for these decisions change frequently as do attitudes about certain types of family violence.

Over the years, community management of these cases has fluctuated, from simply ignoring them and labeling intrafamilial sexual abuse as a "family problem" best handled internally by family members, to framing them strictly as crimes, to be dealt with by removing children from their homes, isolating them from the offending parent and possibly other family members, and working vigorously to prosecute and incarcerate the offenders. Parent offenders may be seen as "all bad" (offender) or "a good parent with a problem" (parent). At times, these opposing responses may be pursued simultaneously by different societal agents. One community agency may be seeking to incarcerate the parent offender while another is seeking to reunite the family. The mandates of intervening agencies can clash, resulting in muddled and inconsistent messages' being sent to child victims, parent offenders, and other family members.

Of course, parent-child sexual abuse, like all forms of family violence, is both a complex family problem *and* a serious crime with lasting negative effects for victims. Neither the crime nor the family issues should be ignored by abuse professionals or the community. The presence of the offender-victim relationship does not eliminate the psychological reality of the parent-child relationship for the child, nor vice versa. Both relationships are present and operating in the lives of abused children, and both will continue to have an impact over their life course. Sexual assault is a serious crime, yet parents, even abusive parents, are enormously important to children. Some parent offenders are not "all bad" and, over time, may have much to offer their children, with appropriate intervention. Therefore, one considerable challenge facing the community systems charged with responding to these cases is how to recognize the importance of both of these relationships (parent-child and offender-victim) to children and how to take them both into account when intervening for the good of children. Getting locked into only a criminal justice response or only a family preservation model ignores half of the reality of the entire situation. A sophisticated community response to parent-child sexual abuse must accommodate the multifaceted and complex nature of the relationships in these families for the good of child victims.

SEXUAL ABUSE AND FAMILY DEVELOPMENT

A second challenge for abuse professionals is to view intrafamilial sexual abuse cases in a longitudinal, life course, and developmental context. Individuals and family systems undergo developmental growth over time.[6] Therefore, sexual abuse cases must be viewed in a temporal as well as a social context. The efforts of the agencies commonly involved with these cases (e.g., child protective services, law enforcement, criminal justice system, medical system, mental health system) primarily are directed towards three goals: (1) investigating and adjudicating abuse charges, (2) developing immediate and relatively short-term protection plans for the children involved, and (3) engaging victims, offenders, and family members in appropriate treatment and treating the emergent problems associated with the abuse. Obviously, these are all important tasks that require sensitive and skillful work by professionals. However, these professional efforts usually involve a relatively short period of time in the total life course of individuals and families, and often are limited in their scope. Ultimately, intervention by abuse professionals will be simply a memory for child victims, parent offenders, and other family members, while familial relationships of some sort likely will continue for many years.

Many difficult, long-term concerns face abusive families, and these long-term problems are often overlooked by the intervening systems. The work associated with the immediate crisis of discovery, investigating a case, founding a case, developing protection plans, engaging victims and offenders in treatment, and conducting prosecution may overshadow the less urgent long-term tasks. Will this family reunite if some sort of separation of offender and victim has occurred? How will decisions about reunification or dissolution be made? How will these families function when the investigation and adjudication of the case is over? How will family members relate to one another after treatment is completed? What kind of relationship will the child and offending parent have in the long term? If the parent offender has been incarcerated, how will the family function when he or she is released? How can the safety of children be maintained when professionals are no longer involved with the case? How will this family meet the inevitable developmental challenges ahead? How will this family function 2 years, 5 years, 15 years, even 30 years after the discovery of abuse by professionals? Over the years, these long-term issues may actually be more important to the welfare of the child than many of the immediate crisis problems that receive so much professional attention in the aftermath of disclosure.

Although there is a growing body of research on the characteristics of incestuous families,[9,17,18,22,26,27] no longitudinal study has examined how these families change, function, and naturally resolve these family relationship tasks over time. In addition, no longitudinal study has investigated the long-term familial and relational effects of interventions commonly used in sexual abuse cases. Consequently, at this point little guidance is available from the empirical research literature. However, it is clear that these families do not cease to exist when a child abuse case is closed by professionals or a parent offender is sentenced to prison. It is likely that in most cases of parent-child sexual abuse, families will persist in one form or another long after the professionals have exited their lives. Even if the offender is incarcerated, he likely will be released within five years,[16] and most probably will return to the family. Therefore, a second task of intervention is to consider all the problems incestuous families will face over time, to help them develop ways of anticipating and managing these problems, and to achieve some form of long-term family resolution in the best interest of child victims.

FAMILY RESOLUTION

The term *family resolution* is used in this chapter to denote the process of helping to develop a long-term familial outcome that will serve the best interests of a child victim over his or her life course. Neither family preservation, family reunification, family separation, nor family dissolution is the purpose of family resolution therapy. Rather, the goal of intervention is to develop an individualized, long-term resolution of familial relationships and related issues that takes into account both the offender-victim and the parent-child relationships that are present in incestuous families and to work for the welfare of the child victim. Child safety and welfare is of paramount concern in family resolution, but the potential benefits to child victims of maintaining relationships with parents when significant emotional bonds exist is also recognized.

These resolved parent-child relationships will function very differently from how they operated during the abuse period. They will not be "normal" or like traditional parent-child relationships, because the parents remain sexual offenders and continue to present an ongoing risk to children. Family resolution therapy seeks to develop familial and relationship structures and processes that offer reasonable levels of child protection, while allowing child victims access to their parent offenders and other family members. In addition to common components of victim, offender, and family therapy, these structures and processes will incorporate family contact and operational rules, ongoing supervision of the offender, relapse prevention techniques and other restrictions that are quite unlike the way normal families operate.[23] Though these procedures are complicated and difficult to implement, they allow children to benefit from an altered and improved relationship with their parents in an abuse-inhibiting environment.

Flexibility is the hallmark of successful family resolution, since no one family structure is best for every abused child. The prospects for family resolution exist on a continuum of potential family structures, with the level of parent offender contact with the child victim being the construct of interest. This structural continuum can range from parental divorce with no contact between offender and victim, to family reunification with daily contact under protective restrictions. Resolution can also result in a variety of other "middle ground" family situations that incorporate different levels of contact. Some couples may divorce and only limited supervised contact between the child victims and their parent offenders may be judged beneficial to the children. In other families, the offending parent may live outside the home but have frequent supervised contact with the child victim. The goal of family resolution therapy is to develop an individualized structure that provides the level of contact that is best for the child. For some children, no contact may be what is in their best interest. For others, family reunification serves them best. And for still other children, a structure that offers limited contact with parent offenders is best. As children grow and families change, family structures and protection procedures may change over time as the needs of the children change.

PARENT-CHILD EMOTIONAL ATTACHMENT

Critical to family resolution decisions and therapy is the issue of whether or not any sort of emotional attachment ever existed between a parent offender and a child victim. In cases where stepparents or cohabiting partners of biological parents are the offenders, it is not uncommon for child victims to have relatively little emotional connection to the offending adults. The offending adult may be simply "Mom's boyfriend" or "Dad's wife" rather than an emotionally attached parental figure of significance to the victim.

On the other hand, children may be highly attached to their offending parents, view them as supportive and good parents apart from the abuse, and want to continue the relationship. Professionals must remember that the quality of the emotional attachment of a child to an offending parent cannot be inferred from the strict legal relationship that exists between the two. Despite the frequently assumed power of "blood" relationships, a child may have little or no emotional attachment to a persistently abusive biological parent. However, a child may be emotionally bonded to "Mom's boyfriend" or a stepparent who, from the child's perspective, functioned as a good parental figure apart from the abuse. Therefore, the quality of the relationship before abuse and the current emotional attachment of the child to the offender should be thoroughly assessed and given significant weight in resolution decision making. Too often, only the legal relationship of the offender to the child is considered in professional decision making. Most of the following points assume that a significant emotional bond existed between the offender and the victim prior to and even during the abuse, and that the attachment persists during the professional intervention period after the disclosure of abuse.

RESOLUTION ISSUES DURING THE IMMEDIATE AFTERMATH OF DISCLOSURE

For professionals, a sexual abuse case begins with the report of abuse and ends when the case is officially closed. However, for families the sexual abuse and the relational dynamics associated with it have been ongoing for some time prior to the report, and its impact will continue over the life of the family long after the last abuse professional is seen. For families, disclosure is a midpoint, not a beginning—their family life does not end when the case is closed by professionals.

The immediate aftermath of disclosure is the beginning of the long-term family resolution program, and decisions and interventions by professionals at that time can either aid or hinder a successful resolution. However, decisions made by professionals during this period typically are based on current, emergent needs, with little thought about how those decisions might affect the family in the long run. Therapy for child victims, parent offenders, and other family members is usually directed towards individual needs and immediate problems. Long-term resolution issues usually are of secondary importance. If professionals consider the potential long-term implications of their interventions in addition to the immediate impact, they can maximize the effectiveness of their efforts. Examples of some of these immediate resolution issues and ways in which their long-term consequences can be understood are discussed below.

Offender's Acknowledgment or Denial of Sexual Abuse

The most critical concern for long-term resolution is whether or not the offender acknowledges the sexual abuse. This issue has obvious immediate consequences, but the importance of offender acknowledgment for the long-term welfare of the victim and the family cannot be overemphasized. The necessary activities of investigation, case founding, arrest, and prosecution should be conducted in a manner that encourages acknowledgment of the abuse by the parent offender. Beyond the fact that it simplifies many of the initial efforts by professionals, acknowledgment of the abuse is also the single most important step in successful family resolution. Without acknowledgment of the abuse by the offender, establishing any form of functional parent-child relationship is extraordinarily difficult, if not impossible.

Unfortunately, too often, only the offender-victim roles are considered in the initial stages of a parent-child sexual abuse case. Investigations often are conducted in a confrontational and adversarial manner that does not encourage an acknowledgment from the parent offender. Criminal investigation and prosecution are important parts of society's response to sexual abuse and need to occur. However, if they are the only response, then children and families will be poorly served. Relatively few parental sexual offenders are incarcerated, and those that are will spend less than five years in prison on average.[16] Also, parent-child relationships do not end just because a parent is in prison. Therefore, if investigations can be conducted with the long-term implications for the parent-child relationship in mind and with an eye toward gaining an early acknowledgment, family resolution will be greatly aided.

Offender's Discrediting of Victim

After a disclosure or discovery of parent-child sexual abuse, it is not uncommon for the parent offender not only to deny the abuse but also to attempt to discredit the child victim. One of offenders' greatest fears is disclosure by victims.[7] Consequently, they frequently take steps during the abuse period to be prepared to defame the victim and encourage others to discount the victim's statements about the abuse. For example, a parent offender's contingency plans during the abuse period might include: (1) frequently pointing out the victim's faults to others, particularly the nonoffending parent; (2) emphasizing to others how much the victim lies about many things; (3) drawing attention to any lie or misunderstanding associated with the victim; (4) harshly disciplining the victim in front of family members, so that if the child victim tells someone about the abuse, the parent offender can say revenge was the motive; (5) sharply restricting the victim's activities, to isolate the victim from others and to provide a revenge excuse if needed; (6) drawing attention to anything the victim does that could be construed as sexual (e.g., too much makeup, tight jeans) to portray the victim as seductive or overly sexualized; (7) calling victims sexually derogatory names in front of others; or (8) asking victims about their sexual activities in front of others.

Through activities such as these, offenders can set up victims not to be believed or trusted if they disclose the abuse. These strategies also build a fear within the child victim that he or she is not likely to be believed by others. By conducting a preemptive strike on the child's character or setting up a plausible explanation for why a child would make a false accusation, a parent offender can reduce the likelihood that the child will tell, and can have a ready explanation for the "false" report if the child does tell. These discrediting activities are very painful and confusing for child victims and must be appropriately clarified and resolved for the parent-child relationship to continue for the benefit of the child.

Immediate Separation and Visitation

In cases of parent-child sexual abuse where the nonoffending parent is judged to be protective, parent offenders are often asked to leave the home rather than the children being removed. If nonoffending parents are judged not protective, child victims may be removed from the home. These interventions are made primarily for the safety and protection of the children. Offender removal usually is preferred, because it is less disruptive to children.

There also are long-term therapeutic reasons for preferring offender separation over child removal. For successful long-term resolution to occur, child victims and other family members need a significant period of not only physical distance from the offender, for safety, but psychological and emotional distance as well.[23] With separation of the offender, the victim, nonoffending parent, and nonabused siblings have the time and psychological space to assess how the offender managed to manipulate them psychologically and emotionally to create an environment conducive for abuse. With therapeutic guidance, they can work on better ways of functioning and operating as a family system without this manipulation, a critical task for successful family resolution. The family can develop new processes and ways of functioning that do not include the offender's orchestration of the family environment. Over time, these new ways of functioning become part of a new, healthier homeostatic level for the family system.

With parental separation comes the issue of visitation. Often parent offenders may agree to leave the home but then demand immediate visitation with their children. Because the immediate concern of the community response system is protection of the child from re-offense, often only supervised visitation is granted. The belief is that the children will not be in physical danger if the visits are supervised. Unfortunately, the offender's significant emotional and psychological control over the child victim, nonoffending parent, and nonabused siblings may be the greatest threat in the long run. Even in supervised visits, parent offenders have great potential for manipulating victims into minimizing, discounting, and even recanting their disclosure of sexual abuse, often out of fear, love, or sympathy for the abusive parent. Parent offenders also can coerce nonabusing parents into attempting to rescue them, assuming indirect responsibility for the abuse, or even punishing the child victim. Offenders can maneuver nonabused siblings into projecting blame and anger onto victims. Therefore, continued contact immediately after disclosure, even if it is supervised, allows parent offenders the opportunity to continue to manage and manipulate the offense system they created within the family.

Disclosure usually stops the sexual abuse and alters the status quo between the child victim and the parent offender. Relationships among other family members and the parent offender also are changed, and the family system is challenged by this crisis to develop new ways of functioning. The natural homeostatic inclination of family systems faced with such significant change is to attempt to return to the previous state of functioning.[11] Families seek to maintain and/or return to the old ways of operating and to reestablish prior processes. Therefore, interventions must combat the homeostatic push and promote dramatic morphogenic change in the family system. Towards this goal, all family members need distance and time away from the parent offender in order to consider the significance the abuse has had on their relationships and to develop new ways of functioning. This inter- and intrapersonal exploration needs to be done without the offender's self-serving input and ability to manipulate the family. The child victim and other family members need time and distance from the offender in order to reassess the nature of their relationships and their desire to be emotionally invested in the parent offender in the future.

One goal of intervention is to break the abuse-based family systemic processes and promote an abuse-inhibiting environment. Separation from the offender helps this task and ongoing, regular contact with the offender makes it very difficult. Therefore, separation, removal, and visitation decisions should be made not only with the immediate physical safety of the child as the goal; the therapeutic impact on the long-term family change process and ultimate resolution should be considered as well.

Offender Manipulation of the Family System

Intrafamilial sex offenders create offense systems within the family. That is, they attempt to direct and control family members and family processes in order to develop and maintain a noninhibiting family environment that accommodates their molestation of children. Parental child molesters manage their child victims and other family members through emotional and psychological manipulation and, at times, with psychological and physical intimidation. They know their child victims well, and can use their children's psychological pressure points to manage them and gain leverage over them. They have continuous access to their children and a position of power in their lives, so the process can be slow and continual. Through this "grooming" process,[8] parent offenders can isolate the child victim from other family members, develop trust while slowly testing and crossing personal and sexual boundaries, frame their behavior as normal, develop a sense of secrecy with the victim, and create an atmosphere of acceptance of these behaviors within the family system.

To others, specific acts of offender manipulation can seem innocent and unrelated to the abuse. For example, why would a father repeatedly tell his slim 11-year-old stepdaughter that she was fat? What kind of leverage would those comments give an offender over a victim? They might make her less sure of herself, less confident in her perceptions and judgment. They might even make her question her own sense of reality, because this is her father saying these things. They may hurt her and move her to seek her father's approval and love. When the child victim believes what the parent offender says, and incorporates it into her self-image, this simply reflects the influence he has over her. Further, his manipulative statements gain credibility if they are not refuted by other family members. In fact, they may even come to be believed by other family members and become part of a shared familial "reality." Such influence can be constant, pervasive, and insidious, even though individual comments and events may seem innocuous, innocent, and even playful. A critical task of family resolution is for all the family members to understand exactly how parent offenders created and maintained the noninhibiting offense system through manipulation, grooming, management, and intimidation. These must be exposed within the family, acknowledged by the parent offender, clarified for the child victim, and corrected within the family process.

Shared Familial Cognitive Distortions

Individual therapy for sexual offenders typically includes treatment components for identifying and changing cognitive distortions.[1,4] However, the content and nature of these distortions are relevant not only to offender treatment but to intervention with victims and family members as well. As noted above, many of these cognitive distortions often are held by family members and may constitute a shared familial reality. They can serve as the basis for much of the manipulation, management, and intimidation of the family by the parent offender. Therefore, a critical step in family resolution is identifying and correcting, not only misguided thinking by the offender, but distorted cognitions by victim and family members as well.

Parent offenders' responsibility to their victims and families requires that they acknowledge their sexually abusive behavior as not capricious or accidental in nature but as a well-planned endeavor, implemented with great care and forethought. In sexual offender therapy, offenders must break through their internal cognitive justifications and explanations that have been maintained and defended over a period of time. Sharing this contorted thinking with victims and family members and connecting it to the abusive behavior aids their therapy. By understanding offenders' thinking errors, victims and family members can better understand their own thinking and behavior that kept them from recognizing signals that abuse was occurring. Therefore, information garnered from parent offenders' therapy can be instrumental in the therapy of victims and family members.

For example, it may become the family "lore" that father molested son because father is an alcoholic, was drunk during the abuse episodes, and acted completely out of character because of his intoxication. This simple one-factor answer seems to explain father's sexually deviant behavior to the satisfaction of the family, and seems plausible on the surface. In fact, friends, neighbors, coworkers, and extended family may agree with this easy explanation and repeatedly reinforce it to the victim and the family. After all, father is a normal, regular person, a good neighbor, a good friend, and a good employee. People were shocked to learn about his sexual abuse of his son, and really still cannot believe it. Obviously he is not a "child molester" like the ones everyone reads about in the newspapers. There must be some explanation.

Family members, friends, and acquaintances are more comfortable viewing father as an alcoholic than as a child molester. They tend to accept such an explanation because it is more socially acceptable and comfortable to those in the offender's social network. They may also hold to a stereotype of a child molester that is inconsistent with their perceptions of father. Father may play on this theme and attempt to gain sympathy from family members and others for his substance abuse disorder and thus shift the focus away from his deviant sexual behavior. Also, holding this belief simplifies treatment and many other issues. Father simply needs to be kept sober and have his alcoholism treated in order to prevent further sexual abuse.

Challenging and changing shared familial cognitive distortions that comfortably explain abusive behavior is not an easy task, because of the sheer systemic weight they often carry in a family. Objectively, they usually can be contested rather easily. In the above example, therapists could discuss with the offender and the family members the fact that many men get drunk and a very, very small proportion of them molest children while intoxicated. Also, many people have very serious substance abuse problems, but a very small percentage of them molest children. Therefore, substance abuse does not seem to be a very good explanation for child molesting. With minimal intervention, most offenders and family members can understand the logical error of their thinking.

More difficult, and more important, is helping the family face the implications of their cognitive inaccuracy. Discrediting and changing any simple shared familial distortion that previously provided a ready and more socially acceptable explanation for the sexually abusive behavior has enormous implications for the long-term functioning of the family.

It means the parent offender really does have a serious sexual deviancy problem. It means the abuse was purposeful and not accidental. It means the family has to face the reality that the parent is dangerous to children. It means the family's prior judgment about the situation was incorrect and calls into question their judgment. It means significant and difficult treatment is needed. Such realizations are serious challenges to the long-term integrity of the family system, and likely will be resisted. Consequently, family members may hold strongly to their cognitive distortions or rekindle them periodically, not because they do not understand the logical inaccuracy of their thinking, but because they cannot bear the implications of not holding to them. Therefore, successful family resolution requires that the shared familial cognitive distortions be exposed and corrected in parent offenders, child victims, and other family members. To accomplish this task, offender, victim, and family therapists must coordinate their efforts, and the importance to the family of changing these thinking errors must be understood by all the professionals involved.

Conflicted Feelings by Victims

Child victims typically have conflicted feelings about their parent offenders. They may talk about how much they love and how much they hate the parent offender in the same sentence. It is not uncommon for child victims to be highly bonded to their parent offenders and view their relationship as emotionally close but also to speak of the betrayal inherent in the abusive relationship.[13] Child victims even may view the offending parent as the better parent and have significant difficulties with the nonoffending parent. At the same time, they are confused as to why this good parent hurt them and may become more confused as they go through treatment. Sorting out these conflicted feelings, not just for the child victims, but for all family members, is a primary task of family resolution.

Upon the disclosure of sexual abuse, child victims frequently are met with a barrage of statements from people significant in their lives indicating how they "must" or "should" feel about their parent offenders. Frequently, victims may not have "permission" from significant others to have positive regard for their parent offenders or genuine concern for the parent offender's welfare. Instead, others expect and even demand that victims express negative feelings toward or even hate the parent offender. The opposite may be true as well. That is, victims may be told they cannot feel negative toward their parents, even if they are offenders. They may be told they should still love and respect parent offenders, simply because they are parents. When child victims are confronted with such a barrage of emotional demands from other people, their ability to clarify their own feelings is confounded. Child victims may be confused if they do not feel the same degree of loathing or love for the offending parent that is being demanded by others. Child victims might make the interpretation that something must truly be wrong with them if they do not have the required positive or negative feelings for the offender. Therefore, therapists must not only assess the conflicted feelings held by victims and family members individually, they should also evaluate the emotional pressure put on them by significant others such as extended family, friends, and even other professionals.

Family resolution therapy focuses on dissecting, clarifying, and translating the parent offender's behavior and the child victim's responses to the offender's behavior. One key question in this process is, What was honest in the parent child relationship and what was manipulation in order to offend and maintain control? Child victims and family members often will reexamine every positive thing parent offenders have done over the years and ask themselves, were these acts honest, genuine expressions of caring or simply selfish, manipulative, offense-driven grooming behaviors. The goal of family resolution therapy in this process is to capitalize on the genuine caring parts of the relationship but provide a reality check on the manipulative, grooming parts. Abusive parents can love their child victims and do loving and caring things for them. However, the abuse was not about love, regardless of the justifications offered by the offender. Rather, it was about establishing and maintaining a deviant sexual outlet.

The therapy process for conflicted feelings can be slow. The focus can swing wildly from the parent-child relationship to the offender-victim relationship. Both relationships are present and need to be thoroughly examined, clarified, and resolved in therapy. Therapists need to recognize victims' conflicted feelings and distorted cognitions about parent offenders. Therapists should be supportive of the victims' feelings, however conflicted they may be, because conflicted feelings are the norm and are valid. Therapists should guard against being overtly directive or condemning of the parent offender while gently challenging victims' cognitive distortions about the abuse behavior. The positive parts of the parent-child relationship can be affirmed, while the offender-victim relationship should be challenged. The therapeutic challenge is to keep these role definitions separate and distinct. Resolution therapy is a fluid process that can go through various stages over time. Enabling child victims, family members, and parent offenders to explore their conflicted feelings and cognitions, and helping them test different ways of thinking about what happened and the future, is critical to the resolution therapy process.

Forgiveness of the Parent Offender

The issue of child victims "forgiving" their parent offenders is controversial.[23] Whatever stance one takes, a clear complication for the recovery of child victims and for long-term family resolution arises when significant others quickly forgive the parent offenders. It is interesting that people whom the parent offender has never victimized often immediately rally to forgive or to make excuses for the parent offender, apparently with little thought about the discounting impact this response might have on child victims. Immediate forgiveness of the parent offender by significant others tends to leave child victims feeling demeaned and emotionally abandoned. Children in this situation also are likely to feel strong pressure to forgive the offender when they are not emotionally or cognitively prepared to do so. They may be confused by the forgiving actions of others and regret that they do not feel the same sense of forgiveness.

As with the problem of conflicted feelings, therapists should make a point of assessing the attitudes of significant others towards the offender and how these attitudes might affect the victim. The therapy should give the child the time and emotional space to sort out his or her own conflicted feelings about possible forgiveness and help place the attitudes and actions of others in perspective for the child. Family therapy can help others understand the impact of their actions on the child. The goal of therapy is neither to encourage nor discourage forgiveness by the child. Rather, family resolution therapy seeks to enable the child to examine his or her feelings over time and with the changes that come with therapy, and to arrive at an independent decision regarding forgiveness. For some children feeling and expressing forgiveness will be a necessary component of their recovery. For others, such a response would not be helpful. In either case, a premature push for forgiveness by family members, friends, or even professionals makes recovery and genuine family resolution more difficult.

Personal Independence

After disclosure, victims are emotionally vulnerable to other people. The absence of the offending parent often leaves an emotional void in their lives and they may feel guilty about having revealed the abuse. They also are confronted with the enormous stress of coping with all the things that happen after the disclosure of abuse. Some victims have been conditioned by offenders to be influenced by others. Victims frequently are unsure of themselves. The offender may have created a set of false beliefs about others and the actions of others that the victim may not know how to manage. Personal independence and independent thinking, particularly by victims, often have been discouraged in the family.[26] Therefore, the development of age-appropriate personal independence in child victims is necessary to long-term family resolution. Personal independence is necessary for decision making about the nature of the relationship the child victim wants ultimately to have with the parent offender. It is also mandatory for safety and protection. Resolution decisions cannot be made if the child continues to be emotionally dependent upon or unduly influenced by the parent offender.

Therapists and other professionals should avoid stepping in where the parent offender left off by immediately telling the victim how to think and feel. Rather, therapists should teach child victims how to receive information, process it independently, form their own conclusions, and develop their own appropriate thinking about the abuse, their relationship to the offender, and their relationships with other family members. A therapist can offer challenges when the child's thinking continues to be influenced by the offender or is clearly distorted or inaccurate. Therapy may even include using clarifying information from the parent offender that specifically identifies how he or she influenced certain beliefs held by the child victim. However, simply changing the content of distorted cognitions is not enough. Victims need to learn the process of personal independence and unlearn the conditioned influences used by the parent offender. As a sense of personal independence grows, meaningful decisions about family resolution can be made by the child.

Response of the Nonoffending Parent

Nonoffending spouses are critical to the recovery of abused children[10] and the key to successful, long-term family resolution. Successful resolution depends upon these parents' being able to function in a supportive and protective manner with the child victim and to monitor and mediate the quantity and nature of contact parent offenders have with children, if such contact is deemed useful for children. Throughout treatment, these parents will need to

- believe the child's description of the abuse,
- be emotionally supportive of the child,
- be instrumentally supportive of all the children in the family,
- develop a sense of personal independence from the offending parent,
- develop an understanding of the ongoing threat the parent offender presents to children, and
- be able to intervene when necessary to protect their children.

Developing these responses in nonoffending spouses is a primary task of family resolution therapy. Without an assertive, independent, and protective nonoffending parent, any significant contact between the parent offender and the child victim will be difficult to monitor for safety.

It is difficult to underestimate the traumatic impact the disclosure of parent-child sexual abuse has on nonoffending parents. The disclosure and its aftermath is a genuine, major crisis. It is a life threat to their whole world—their family, marriage, children, privacy, economic subsistence, sense of self-efficacy, and emotional welfare. Nonoffending parents immediately have a sense of divided loyalty between their spouse and their child, fear of the consequences, confusion about what actually happened, and more confusion about what to do. Consequently, these parents tend to react in a crisis-survival mode. They frequently act in ways difficult for even seasoned abuse professionals to understand. Professionals may even find themselves getting angry with and condemning these parents when they are unsupportive of child victims, side with parent offenders, and act in ways that are harmful to their children. Some professionals may find themselves being angrier at the unprotective nonoffending parent than at the parent offender.

However, these parents need understanding, compassion, and support from professionals, not condemnation and anger. For most of these parents, the disclosure of child sexual abuse is the single biggest crisis of their lives. They are not prepared for it and frequently have emotional difficulties of their own that make reacting appropriately even more difficult. Professionals need to remember the long-term importance of these parents to child victims and structure intervention programs to help move them toward being supportive and protective parents. Understanding the impossible position in which these parents are placed and placing their reactions in context is a first step in this process.

Reactions by nonoffending parents are varied and reflect the highly emotionally charged nature of the significant threat to survival they perceive. For some, survival means responding with disbelief or even condemning the child victim, and giving strong support to the parent offender. For others, even though they may believe the child, survival demands that they minimize the extent or impact of the abuse. Some may direct their anger to the intervening professionals, and some simply may remain ambivalent. Still others react with anger and hatred toward the offender and demand that everyone, including the child victim, hate the offender. They frantically attempt to limit the damage the disclosure has created in the family and desperately seek the aid or influence of the child victim to accomplish this. Their responses may be impulsive, erratic, confused, contradictory, and disturbing. Often, things are said and done that hurt the child victim.

Common complicating responses by nonoffending parents that need to be dealt with early in treatment include

- being skeptical about the abuse because they do not believe it could have happened without their knowing about it ("He was never really alone with her"),
- repeatedly questioning victims about why they did not tell sooner ("Why didn't you tell me as soon as it happened?"),
- minimizing or discounting the severity and long-term impact of the sexual assaults ("He only touched her a few times. How much could that hurt her?"),
- making justifying excuses for the offender ("He was sexually abused too," "He does crazy things when he gets drunk," "He just got fired"),
- assuming responsibility for the abuse ("I wouldn't have sex with him," "I should never have gone back to work"),
- making premature definitive statements about their decision to stay with the offender ("He's my husband and I have to stand by him no matter what"),

- telling the victim not to tell other family members or friends about the abuse ("It will hurt your father if you tell everyone"),
- telling young victims about their concerns about financial worries ("I don't know how we are going to make it if your dad has to get an apartment"),
- telling victims about their fears about the legal consequences the offender is facing ("He will go to jail for 30 years for this").

These and other immediate complicating reactions by nonoffending parents should be assessed, and limited when possible.

At the time of disclosure, nonoffending parents should be directed away from focusing on the parent offender and encouraged to focus on the needs of the child victim and other children in the family. The pull for the nonoffending spouse is usually toward the offender. Spouses often are desperate for some explanation. How could the person they are married to be capable of molesting their child or any child? Their first thought is, there must be some misunderstanding. The message this reaction tends to send to the child victim and the intervening professionals is that the spouse does not believe the child and probably will not be protective. In fact, the nonoffending spouse simply may be acting normally, as most people would when told a story that is completely outside their reality.

In addition, as described above, the offender may have prepared contingency plans to use if and when the sexual offending was disclosed. At the time of disclosure, the non-offending spouse is open to—even desperate for—some explanation other than the reality of sexual abuse. Therefore, the offender's justifying explanations and excuses may be readily embraced by the spouse. Offenders know their spouses well, and can conceive effective ways to influence them. Consequently, it is often not difficult for them to keep their spouses aligned with them after disclosure.

Professionals need to understand that disbelief of child victims and alignment with parent offenders by nonoffending parents is not necessarily due to a lack of caring, empathy, love, or desire for safety for the child victim. These parents rarely make harmful comments or poor decisions out of malice, but out of confusion, ignorance, and fear. These behaviors may be due to a confluence of factors including:

- the nonoffending spouses' personal and emotional deficits,
- their fears about the survival implications of the disclosure,
- their own sense of guilt for not preventing the abuse,
- the difficulty of believing an incredible story,
- the parent offender's contingency planning for discovery, and
- the parent offender's ongoing manipulation of the situation after disclosure.

A task of family resolution therapy is to help nonoffending spouses deal with all of these issues and work to help them become assertive, supportive, and protective of the child victim.

The support and building up of nonoffending spouses should begin immediately after the disclosure. As noted above, nonoffending spouses need time and distance from parent offenders in order to avoid further manipulation and to get some clarity about the abuse and how the abuse system was managed. Until the nonoffending spouse sorts out the disparity between the sexually abusive behavior and that of the spouse they thought they knew, it is best that the parent offender be gone from the home and have no contact with any of the children.

These parents also need prompt help and support with managing the trauma to the child victim, other children in the family, and themselves. They need information about the legal system, the expectations of the child protective system, the impact of sexual victimization on children, and treatment availability. When there is a therapy group for nonoffending parents, they should begin attending as soon as possible. The spouses need support, both practical and emotional. Disclosure of the abuse generates enormous demands on nonoffending spouses, such as additional expenses for therapy, transporting the children to therapy and other meetings within the child protection and criminal justice systems, dealing with the multitude of professionals who are suddenly in their lives, and having to immediately finance a separate household with their current income. Alone, these responsibilities are enormous. When the emotional stress of helping a traumatized child is included, it is no wonder that these nonoffending parents often make inappropriate decisions and behave in ways that tend to disappoint and anger the very professionals on whom they need to rely.

The community response system should view nonoffending parents as lifetime resources for children who need to be understood and supported. Successful family resolution is dependent upon helping these parents become supportive and protective. Intervention should not be confrontational or adversarial, even when the actions of nonoffending spouses are not supportive of child victims. Confrontation and anger isolates and disengages nonoffending spouses from the helping professionals, enables the offender to be more successful in manipulating the nonoffending spouse, makes the tasks of family resolution more difficult, and hinders the development of a primary support system for child victims. Therefore, abuse professionals should have a clear idea of why nonoffending parents act the way they do, view them as long-term supportive resources for the child, help these people deal with the tremendous crisis they are going through, and help them become supportive and protective parents.

Nonabused Siblings

Nonabused siblings of victims of parental sexual abuse typically get only minimal intervention when the abuse is disclosed. Once it is determined by child protective services or law enforcement that these children were not directly victimized, their needs usually get the least priority. However, these children typically do have important needs, and dealing with these needs is critical to family resolution. Unfortunately, nonabused siblings tend to become committed to the notion that the abuse had nothing to do with them, that it did not affect them in any way, that they were never at risk, and that the abuse is really not their business. If the community response system ignores them, this cognitive and emotional disengagement is reinforced. These children tend to be all too willing to be out of the loop and disconnected from the aftermath of disclosure. Therefore, engaging them in treatment can be difficult, when it is attempted at all.

It is not unusual for nonabused siblings to be angry at the victim for disclosing the abuse. The siblings may believe that they are being unfairly inconvenienced by the consequences of disclosure. In particular, if the parent offender is removed from the home, if contact with the offending parent is not permitted, if the nonoffending parent is distracted and less available because of the crisis of disclosure, or if the family suffers financial or other hardship after disclosure, siblings may blame the victim for telling. This rift in the sibling subsystem must be corrected for successful family resolution to occur.

Because these children were not identified as victims, it is not unusual for their contact with the parent offender to continue. The court process may take several months, leaving the offender with access to these children. Unfortunately, ongoing contact with the offender not only places the siblings at risk for abuse but also makes it difficult for them to have the distance from the offender that they need to sort out their issues, such as anger towards the victim. Nonabused siblings need physical and emotional distance from the parent offender just as victims and nonoffending spouses do. Also, sibling contact with parent offenders tends to isolate child victims from their sibling group, gives the impression that somehow victims are different from other children, and suggests there is something wrong with them. The rift between the abused and nonabused siblings is bolstered.

There are other concerns about premature contact between the parent offender and the nonabused children. These children may actually have been victimized and simply are not disclosing because they are afraid, especially after witnessing the response to the disclosing victim. Ongoing contact with the offender reduces the likelihood that siblings who may also have been abused will ever reveal it. Contact gives the impression that the parent offender is only a risk to the disclosing child victim and not to other children. This impression is a serious problem to long-term family resolution, where a key component is understanding the ongoing risk offenders present to all children. If the professionals do not act as if the parent offender is potentially dangerous to all children, it is difficult to build this belief in family members.

Siblings often are confused, embarrassed, and emotionally distraught over the accusations against the offending parent. Therefore, in a self-protective bent, they rarely ask questions about the abuse. It is important to keep these children informed about and included in the protective service and judicial process and the treatment process. These children have been affected by the abuse. They need information and help in defining the emotional impact the abuse has had on their lives and how it has affected their thinking about the parent offender. They also need information about their victimized sibling and how the abuse may have affected him or her. They have questions about the abuse and about their response to the disclosure. What is sexual abuse? Do they need to take sides? Who is telling the truth? What really happened? Is Dad really a sex offender? As nonoffending spouses do, nonabused siblings often align with the parent offender, for many of the same reasons. Disclosure of sexual abuse is a significant threat to them and their lives. Therefore, it is crucial to the family resolution process that nonabused siblings, as well as other family members, be kept informed about the intervention process and that they receive treatment to help them sort out these questions, deal with their distorted thinking, and resolve conflicted feelings.

Under some circumstances, it is in the nonabused siblings' best interests to have some sort of contact with the parent offender. Such a decision should be made on the basis of what is in the best interests of the children, not because the parent wants it, or because of an arbitrary legal argument disconnected from the physical and psychological welfare of the children. In some cases, contact with the parent offender can serve to reassure children that the absent parent is healthy and safe, even though they are not seeing him or her. Contact can decrease the resistance these siblings have to being included in the treatment process. Contact through a clarification process[19] can give the siblings an opportunity to hear the parent offender assume full responsibility for the trouble the family is experiencing.

Contact does not necessarily have to be face-to-face. It can often be accomplished by using a letter from the parent offender or a videotape of the parent offender speaking to the children. These mechanisms are useful because the contact can be monitored and controlled for the benefit of the children. In rare cases, an in-person, professionally supervised contact is best for the children. Professionals should be conservative when making decisions about contact between parent offenders and their children and should not underestimate the potential harm of even brief, supervised visitation. As noted above, parent offenders can cause problems in ways that are undetectable even by professionals. Decisions should be made based not only on immediate concerns; the impact on long-term family resolution should be considered as well.

CONCLUSION

Children molested by emotionally attached parents necessarily have conflicted feelings about their parent offenders. The stronger the emotional bond to the parent, the more taxing are those conflicted feelings to the child. Victims express these feelings in therapy in many ways, but the depth of their confusion and distress frequently is revealed most poignantly in their letters to their abusers. As one victim wrote, "You know that I hated people who would molest kids—cuz we talked about it—if you weren't my dad I would think you should be punished a lot. But cuz you're my dad, it's harder." Another wrote, "I remember one time when a friend said you touched her when you were wrestling. I stuck up for you and said 'he did not'. Then I didn't think you did, and I am mad!" The commitment child victims have to their parent offenders is often very strong, even when the abuse has been severe. As one child wrote in a letter to a judge, "I love him so much because I could always turn to him when I needed someone. Dad is the specialist guy I know. He is the cuddliest, the funniest. I just can't stand being without him." Child victims' conflicted feelings parallel the conflicted societal values often reflected in the community response to intrafamilial violence.

Resolving the tangled emotional mass created by a parent's sexual abuse of his or her child is a lifelong endeavor for child victims, parent offenders, nonoffending parents, and nonabused siblings. Helping incestuous families achieve some sort of long-term resolution to these important family relationship issues is the responsibility of abuse professionals and the community response system. Although many urgent tasks must be completed after the discovery of sexual abuse, case decisions should not be based solely on the demands of the emergent situation. Rather, the potential long-term impact of these decisions should be considered and given equal weight in the decision-making process. Abuse professionals need to understand that the time period of professional intervention with incestuous families is relatively short compared to the family developmental life cycle, and that family relationships rarely end because of abuse or the disclosure of abuse. Most incestuous families are going to achieve some sort of family resolution with or without the help of professionals. That is just the nature of families, even abusive ones. The goal of family resolution therapy is to develop a family structure and a level of family functioning that promotes the safety of children and enables children to benefit from parental relationships when possible. Considering the issues raised in this chapter will help families achieve this goal.

R E F E R E N C E S

1. Abel GG, Becker JV, Cunningham-Ratherner JC, et al. *The treatment of child molesters.* Atlanta: Privately printed. 1984.

2. Alexander, PC. A systems theory conceptualization of incest. *Fam Process* 1985;24:79–88.

3. Arnold C II. Family preservation and reunification in intra-familial sexual abuse cases: A CPS attorney's perspective. *Child Sexual Abuse* 1993;2(2):109–111.

4. Association for the Treatment of Sexual Abusers. *Ethical standards and principles for the management of sexual abusers.* Beaverton, OR: Association for the Treatment of Sexual Abusers. 1997.

5. Burr WR, Hill R, Nye FI, Reiss IL. *Contemporary theories about the family: Research-based theories, Volume I.* New York: Free Press. 1979.

6. Carter EA, McGoldrick M. *The family life cycle: A framework for family therapy.* New York: Gardner Press. 1980.

7. Conte JR, Wolf S, Smith T. What sexual offenders tell us about prevention strategies. *Child Abuse Negl* 1989;13(2):293–301.

8. Christiansen JR, Blake RH. The grooming process in father-daughter incest. In AL Horton, BL Johnson, LM Roundy, and D Williams (eds.), *The incest perpetrator: A family member no one wants to treat,* 88–98. Newbury Park, CA: Sage. 1990.

9. Dadds M, Smith M, Webber Y, Robinson A. An exploration of family and individual profiles following father-daughter incest. *Child Abuse Negl* 1991;15:575–586.

10. Deblinger E, Heflin AH. *Treating sexually abused children and their nonoffending parents: A cognitive behavioral approach.* Thousand Oaks, CA: Sage. 1996.

11. Dell P. Beyond homeostasis: Toward a concept of coherence. *Fam Process* 1982;21:21–41.

12. Ewing CP. Family preservation and reunification in intra-familial sexual abuse cases: A justice perspective. *J Child Sexual Abuse* 1993;2(2):113–115.

13. Finkelhor D. The trauma of child sexual abuse: Two models. In GW Wyatt and GJ Powell (eds.). *Lasting effects of child sexual abuse,* 61–82. Newbury Park, CA: Sage. 1988.

14. Friedrich WN. *Psychotherapy of sexually abused children and their families.* New York: W. W. Norton. 1990.

15. Gill E. *Systemic treatment of families who abuse.* San Francisco: Jossey-Bass. 1996.

16. Greenfeld LA. *Sex offenses and offenders: An analysis of data on rape and sexual assault.* Washington, DC: Bureau of Justice Statistics, NCJ-163392. 1997.

17. Hanson RF, Lipovsky JA, Saunders BE. Characteristics of fathers in incest families. *J Interpers Viol* 1994;9(2):155–169.

18. Hoagwood K, Stewart JM. Sexually abused children's perceptions of family functioning. *Child Adolesc Soc Work* 1989;6:139–149.

19. Lipovsky J, Swenson CC, Ralston ME, Saunders, BE. The abuse clarification process in the treatment of intrafamilial child abuse. *Child Abuse Negl* 1998;22:729–741.

20. Maddock JW, Larson NR. *Incestuous families: An ecological approach to understanding treatment.* New York: W. W. Norton. 1995.

21. Minuchin S. *Families and family therapy.* Cambridge: Harvard University Press. 1974.

22. Morris T, Lipovsky JA, Saunders BE. The role of perpetrator acknowledgment in mediating the impact of child sexual assault: An exploratory study. *J Child Sexual Abuse* 1996;5(3):95–102.

23. O'Connell MA. Reuniting incest offenders with their families. *J Interpers Viol* 1986;1(3):374–386.

24. Patton MQ. *Family sexual abuse: Frontline research and evaluation.* Newbury Park, CA: Sage. 1991.

25. Pence DM. Family preservation and reunification in intra-familial sexual abuse cases: A law enforcement perspective. *Child Sexual Abuse* 1993;2(2):103–108.

26. Saunders BE, Lipovsky JA, Hanson RF. Couple and familial characteristics of father-child incest families. *Fam Social Work* 1995;1(2):5–25.

27. Smith DW, Saunders BE. Personality characteristics of father-perpetrators and non-offending mothers in incest families: Individual and dyadic analyses. *Child Abuse Negl* 1995;19(5):607–617.

28. Trepper TS, Barrett MJ. *Systemic treatment of incest: A therapeutic handbook.* New York: Brunner/Mazel. 1989.

Chapter 4

The Long-term Medical Consequences of Sexual Abuse

Carol D. Berkowitz, M.D.

Women and men who have a history of childhood sexual abuse often experience particular medical problems later in life. Internists and family practitioners treating these patients are frequently unaware of the sexual abuse history. Common complaints include irritable bowel syndrome, chronic pelvic pain, headache, pain syndromes, eating disorders, and disorders characterized as somatization. A history of sexual abuse is also associated with overutilization of medical services. In many cases, the secretive nature of sexual abuse makes it difficult for the physician to elicit affirmation of this history from the patient. However, obtaining an accurate history of prior sexual abuse may avoid costly and unnecessary medical work-up and help get the patient referred to appropriate mental health resources.

GENERAL CONSIDERATIONS

Although the pediatric community deals with the immediate diagnostic and medical problems associated with child sexual abuse, internists and family practitioners care for women and men who experience the long-term medical consequences of their childhood experiences. Yet, a history of sexual abuse in a patient may not be readily apparent, because of the secrecy that is often associated with the condition.

The real scope of the problem of long-term medical sequelae may be more accurately estimated by noting the estimated overall prevalence of sexual abuse. Reports suggest that between 20 percent and 75 percent of women seeking medical attention have been either sexually or physically victimized.[13,57,63] Other studies, focusing on sexual abuse during childhood, have consistently reported that 20–25 percent of women and 10–15 percent of men have been sexually abused before reaching adulthood.[18,32,70]

Another way to assess the number of individuals who may have been victims of sexual abuse is to note that there were 217,700 reported cases of suspected child sexual abuse in 1993.[46] Even this figure may represent too low an estimate, since some investigators claim that up to 98 percent of cases of abuse go unreported.[2,38,52]

Regardless of which figure one subscribes to, sexual abuse is prevalent. Some affected individuals experience psychological, psychosexual, and interpersonal difficulties, which are discussed in greater detail in chapters 2 and 3. It is important to note, however, that medical and psychological problems are interrelated, especially in conditions with a functional rather than an organic basis.

Psychological problems noted to occur at increased incidence in individuals with a history of sexual abuse include

- severe depression[5,12,17,23,58]
- anxiety disorders[3]
- substance abuse[42,51,65]
- multiple personality disorder[24]
- posttraumatic stress disorder[12]
- eating disorders, particularly bulimia nervosa[26] and somatization[7,8,43]

Psychosexual dysfunction, reported more frequently among women who have been sexually abused, is associated with both chronic pelvic pain and sexual dysfunction.[65] Promiscuity,[28,31,39,40] prostitution,[30,45] and adolescent pregnancy[28] are also reported with increased frequency in women who have been sexually abused as children.

DIAGNOSTIC CONSIDERATIONS

Assessing the association between a given medical condition and child sexual abuse is inhibited by the secretive nature of sexual abuse. Rarely is the abuse history spontaneously elicited during the course of a medical evaluation.[13] One study (Drossman et al.) found that 59 percent of women with a history of abuse had never discussed the abuse with anyone other than family members, and a third had never told anyone of the abuse. Only 17 percent had ever discussed the abuse with a physician. Another survey[33] reported that only 5.1 percent of women studied ever disclosed information about their sexual abuse to a physician. Patients with symptoms related to abuse may be misdiagnosed and be subjected to multiple, often invasive and unnecessary diagnostic studies in a search for an organic etiology.[17]

Medical conditions identified as being associated with sexual abuse include

- gastrointestinal disorders
- gynecologic complaints
- neurologic conditions
- pain syndromes
- eating disorders
- disorders that can be characterized as "somatization"

Gastrointestinal Disorders

The association between gastrointestinal disturbances and sexual abuse has been reported in a number of studies.[12–15,34,53,59,60,62,65,67,68] An association between stressful events and gastrointestinal disorders is understandable, given the effects of stress on gastric secretion and gastrointestinal motility.[69] As early as 1929, an alteration in gastric secretion during the digestive process when an individual receives disturbing information was noted.[9] Similarly, anxiety can increase gastrointestinal motility, as is noted when individuals taking academic examinations experience diarrhea.

Most of the gastrointestinal disorders associated with child sexual abuse are classified as functional, that is, conditions with no structural, infectious, or metabolic basis. Functional gastrointestinal disorders include irritable bowel syndrome, nonulcer dyspepsia, and chronic abdominal pain.

Irritable bowel disease affects 8–17 percent of the general population.[14,37,62] It is second only to the common cold as a reason for absenteeism from work.[68] The disorder is reported to occur 2.5 times more frequently in women than in men and to be common not only in Western countries but also in developing nations of the world.[19] The symptoms include abdominal pain, abdominal distention, and an alteration in bowel habits. The pain is of variable intensity, but in some cases it is so severe that it has been likened to labor pains. The pains arise from both the small and large intestines. Gaseous abdominal distention is also of varying degrees; it tends to be mildest early in the day and increase as the day progresses. Stooling problems are also variable. In some patients there are frequent loose stools, while in others frequent stooling is characterized by pellet-like movements. Constipation with infrequent defecation is noted in other cases, and many patients fluctuate between periods of diarrhea and periods of constipation. Although mucus may be passed during a bowel movement, blood is not present.

The diagnosis of irritable bowel syndrome is a clinical one, since there are no confirmatory laboratory studies. The diagnostic criteria for irritable bowel syndrome, referred to as the Rome criteria, are three or more months of continuous or recurrent abdominal pain, usually relieved by defecation, associated with a change in frequency or consistency of stool and/or disturbed stooling at least 25 percent of the time (i.e., two or more of the following: altered stool frequency, form, or passage), usually associated with bloating or sensation of abdominal distention.[61] Patients with irritable bowel syndrome may also experience noncolonic symptoms which may have a functional or somatic component. These include

- nausea
- early satiety
- dysphagia
- lethargy
- back pain
- thigh pain
- urinary frequency
- urinary urgency
- dyspareunia
- the pain and fatigue associated with fibromyalgia[19]

The link between irritable bowel syndrome and sexual abuse has been supported by several studies. An initial study, reported in 1990, used a self-administered questionnaire that asked for information about demographics, symptomatology, and health care utilization as well as a history of abuse.[13] Questions about sexual abuse included inquiries about exposure, threats of abuse, and touching. Overall, 44 percent of the women followed in this gastroenterology practice reported they had been abused. When the patients were divided into those with functional complaints, 53 percent had been sexually abused compared to 37 percent of those with organic diagnoses. In a study that used a face to face interview and compared patients with irritable bowel syndrome with those with inflammatory bowel disease,[67] patients with irritable bowel disease were significantly more likely to have suffered from either severe childhood abuse or severe adult sexual trauma (54 percent versus 5 percent with inflammatory bowel disease).

Felitti reported a similar association between abuse and irritable bowel syndrome in an HMO-based population. He studied 131 sequential adult patients who acknowledged a history of incest, molestation, or childhood rape on a lengthy medical questionnaire. He noted gastrointestinal distress in 64 percent of the study group compared to 39 percent of the controls using a retrospective chart review.[17] The most common gastrointestinal disturbance was irritable bowel syndrome (chronic constipation, intermittent diarrhea, and recurrent cramping). There were also other undiagnosed chronic recurrent gastrointestinal disturbances. The average duration from sexual abuse to medical assessment was 30 years.

The association between bowel symptomatology and child sexual abuse exists even in a nonclinic population. One study[60] of a population-based sample using a mailed self-administered questionnaire found that 41 percent of women and 11 percent of men reported some type of abuse. Gastrointestinal symptoms were highly associated with abuse. Fifty percent of patients with irritable bowel syndrome had a history of abuse, compared to 23 percent of responders who did not have irritable bowel syndrome.

A history of prior sexual abuse has also been noted with increased frequency among patients diagnosed with nonulcer dyspepsia compared to those with ulcer disease.[13] Nonulcer dyspepsia is characterized by chronic unexplained upper abdominal pain or discomfort. The condition appears to be related to the interaction of impaired motor and sensory function (disordered gastric emptying, increased visceral sensitivity, increased gastric acid secretion), psychosocial factors, and infection with *Helicobacter pylori.*[54,59]

Symptoms related to recurrent lower abdominal pain are also associated with a history of childhood sexual abuse, and an odds ratio has been reported of lower abdominal pain between abused and nonabused patients as 1.58 (0.82 to 3.05, 95% CI).[13] An association has also been observed between chronic lower abdominal pain (as a gastrointestinal condition), chronic pelvic pain (as a gynecologic disorder), and child sexual abuse.[64] Although disturbances of the reproductive organs may give rise to chronic pelvic pain, one study[48] noted that 7–60 percent of the referrals to gynecologists for chronic pelvic pain were attributable to irritable bowel syndrome. The relationship between chronic abdominal pain in children (a complaint noted in about 10 percent of school age children) and child sexual abuse appears less well established.[1,56]

Psychiatric disorders are also correlated with irritable bowel syndrome and prior abuse, and these appear to be co-morbid conditions. One study[37] found that 94 percent of 35 patients with irritable bowel syndrome had a lifetime prevalence of any DSM-IIIR Axis I disorder, with mood and anxiety disorders being most prevalent.

Gynecologic Disorders

An association between child sexual abuse and a number of gynecologic disorders—most notably chronic pelvic pain—is also reported. Chronic pelvic pain (CPP) is defined as noncyclic lower abdominal and pelvic pain of at least six months duration. The prevalence of CPP is about 12 percent and the lifetime occurrence rate is 33 percent.[41] The condition usually affects women between adolescence and their midthirties. The differential diagnosis of pelvic pain is lengthy and includes disorders such as pelvic inflammatory disease, pelvic adhesions, urinary tract problems, endometriosis, leiomyomas, endometritis, and cervical stenosis.[36] In addition to chronic pelvic pain, many women with this complaint also experience other abdominal pain, dysmenorrhea, gastrointestinal symptoms, shortness of breath, and menstrual irregularities.[66] In general, these women demonstrate a high degree of somatization. Although a complete history and physical evaluation are key to the diagnosis, laparoscopy is a popular diagnostic modality used to assess patients with CPP.[47]

Chronic pelvic pain accounts for substantial utilization of medical resources, and other associated costs. Five to 25 percent of all diagnostic laparoscopies are performed for chronic pelvic pain.[35,56] In the 1980s, the average cost per procedure was $1,500. The rate of detecting pelvic pathology in women with chronic pelvic pain ranges from 8 percent to 83 percent.[27,66] In addition, 10–19 percent of hysterectomies are performed because of chronic pelvic pain. In 1991, about 78,000 hysterectomies were performed for this complaint.[50]

The cost of chronic pelvic pain is measurable not only in terms of the diagnostic and operative procedures but also in time lost from work and lower earning potential. One study[27] noted that women with chronic pelvic pain had significantly lower occupational status in spite of a similar education when compared to controls.

The etiology of CPP is elusive. The major focus of the diagnostic work-up is differentiating anatomic from functional pain and determining what psychosocial and sexual factors may be contributing to the patient's symptomatology. Numerous studies have proposed a link among chronic pelvic pain, adult sexual adjustment problems, and childhood sexual abuse.[4,16,21,25] In one report,[66] 64 percent of women with chronic pelvic pain had experienced some type of sexual abuse before the age of 14, compared to 23 percent of the women in the comparison group. (The comparison group were women being evaluated for fertility problems or for bilateral tubal ligation.) However, this association is not clear and some investigators have questioned the link between child sexual abuse and chronic pelvic pain.

One investigator suggested that women with somatic complaints are more likely than others to exaggerate or even fabricate stories of prior sexual trauma.[50] Some studies have failed to show a higher incidence of child sexual abuse among women with chronic pelvic pain compared to all women using a gynecology clinic.[20] The difference between these studies may reflect a number of factors: lack of appropriate control groups, biased sampling, use of inadequate questionnaires and psychiatric interviews, variable assessments of organic pathology, small sample size, and varying operational definitions. For instance, some investigators use three months as evidence of chronic pain,[27,66] while others maintain that the pain must have been present for at least six months.[50]

Somatization

Somatization is a term that was first used by Stekel in 1943 to describe a bodily disorder that arises as an expression of a deep-seated neurosis.[29] It appears that there is no accepted definition of the term somatization, since it does not represent a specific illness or pathophysiologic process. The term is used to characterize a variety of illnesses and diagnostic entities. Overall, 10–30 percent of all adult patient visits to primary care providers and 10–20 percent of the American medical budget are related to somatization.

Whether pelvic pain is a symptom of somatization or is related to venous congestion in the pelvic area is unresolved. Although the pathophysiology of somatization is not well understood, it appears that people who somaticize perceive bodily sensations differently than others and amplify symptoms. A genetic predisposition is noted in some families. There is also a psychophysiologic basis, as evidenced by the somatic symptoms associated with panic attacks and stress.

In a number of patients, somatization appears to be related to prior childhood sexual abuse.[43] Briere and Runtz[7,8] attribute somatization following child sexual abuse to a preoccupation with bodily processes. In addition to symptoms involving the gastrointestinal tract or pelvic area, pain-related symptoms may also be a manifestation of somatization. Somatic symptoms may have their onset during childhood and adolescence. Somatic symptoms that occur as a result of childhood sexual abuse have been studied more in children than in adults.[20] Psychobehavioral problems that include enuresis, encopresis, anxious behavior, tics, and disturbed sleeping and eating patterns, as well as somatic complaints related to the gastrointestinal and genitourinary systems are reported. Headaches, fainting, and dizziness are particularly noted in adolescent rape victims, who frequently seek medical care for these complaints yet do not mention their prior sexual assault.[3]

Similarly, a history of childhood sexual abuse is reported with increased frequency in adult patients suffering from neurologic complaints, including headache and backache. Felitti[17] reported chronic headache in 45 percent of the sexually abused group compared to 25 percent of the control group.

Childhood sexual abuse should be considered as a possible predisposing event in the assessment of the adult headache patient.[11] Headaches are the seventh most common symptom for which adult patients seek medical care, and account for 2 percent of all visits to family practitioners, internists, and general practitioners.[44] The differential diagnosis of headache involves a long list of disorders including migraine, cluster headache, tension-type headache, and disorders related to structural disturbances of the cerebral parenchyma, meninges, and extracranial structures. Psychogenic headaches probably compose a large component of chronic or recurrent headaches followed in a primary care setting.

Eating Disorders

The relationship between childhood sexual abuse and adult obesity is worth noting. Approximately 40 million Americans are at least 20 percent heavier than their ideal weight.[22] Forty percent of these individuals are 40 percent over their ideal weight. The medical complications of obesity are multiple and include premature atherosclerotic disease, hypertension, sleep apnea, gout, non-insulin-dependent diabetes, hyperlipidemia, cholelithiasis, degenerative joint disease, breast cancer, and low self-esteem, and there is increased morbidity and mortality among obese individuals. The etiology of obesity is multifactorial, but a link between obesity and child sexual abuse was recently reported.[17] This study noted that 60 percent of previously abused patients were fifty or more pounds over their ideal weight compared to 28 percent in the control group. Both the frequency and the severity of the obesity were greater in the abused versus the nonabused groups. Twenty-five percent of the abused group were more than 100 pounds over ideal weight compared to only 6 percent of the nonabused group. The onset of obesity followed the sexual abuse and was noted to be proximate in time. In addition, two-thirds of the abused morbidly obese individuals had been victims of incest. The association between adult obesity and childhood sexual abuse has not been adequately explored by other investigators.

Other Medical Conditions

Other conditions that have been reported in association with child sexual abuse include learning disabilities, breast disease, bladder infections, disorders of the immune system, yeast infections, and the perception of oneself as being overweight.[17,57] Asthma has also been noted by a number of investigators to occur with increased frequency among sexual abuse victims,[16,17]occurring in 13 percent of the sexually abused group, compared to 8 percent in the control group.

For the most part, studies to date have assessed the history of abuse in a disease afflicted population. In general, the populations studied attended specific practices or clinics and were selected for the presence of symptoms that are often considered functional in origin. Included among these symptoms are gastrointestinal complaints such as abdominal pain and diarrhea, chronic pelvic pain, headache, and nonspecific skeletal pain. Some of the studies were conducted with a psychiatric focus to determine the relationship between functional symptomatology and psychiatric conditions.

Most studies attempt to separate the physical from the psychological sequelae of abuse. Although the purist will maintain that it is important to define the medical sequelae of childhood sexual abuse, such a distinction is both artificial and not clinically useful. The body and the psyche of the patient are inseparable. The studies to date have suggested with a high degree of probability that certain medical as well as psychological disturbances are associated with childhood abuse. Briere[6] specifically comments on the overlap between psychological and somatic factors and questions the functioning of one independently of the other.

Adjusting or reacting to the sexual abuse has been associated with an increase in certain behaviors which themselves are associated with medical sequelae. Promiscuity, substance abuse, and smoking all introduce additional medical concerns into the health evaluation.[57] Each of these behaviors is associated with specific health care risks, such as sexually transmitted diseases, including AIDS, and alcoholism, cirrhosis of the liver, emphysema, lung cancer, and heart disease.[6] It is of interest to note that while there is high use of health care resources, there is a low frequency of Pap smears,[57]another sign of high-risk behavior.

OVERUTILIZATION OF MEDICAL RESOURCES

The frequent use of health services might skew the association between child sexual abuse and certain medical conditions. A study of 51 women[55] found that health care usage was twice as high in college women who had reported being sexually abused as children than in a control population. Another investigation[17] also noted an increased number of doctor office visits in the sexually abused group. The average number of visits in the United States is 4.3 per year. High utilization is 10 or more visits per year. Twenty-two percent of sexually abused patients—compared to 6 percent of the control population—visited a doctor 10 or more times a year.

Surgical procedures are also reported to occur with increased frequency among adult patients who have been sexually abused. Arnold et al.[2] note that the indications for the procedures were often questionable and the abnormal or objective findings were often lacking. The seven patients in their study had a mean number of eight operations with 66–70 percent resulting in normal findings. This admittedly small sample does not provide sufficient data, however, to conclude that surgical procedures are commoner in sexually abused individuals.

Health resources utilization or health consulting behavior may be related to one's perception of well-being and self-esteem. The conception of oneself as "damaged goods" appears to contribute to a patient's sense of not being well.[33] Discontent with one's own body may increase health services utilization. Felitti[17] reported augmentation mammoplasty in 5 percent of patients with a history of sexual abuse compared to none of the controls.

MALE PATIENTS

Most studies on medical conditions associated with prior sexual abuse have had a predominance of female subjects. It is easy to understand how gynecologic studies such as those on chronic pelvic pain would involve women. Even Felitti,[17] however, dealing with a broader range of conditions, noted that 96 percent of the patients in his study were women.

There is little written about men who were sexually abused as boys or adolescents. Ray,[49] in a study of male incest survivors, described the presence of negative self-concepts but did not comment on any specific medical conditions. This remains an area for future investigation.

EVALUATING ADULT PATIENTS FOR PRIOR ABUSE

The challenge for the healthcare worker will be to recognize which symptoms may be related to childhood sexual abuse and to give the patient the opportunity to disclose such events. The ease with which such a history is obtained is influenced by the experience and comfort of the interviewer while discussing sexually related issues with the patient. Drossman[12] notes he does not ask directly whether a patient has been sexually abused but queries if there is anything else that the patient feels is important to discuss. Eliciting a history of prior sexual abuse in a patient with functional complaints may not only abort an unnecessarily costly and invasive medical work-up but, more important, may get the patient referred to the appropriate mental health resources.

CONCLUSIONS AND FUTURE IMPLICATIONS

Although there is some information about the long-term medical sequelae of childhood sexual abuse, there are many unanswered questions. Can pediatricians identify those children who, after being abused, are at risk for developing medical problems related to the abuse? Does medical and psychologic intervention during childhood alter the long-term outcome? Should a history of abuse be incorporated into every adult medical assessment, the same way that a history of smoking or prior surgeries is included? It has taken a number of years for the pediatric community to become cognizant of the problem of child sexual abuse. The challenge will be for health care providers managing adults to become equally aware.

REFERENCES

1. Antonson DL. Abdominal pain. *Gastrointest Endosc Clin N Am* 1994;4:1–21.
2. Arnold RP, Rogers D, Cook DAG. Medical problems of adults who were sexually abused in childhood. *Br Med J* 1990;300:705–708.

3. Bachmann GA, Moeller TP, Bennett J. Childhood sexual abuse and the consequences in adult women. *Obstet Gynecol* 1988;71:631–642.

4. Beard R, Belsey E, Lieberman B, et al. Pelvic pain in women. *Am J Obstet Gynecol* 1977;128:566–570.

5. Bernstein G. Office management of the incest victim. *Medical Aspects of Human Sexuality* 1979;Nov.:67–87.

6. Briere J. Medical symptoms, health risk, and history of childhood sexual abuse. *Mayo Clin Proc* 1992;67:603–604.

7. Briere J, Runtz M. Multivariate correlates of childhood psychological and physical maltreatment among university women. *Child Abuse Negl* 1988;12:331–341.

8. Briere J, Runtz M. Symptomatology associated with childhood sexual victimization in a nonclinical adult sample. *Child Abuse Negl* 1988;12:51–59.

9. Cannon WB. Bodily changes in pain, hunger, fear and rage. 2nd ed. New York: Appleton. 1929.

10. Cunningham J, Pearce T, Pearce P. Childhood sexual abuse and medical complaints in adult women. *J Interpers Viol* 1988;3:131–144.

11. Domino JV, Haber JD. Prior physical and sexual abuse in women with chronic headache: Clinical correlates. *Headache* 1987;27:310–314.

12. Drossman DA. The link between early abuse and GI disorders in women. *Emerg Med* 1992;April:171–175.

13. Drossman DA, Leserman J, Nachman G, et al. Sexual and physical abuse in women with functional or organic gastrointestinal disorders. *Ann Intern Med* 1990;113:828–833.

14. Drossman DA, Sandler RS, McKee DC, et al. Bowel patterns among subjects not seeking health care. *Gastroenterology* 1982;83:529–534.

15. Drossman DA, Talley NJ, Leserman J, Olden KW, Barreiro MA. Sexual and physical abuse and gastrointestinal illness: Review and recommendations. *Ann Intern Med* 1995;123:782–794.

16. Duncan L, Taylor H. A psychosomatic study of pelvic congestion. *Am J Obstet Gynecol* 1952;64:1–12.

17. Felitti VJ. Long-term medical consequences of incest, rape, and molestation. *South Med J* 1991;84:328–331.

18. Finkelhor D. *Sexually victimized children.* New York: Free Press. 1979.

19. Francis CY, Whorwell PJ. The irritable bowel syndrome. *Postgrad Med J* 1996;73:1–7.

20. Fry RP. Adult physical illness and childhood sexual abuse. *J Psychosom Res* 1993;37:89–103.

21. Fry RP, Crisp AH, Beard RW, McGuigan S. Psychosocial aspects of chronic pelvic pain, with special reference to sexual abuse: A study of 164 women. *Postgrad Med J* 1993;69:566–574.

22. Gately A. Obesity. In RH Rubin, C Voss, DJ Derksen, A Gateley, RW Quenzer (eds.), *Medicine: A primary care approach,* 408–411. Philadelphia: W. B. Saunders. 1996.

23. Gelinas DJ. The persisting negative effects of incest. *Psychiatry* 1983;46:312–332.

24. Goulding RA, Schwartz RC. *The mosaic mind: Empowering the tormented selves of child abuse survivors.* New York: W. W. Norton. 1995.

25. Haber J, Roos C. Effects of spouse abuse and/or sexual abuse in the development and maintenance of chronic pelvic pain in women. In Fields HL, Dubner R, Cervero F (eds.), *Advances in pain research and therapy,* vol. 9, pp. 889–895. New York: Raven Press. 1985.

26. Hall RC, Tice L, Beresford TP, Wooley B, Hall AK. Sexual abuse in patients with anorexia nervosa and bulimia. *Psychosomatics* 1989;430:73–79.

27. Harrop-Griffiths J, Katon W, Walker E, et al. The association between chronic pelvic pain, psychiatric diagnosis, and childhood sexual abuse. *Obstet Gynecol* 1988;71:589–594.

28. Herman J. *Father-daughter incest.* Cambridge: Harvard University Press. 1981.

29. Hollifield M, Vogel AV. The somatizing patient in medicine: A primary care approach. In Rubin RH, Voss C, Derksen DJ, Gateley A, Quenzer RW (eds.), *Internal medicine: A primary care approach,* 389–392. Philadelphia: W. B. Saunders, 1996.

30. James J, Meyerding J. Early sexual experience and prostitution. *Am J Psychiatry* 1977; 134:1381–1385.

31. Kaufman I, Peck AL, Tagiuri CK. The family constellation and overt incestuous relations between father and daughter. *Am J Orthopsychiatry* 1954;24:266–279.

32. Kinsey AC, Pomeroy WB, Martin CE, Gebhard PH. *Sexual behavior in the human female.* Philadelphia: W. B. Saunders. 1953.

33. Lechner ME, Vogel ME, Garcia-Shelton LM, Leichter JL, Steibel KR. Self-reported medical problems of adult female survivors of childhood sexual abuse. *J Fam Pract* 1993;36:633–638.

34. Leserman J, Drossman DA, Li Z, et al. Sexual and physical abuse history in gastroenterology practice: How types of abuse impact health status. *Psychosom Med* 1996;58:4–15.

35. Levitan Z, Eibschitz I, Devries K, et al. The value of laparoscopy in women with chronic pelvic pain and a "normal" pelvis. *Int J Gynaecol Obstet* 1985;23:71–74.

36. Lipscomb GH, Ling FW. Chronic pelvic pain. *Med Clin North Am* 1995;79:1411–1425.

37. Lydiard RB, Fossey MD, Marsh W, Ballenger JC. Prevalence of psychiatric disorders in patients with irritable bowel syndrome. *Psychosomatics* 1993;34:229–234.

38. Markowe HIJ. The frequency of childhood sexual abuse in the UK. *Health Trends* 1988; Feb.:2–6.

39. McCary JL. My most unusual sexual case: Nymphomania. *Med Aspects Human Sexuality* 1979;May:74–75.

40. Meiselman K. *Incest: A psychological study of causes and effects with treatment recommendations.* San Francisco: Jossey-Bass. 1978.

41. Milburn A, Reiter RC, Rhomberg AT. Multidisciplinary approach to chronic pelvic pain. *Obstet Gynecol Clin North Am* 1993;20:643–661.

42. Miller BA, Downs WR, Gondoli DM. The role of child sexual abuse in the development of alcoholism in women. *Violence Vict* 1987;2:157–172.

43. Morrison J. Childhood sexual histories of women with somatization disorder. *Am J Psychiatry* 1989;146:236–241.

44. Murata GH. Headache in medicine: A primary care approach. In Rubin RH, Voss C, Derksen DJ, Gateley A, Quenzer RW (eds.), *Internal medicine: A primary care approach,* 357–360. Philadelphia, W. B. Saunders, 1996.

45. Nakashima I, Zakus G. Incest: Review and clinical experience. *Pediatr for the Clin* 1977; 60:696–701.

46. National incidence study: Implications for prevention. National Committee to Prevent Child Abuse. [Online]:http://www.childabuse.org/fs13.html.

47. Nolan TE, Elkins TE. Chronic pelvic pain. *Postgrad Med J* 1993;94:125–138.

48. Rapkin AJ, Mayer EA. Gastroenterologic causes of chronic pelvic pain. *Obstet Gynecol Clin North Am* 1993;20:663–683.

49. Ray S. Adult male survivors of incest: An exploratory study. *J Child Sexual Abuse* 1997; 5:103–114.

50. Reiter RC, Shakerin LR, Gambone JC, Milburn AK. Correlation between sexual abuse and somatization in women with somatic and nonsomatic chronic pelvic pain. *Am J Obstet Gynecol* 1991;165:104–109.

51. Rosenhow DJ, Corbett R, Devine D. Molested as children: A hidden contribution to substance abuse. *J Subst Abuse Treat* 1988;5:13–18.

52. Russell DEH. *The secret trauma: Incest in the lives of girls and women.* New York: Basic Books. 1986.

53. Scarinci IC, McDonald-Haile J, Bradley LA, Richter JE. Altered pain perception and psychosocial features among women with gastrointestinal disorders and history of abuse: A preliminary model. *Am J Med* 1994;97:108–118.

54. Scolapio JS, Camilleri M. Nonulcer dyspepsia. *Gastroenterologist* 1996;4:13–23.

55. Sedney MA, Brooks B. Factors associated with a history of childhood sexual experience in a nonclinical female population. *J Am Acad Child Adolesc Psychiatry* 1984;23:215–218.

56. Seidel JS, Elvik SL, Berkowitz CD, et al. Presentation and evaluation of sexual misuse in the emergency department. *Pediatr Emerg Care* 1986;2:157–164.

57. Springs FE, Friedrich WN. Health risk behaviors and medical sequelae of childhood sexual abuse. *Mayo Clin Proc* 1992;67:527–532.

58. Summit R, Kryso J. Sexual abuse of children: A clinical spectrum. *Am J Orthopsychiatry* 1978;48:237–251.

59. Talley NJ, Fett SL, Zinsmeister AR. Self-reported abuse and gastrointestinal disease in outpatients: Association with irritable bowel–type symptoms. *Am J Gastroenterol* 1995;90:366–371.

60. Talley NJ, Fett SL, Zinsmeister AR, Melton LJ. Gastrointestinal tract symptoms and self-reported abuse: A population-based study. *Gastroenterology* 1994;107:1040–1049.

61. Thompson WG, Dotevall G, Drossman DA, et al. Irritable bowel syndrome: Guidelines for the diagnosis. *Gastroenterology* 1980;79:283–288.

62. Thompson WG, Heaton KW. Functional bowel disorders in apparently healthy people. *Gastroenterology* 1980;79:283–288.

63. Toomey TC, Hernandez JT, Gittelman DF, Hulka JF. Relationship of sexual and physical abuse to pain and psychological assessment variables in chronic pelvic pain patients. *Pain* 1993; 53:105–1099.

64. Walker EA, Gelfand AN, Gelfand MD, Green C, Katon WJ. Chronic pelvic pain and gynecological symptoms in women with irritable bowel syndrome. *J Psychosom Obstet Gynecol* 1996; 17:39–46.

65. Walker EA, Gelfand AN, Gelfand MD, Katon WJ. Psychiatric diagnoses, sexual and physical victimization, and disability in patients with irritable bowel syndrome or inflammatory bowel disease. *Psychol Med* 1995;25:1259–1267.

66. Walker E, Katon W, Harrop-Griffiths J, et al. Relationship of chronic pelvic pain to psychiatric diagnoses and childhood sexual abuse. *Am J Psychiatry* 1988;145:75–80.

67. Walker EA, Katon WJ, Roy-Byrne PP, Jemelka RP, Russo J. Histories of sexual victimization in patients with irritable bowel syndrome or inflammatory bowel disease. *Am J Psychiatry* 1993; 150:1502–1506.

68. Whitehead WE, Schuster MM. *Gastrointestinal disorders: Behavioral and physiological basis for treatment.* New York: Academic. 1985.

69. Wolf S. *Educating doctors: Crisis in medical education, research and practice.* New Brunswick, NJ: Transaction. 1997.

70. Wyatt GE. The sexual abuse of Afro-American and white American women in childhood. *Child Abuse Negl* 1985;9:507–519.

71. Wyatt GE, Peters SD. Issues in the definition of child sexual abuse in prevalence research. *Child Abuse Negl* 1986;10:231–240.

72. Wyatt GE, Peters SD. Methodological considerations in research on the prevalence of child sexual abuse. *Child Abuse Negl* 1986;10:241–251.

Chapter 5

Discovery of Childhood Sexual Abuse in Adults

Thomas A. Roesler, M.D.

Primary care physicians are likely to encounter adult victims of childhood sexual abuse in their practices, although often the history of abuse will not be volunteered by the patient but must be drawn out by the clinician. The abuse survivor is often a patient with multiple unexplained complaints, all of which may be related to underlying depression or anxiety. Posttraumatic stress disorder is a significant feature in this group of patients, occurring in nearly three-quarters. The physician should communicate that abuse information is relevant to medical treatment and that support and therapy are available. While reporting of abuse is mandatory, that consideration may be irrelevant to the discovery of childhood abuse in adults, although many victims may wish some sort of disclosure, particularly when the abuser continues to have contact with children.

GENERAL CONSIDERATIONS

Childhood sexual abuse can have serious long-term consequences in adults. The sequelae of sexual abuse affect numerous people coming to the primary care physician for physical and emotional problems in adult life. Evidence is growing, for example, that childhood sexual victimization may be the largest single preventable cause of adult mental illness.[9,39] Considerations for the primary care physician treating these patients include

- who is affected,
- the long-term physical and emotional consequences,
- how to approach patients with histories of abuse,
- what kind of treatment is helpful,
- special issues in the physical exam, and
- how to deal with the legal system.

THE POPULATIONS AT RISK

Sexual abuse is experienced across all racial, ethnic, and socioeconomic lines. It can and has occurred in all varieties of families. However, certain factors place particular individuals at higher risk. Finkelhor,[16] working retrospectively in 1979 with college undergraduates, found eight predictors of sexual victimization. The factors were additive and each represented an approximately 10 percent increase in risk. They were

- presence of a stepfather in the home
- having lived without mother
- defining self as not close to mother
- mother with less than a high school education
- sexually punitive mother
- lack of nonsexual physical affection from mother
- having an income less than $10,000
- having few friends in childhood

In another retrospective study, living with a stepfather increased by seven times a woman's risk of having been victimized.[38]

Adults victimized as children may display no discernible effects. Those without sequelae are likely to be individuals whose abuse was less extensive and who received significant support.[15,18] Yet we also know that effects can be severe. In the Los Angeles Epidemiologic Catchment Area Study,[9] people sexually molested as children had two to four times higher risk of depression, alcohol or drug abuse, and anxiety disorder than nonabused subjects.

When special populations are surveyed to determine the incidence of people having been sexually abused, the numbers are impressive. Psychiatric inpatients,[7,8] outpatients,[24] and adolescents and adults in alcohol and drug treatment facilities[13,26,37] show higher than expected incidence of childhood sexual abuse histories. People attending headache[14] and pelvic pain clinics[46] also have higher frequencies of childhood sexual abuse (see chapter 4). No epidemiologically based study has been done to determine which physical symptoms are seen most frequently in adults victimized as children. Clinical experience suggests that symptoms associated with anxiety and depression are also seen in this population.

Recently, 80 percent of adult patients with vocal cord dysfunction, which can mimic asthma, were found to have a child abuse history.[27] Although considerable attention has been paid to a link between childhood sexual abuse and eating disorders, the relationship is still not clear.[30]

In the physician's practice, the most likely abuse survivor is the man or woman who has multiple unexplained complaints, all of which might be related to underlying depression or anxiety. The treatment never seems to be definitive for these patients, and they may be frequent users of medical services. Patients diagnosed as chronically depressed, having chronic fatigue syndrome, or borderline personality disorder are likely candidates for having an abuse history. Individuals diagnosed as borderline personality disorder have been found to have abuse histories in up to 71 percent of cases.[29] Although none of these potential presentations is diagnostic of a history of childhood abuse, abuse should be included in the differential diagnosis.

One red flag that should alert the physician to the possibility of earlier sexual abuse is the female patient who has difficulty with pelvic exams. Patients with unexplained pelvic pain were three times more likely to report a history of sexual abuse than patients whose pelvic pain had an organic explanation.[46] Other, less obvious indications include the patient who needs to be in control of the physical exam process or requests body-image surgery[28] or exhibits excessive gag reflex or unexplained gagging, or a significant lack of childhood memories.

How does one discover if the patient has been sexually abused? By asking. In rare instances individuals will announce during the first office visit that this is an issue in their lives. More often, people are uncomfortable talking about their abuse, have sketchy memories about what happened to them, or have been waiting for someone to ask. A physician who did an anonymous survey of his practice found that 47 percent of the women admitting to childhood abuse had never told anyone.[22]

Friedman and colleagues[17] surveyed patients to see if they wanted to be asked by their primary care physicians about abuse and if they felt physicians could be helpful in the event such information was revealed. Sixty-eight percent of those asked favored routine inquiry about sexual abuse, and 89 percent felt their physician could be helpful. However, only 6 percent had been asked. On the physician side, one-third of doctors surveyed favored routine inquiry about sexual abuse, and 74 percent felt they could be helpful. But when asked if they themselves included routine questions about sexual abuse, 89 percent said they never asked at initial visits and 85 percent did not ask during annual visits.

It is important to convey the message that it is acceptable for this information to be part of your relationship with the patient. Our society as a whole has been uncomfortable talking about sexual violation of children. If you have discomfort with information about childhood abuse, it can be unintentionally conveyed to your patient and may reinforce the message received in childhood that she or he is somehow responsible for making others feel bad. Before you ask, some thought should be given to what response you would want if you were in the same circumstance. Most adults with whom I have talked indicate they want their medical provider to be open, to listen to what happened, and to hear how the patient feels about it.

One approach to this area is to include a question about sexual abuse on the screening form most providers use with patients new to the practice. The question might read, "In your childhood, were there any experiences most people would consider traumatic? Examples might be death of a parent, a life-threatening illness or accident, or sexual or physical abuse." This gives the message that you consider such experiences important.

The patient might or might not be prepared to open up about the abuse at the time. Experience indicates that some individuals reveal more to a piece of paper, while others feel more comfortable talking with an interviewer. It has also been shown that the more ways a patient is asked, the greater the probability of a positive answer. Asking sets the expectation that this is something one can discuss with this physician. On the other hand, pressing for an answer runs the risk of making a patient feel compelled to say what the clinician wants to hear or making her or him resist talking about the experience altogether.

Emergency room charts of nonpsychotic, female patients being admitted to a psychiatric facility were reviewed for indications of childhood sexual abuse. The residents doing the emergency room screening were then instructed to ask the next 50 female patients being admitted if they had been sexually abused. The percentage of positive responses increased from 6 percent to 70 percent.[5]

RESPONSE TO DISCLOSURES OF ABUSE

If your patient does disclose a history of sexual abuse, what next? Disclosure of abuse can be an extremely painful process. Ask if this is the first time he or she has told anyone. It is helpful to know who else has knowledge of the abuse, as this will begin to define the support network to which the patient can turn. A study of female incest survivors indicated that children younger than 18 were most likely to tell a parent as the first adult. The parent was likely to react negatively to the revelation. Young adults (mean age 25) tended to tell friends or partners, while older adults (mean age 37) told therapists or other professionals.[35] If one waits until adulthood, the response is significantly more supportive than telling in childhood. Nonetheless, most survivors carry a dread that the first person they tell will be rejecting of them, confirming in their own minds that they were responsible for the actions of the abusers in their childhood.

There is evidence that the reaction a child receives upon disclosing the abuse mediates the severity of symptoms experienced in adulthood.[35] A negative response in childhood was associated with more severe symptoms 25 years later, even when the severity of abuse experienced was similar. In this same study, not telling in childhood and waiting until adulthood before disclosing did not help, as symptom levels were similar with the group who told in childhood.

The role of the clinician is to be supportive and listen but let the patient define the limits of his or her comfort. Victimization is the forceful imposition of one's desires on someone less powerful. The opposite is the respectful recognition of others' needs. Making a survivor of childhood abuse talk about it is often experienced as revictimization. Be sympathetic. Take a good history without pushing. It is sometimes necessary to say, "Can we talk about this more next time you come in? I'm sure there are some things you are not comfortable talking about just now but might want to tell me in a few weeks."

It is not necessary to believe everything the patient tells you, even if studies show that memories of childhood abuse can usually be confirmed.[20] It is more important to listen and suspend disbelief if something your patient says does not ring true. Adults who were sexually abused as children generally have very little to gain, and much to lose, from having anyone know about their secret.

Do people get accused falsely of sexual abuse? Yes, but it happens only rarely. Jones and McGraw reviewed sexual abuse allegations and found only 2 percent of the validated cases represented children accusing someone falsely.[23] In the handful of cases in which children (in each case it was an adolescent) named someone falsely, they did have a history of sexual abuse, but they had been molested by someone other than the accused. In general, one encounters patients whose abuse experience is painful and undeniable, even if all the memories are not clearly focused. It is not the task of the medical practitioner to be a detective bent on discovering the truth about what actually happened 20 years before. Instead, the focus needs to be on the emotional reality for the patient in the present.

In the study cited above about disclosure in incest victims,[35] the average person waited 13 years after the abuse ceased before telling anyone. The reason most often given for not telling was fear of physical harm resulting from the disclosure. The reason given most often for finally telling was "I wanted to heal—get on with my life." Telling one's physician is a significant event in the life of many of these individuals.

For the physician, the important first step upon hearing a disclosure of childhood abuse is to begin the process of constructing a validating, supportive network around the patient. The common denominator of child sexual abuse is the secrecy and isolation experienced by the victim. Reversing the sense of isolation is the first goal.

It is not necessary to recommend psychotherapy immediately. Patients may just need a sympathetic ear. They may want you to help them talk about the abuse to a spouse or other family member. A videotaped interview method has been used to generate a supportive environment around adults worried about abandonment following disclosure.[36]

Revelations by women who were sexually abused in childhood range from disclosure of a one-time event to stories of multiple perpetrators and years of repeated rape. Even a one-time event can be traumatic. For example, a woman was raped at age 13 by a 22-year-old neighbor. Because of her belief that she had allowed herself to be seduced and therefore was responsible for the act, she was unable to tell anyone about the incident until she was in her forties. In the meantime her relationships with men were completely determined by her view of herself as "spoiled goods."

Long-term effects are generally predicted by the severity of abuse. Features of the abuse that are often found to predict later symptoms include

- abuse by a parent,
- penetration,
- use of force, and
- length of the abusive relationship.[4]

In community samples, about 40 percent of the total number of persons reporting abuse indicate that the perpetrator was someone inside the family. Thus, incest is actually less common in the general population than extrafamilial abuse. However, very little sexual abuse of children is by strangers. In 90 percent of cases, the abuse is committed by family members or persons well known to the child.

We see a different picture in individuals seeking psychotherapy. The majority of persons seen in a clinical setting who report childhood sexual abuse are victims of incest. Incest is usually a long process beginning in early childhood and often ending in early adolescence. A typical adult survivor of incest will describe an average length of abuse of seven years, with a beginning age of 6 years and mean age of cessation at 13. This is contrary to a common belief that fathers or stepfathers get attracted to postpubertal adolescents. Indeed, it is the young child who is most vulnerable and most often the object of the child molester.

RECOVERY OF MEMORIES

One issue that is baffling to patients, the general public, and inexperienced clinicians is that adults can have selective amnesia for traumatic childhood events. This is a poorly studied but very common phenomenon. People exposed to trauma during childhood use whatever resources they have available at the time of the trauma to survive. In early childhood, forgetting an event or dissociating oneself from the event is a defense mechanism that is very much available and helpful to the child being victimized. Although data defining the extent of the phenomenon are scant, clinical experience suggests partial or complete blocking of childhood sexual trauma experiences is the rule rather than the exception.[12] In our study,[35] we asked why women had not told someone about their abuse, and 28 percent volunteered that they had not told because they had not remembered the abuse. The number would have been much higher had we asked, specifically, "Is there a part of your experience that you were not able to remember for a significant period of time?"

Although we learned about repressed memories by asking our adult patients, Williams[47] approached the question from a different perspective. Children in whom sexual abuse had been confirmed in childhood were asked 17 years later, during adulthood, about their experience. Thirty-eight percent had no memory of the abuse.

A common presentation for someone remembering childhood sexual abuse is the person who says, "There are some things I remember for sure, others I am having a hard time believing, and still other thoughts which are only vague suspicions." Typically, someone will describe sitting up in bed in the middle of the night with a vivid picture in his or her mind that may or may not be left over from a dream experience. The picture is extremely detailed in some respects but confused around the edges. It may be associated with smells, sounds, or taste sensations which give it a sense of immediacy. It is only later that the picture gets infused with emotions that might be expected to accompany the scene. Patients have described such pictures of abuse scenes with almost clinical detachment. Yet these same memories may later be the material of a flashback experience.

There are numerous examples of events or sensations that trigger the return of repressed memories. One woman returned to the town where she spent her childhood and met an uncle who remarked that he was responsible for her breasts growing to be the same size. Instantly, she was able to remember a long series of abuse experiences with the man, memories that previously had not been consciously available to her. Another woman was in a car accident. When she regained consciousness she was being strapped to a gurney and intubated by the paramedic team prior to transport to a hospital. She began struggling violently and threatened to kill the attendants. Later, she was able to describe a previously repressed episode in which she was held down and gang raped orally and anally when she was 6 years old. Relatives confirmed for her that the event had actually occurred. This woman had overcome a disadvantaged childhood, raised several successful children, and had a productive career before she remembered the abuse. It took five years of therapy subsequent to the reawakening of memories for her to return to her previous level of functioning.

Although we don't know when a memory will emerge or what might trigger it, there is a common understanding among experienced therapists that memories remain buried until the individual is in a position to deal with the reality of the experience. Often, memories emerge within a context of a secure relationship, as with a spouse or good friend, or in therapy.

Sometimes patients ask to be hypnotized in order for their memories to be pulled from them. Although hypnosis can be a powerful tool in the treatment of childhood trauma, a reasonable approach is to advise the patient that hypnosis seldom results in memory recovery faster than good psychotherapy. The limiting factor is the amount of material the person is able to process consciously, which is dependent on self-esteem and the degree of personal security the individual is feeling at the time.

The recovery of memories often evokes feelings of helplessness, shame, guilt, and sometimes suicidal ideation. Involving the support network, with the patient's permission—or without, if a life-threatening condition exists—is something the therapist must be prepared to do. Even though an outpouring of emotions is possible at the time of memory recovery, the more likely scenario is a matter of fact description of childhood scenes that are uncomfortable to discuss. Once again, sympathetic listening is the first response indicated, and, often, the only intervention required.

POSTTRAUMATIC STRESS DISORDER

Posttraumatic stress disorder (PTSD) has only recently been recognized to be significant in survivors of childhood sexual abuse.[25] The signs and symptoms of PTSD constitute a significant response by severely abused adults who may be seen in the primary care office. The syndrome, first delineated among returning Vietnam War veterans, has four basic components:[2]

1. First there must be a stressor that "would be markedly distressing to almost anyone."

2. Next is a component that constitutes a reliving of the experience. This is the flashback or intrusive memory that is perceived by the patient as happening in the present.

3. Another collection of symptoms constitutes a wish to avoid the memories of the trauma. These are the "detachment symptoms."

4. The fourth group of symptoms involves the presence of physiologic responses to recurrent intrusive memories or flashbacks. Examples of anxiety symptoms triggered by flashbacks commonly seen in adult survivors are gagging, tachycardia, rapid breathing, and numbness in fingers and toes. Fibromyalgia or chronic tension headaches sometimes can be interpreted as long-term effects of muscle tension associated with anxiety.

A flashback experience can be terrifying for someone living it. It can also be disconcerting to a clinician, who might see a patient calmly discussing an early life experience become silent, turn inward, assume a fetal position under a desk, and completely disregard the clinician for ten minutes. One might consider the patient to be psychotic. Only later will the flashback experience make sense, when it is placed in the context of the patient's history.

Although the management of flashbacks will not typically fall to the primary care physician, it is helpful to know some general principles. Lenore Terr has written extensively about "traumatic play."[43] She describes how a child who has been traumatized will return to the experience in play, often in an abstracted form, but sometimes very literally, in an attempt to have the event come out differently. She relates, for example, that novelist Stephen King watched as a playmate was killed by a train behind his house when they were both 4 years old.[44] He incorporates numerous images of trains chasing boys or other machines killing people in his fiction. Her interpretation is that he is attempting to undo through his art the painful death he witnessed.

Flashbacks can be thought of as a form of traumatic reenactment. There is always the hope that this time the scene will come out differently. Unfortunately, without help from the outside, a victim may just replay the old scenes with all the terrible feelings still attached. In working with flashback memories, it is important to give them a context, define them as an attempt to survive the abuse in adulthood, and look at them as specific events that have qualities that are subject to change. The circumstances that trigger flashbacks can sometimes be avoided or modified. There are specific cognitive techniques that can alter the course of the memory experience. And once the flashback has run its course, there are ways to make sense of what just happened.

PSYCHIATRIC DIAGNOSES OF ADULT SURVIVORS

As we have seen, the effects of childhood sexual abuse can be extremely variable, from few long-term consequences to catastrophic psychiatric illness. Good epidemiological data about prevalence of psychiatric illness in this population are no more available than good epidemiological data about the frequency of physical illnesses in this group. The experience of finding sexual abuse histories in people with personality disorders has created a tendency to theorize that the result of childhood trauma is felt most strongly in personality development. In a recent study, we did structured psychiatric interviews with 45 consecutive individuals entering treatment for problems associated with childhood sexual assault.[33] The most frequent DSM-III-R diagnosis at the time of evaluation was PTSD. The formal criteria were met by 73 percent of the sample. The next most frequent diagnosis was major depression (22%), followed by obsessive compulsive disorder (13%), and simple phobia (13%). Using lifetime prevalence standards, the frequency of individuals experiencing PTSD increased to 78 percent, and those with major depression increased to 67 percent. Those with a diagnosis of borderline personality disorder (as measured by the Millon Clinical Multiaxial Inventory-II) numbered 20 percent. Thus, major Axis I diagnoses were considerably more frequent than was borderline personality disorder.

An interesting finding of this study was the 62 percent of patients who at some time in their lives had met diagnostic criteria for alcohol or substance abuse or dependence (although only 9 percent were using substances abusively at the time of referral). We reported this as an example of "chemical dissociation," a term borrowed from John Briere.[5] A number of these individuals had had significant long-term drug or alcohol use that met research criteria, yet they were able to change their substance use patterns significantly with a life change. We came to believe that drug and alcohol use in this population had a distinct function and was substantially different from more traditional patterns of addiction.[34]

The last ten years have seen a renewed interest in the diagnosis and treatment of multiple personality (dissociative identity) disorder.[31] This entity, which requires the existence of two or more distinct identities or personality states that "recurrently take control of the person's behavior,"[2] had been felt to be extremely rare until investigators began working intensively with individuals with severe abuse histories. Among the 45 individuals described above, 2 (4%) were diagnosed with dissociative identity disorder (DID). Although no claim is made that DID is a major consequence of childhood sexual abuse, most individuals with DID have histories of significant, longstanding, sexual, physical, and emotional abuse.

Patients will occasionally present with a complaint such as "I seem to be two different people." Unless the patient is already in treatment with a capable psychotherapist and has been diagnosed as having DID, this presentation is invariably *not* dissociative identity disorder, since one of the hallmarks of the disorder is lack of conscious recognition of one personality from the others.

PSYCHOTHERAPY

Good psychotherapy can often result in complete removal or significant diminution of symptoms associated with childhood sexual abuse. There is a growing number of talented therapists who deal effectively with issues raised by survivors of childhood sexual abuse. More and more therapists define what they do with survivors as treating the trauma symptoms directly rather than the underlying personality problems.[5,11] Specifically, this "trauma-focused therapy" involves emphasis on network building, breaking down of the isolation of the victim, treating symptoms as "attempts to cope" with childhood experiences, and giving cognitive help in dealing with intrusive memories. A useful paradigm that pervades this kind of psychotherapy involves telling the patient that he or she did whatever was necessary to survive the abuse while it was occurring. The patient used the means available at the time. As most survivors did not receive help in childhood, were unable to make sense of the experience, and have not dealt with the experience with peers in adulthood, there is a tendency to use the same solutions they relied on during childhood. These solutions now are the source of adult problems. New solutions are in order.

For example, a girl may have discovered at age 4 that by hiding in a closet or under a bed, she could sometimes avoid abuse by her father. When faced with situations that remind her of the abusive relationship, as an adult she may be tempted to hide, either figuratively or literally. Hiding, however, might not serve to push away the memory and could result in problems in her current world. Therapy that deals with her present symptoms and behaviors in the context of the past experiences has the best chance of success.

We discussed earlier how important it is to conduct treatment within a therapeutic web of supporting, validating relationships. The physician is part of this support network. Before looking for support to the patient's natural network of family and friends, individual or group therapy may be indicated.

Individual therapy with someone comfortable with abuse issues and their sequelae can provide the central element in the treatment process. Within the therapeutic relationship the person can admit the awful reality of the abuse and begin to make some sense of it. Current life experience is examined and placed in the context of earlier experience. Together, the patient and therapist can plan for the extension of the therapeutic network to include others.

Group therapy has become a mainstay in the treatment of these patients.[1,21] Groups help break down the sense of isolation. Grown-up victims of abuse may never have met another individual who had similar experiences. They often feel unique. They may consider the shame and guilt they feel are warranted, until they see another victim taking responsibility for behavior imposed at a young age by an adult.

An interest in confronting the perpetrator is common among adults victimized as children. She or he may want confirmation of some detail of the abuse, or acknowledgment that it took place. Often there is a desire for closure, a need to get an answer to the question "Why me?" Other motivations include hope for reconciliation or desire to hear an expression of remorse. Rarely, someone just wants to express how angry they are about the abuse they received. My experience, and that of others, is that confrontations are most appropriate late in the process of therapy and often lead to disastrous consequences if entered into prematurely.[40] Very rarely should the impetus to confront the perpetrator come from a treatment person. In the early and middle stages of treatment it is preferable to focus effort on building a therapeutic network of supportive family and friends around the abuse victim.

USE OF MEDICATION

Use of psychotropic medications in the treatment of the sexually abused population is symptom specific. Depression associated with sleep disturbance, anhedonia, appetite disturbance, and chronic pain will often respond to an antidepressant such as fluoxetine in conjunction with psychotherapy. Anxiety symptoms associated with panic attacks and compulsive behaviors will also respond to appropriate pharmacotherapy. In most cases, however, medication should be seen as an adjunct to psychotherapy. Of course, use of psychotropic medications should follow an accurate assessment of suicide risk in the patient.

THE PHYSICAL EXAM

Some individuals with abuse history have difficulty being touched in any way. The medical examination can trigger unpleasant feelings or memories. The exam involves becoming unclothed in front of others and potentially intrusive touching such as during the mouth, breast, pelvic, and rectal exams. A physician who has obtained a sexual abuse history can conduct the exam in a manner that results in the least discomfort for the patient.

Talking about the exam before actually conducting it can eliminate many difficulties. Making eye contact frequently during the exam can help remind the patient of the present relationship with the physician as opposed to a remembered abuse situation. Sometimes the patient will require a physician of a particular gender. Talking directly about what one is doing during the exam and having a supportive assistant who can reassure the patient with additional information are helpful. The patient might want to be accompanied by a friend or relative for moral support.

Patients who previously had difficulties have described successful pelvic exams after taking an antianxiety medication such as lorazepam. Even with precautions, however, the physician may experience a patient dissociating during the procedure. Many female survivors of sexual abuse can give accounts of "going away" during pelvic exams. They describe out-of-body experiences in which they float in a corner of the room and watch the examination. One woman admitted going to her "secret place" during medical examinations. It consisted of mentally becoming a costumed tightrope walker in a medieval circus as she remembered it from a picture in her favorite childhood book.

Asking about dissociation before the exam can be very reassuring to the patient. For the physician, the patient's ability to physically "not feel" the exam can be understood as just one of the survival tactics the patient has learned over the years. She will "awaken" when the exam is over. Some sensitive physicians have become particularly good at recognizing dissociative phenomena during exams, and they use this knowledge to help people disclose histories of abuse.

Pelvic exams are probably the most intrusive part of the medical examination. One must remember, however, that a person's reaction to the exam is idiosyncratic and may be related to a particular type of abuse. One person may have no difficulty with a pelvic but vomit repeatedly when a tongue depressor is inserted in the mouth. Once again, a careful history is the best guide.

REPORTING ABUSE

All states now have laws mandating reporting of suspected child abuse. Laws vary from state to state, but in all cases, physicians are mandatory reporters, that is, required by law to report suspected abuse. A typical law will read "If there is suspicion of someone's harming the child physically or abusing the child sexually, a mandatory reporting person must notify the proper authorities, who will conduct an investigation." In most jurisdictions the reporting authority will be child protective services.

Most physicians have no difficulty reporting sexual abuse of a child. However, there are times when a physician is tempted not to call social services. The doctor may feel he or she knows the family well and that "it couldn't possibly be true." Or there may be the sense that the authorities will "only mess it up." I have heard of cases in which a physician decided that a 13-year-old could give consent to a 40-year-old and that the situation was therefore not abuse. (Under the laws of most states, a 13-year-old cannot give consent to sexual acts with an adult.) When the situation is not clear but there is "a suspicion," it is always best to let the authorities investigate. Nonreporting practitioners are exposing themselves to significant liability, while reporting physicians are protected by the same mandatory reporting statutes.

The laws mandating reporting do not require you to interview the child you suspect might be in an abusive relationship. The suspicion alone is enough to trigger the report. There is sometimes concern that reporting abuse might ruin the alleged abuser's life. In most cases, if there is no evidence of abuse on investigation, little happens to the accused person. If evidence is found, then the abuse can be stopped.

A different issue arises when adults report past abuse. The abuse may have occurred 30 years prior to the disclosure, the statute of limitations having long since expired. However, we can expect that adults who get sexual gratification from children will continue to do so when the opportunity is available to them. The adult in your office may not be the only child victimized by the perpetrator. It is reasonable to ask if the abuser currently has access to children.

A woman made an appointment with me to discuss her abuse at the hands of her father. She had minimal long-term psychological effects, but a family reunion was planned, and she wanted to know what course to follow. When queried about other children who might be at risk, she responded, "Oh no! Why didn't I think of that!" She came from a large family with many nephews and nieces still living in the small town, regularly being left with their grandparents for child care. She and her husband quickly concluded that as many as ten children might be at risk. We made a plan to report the abuse she had experienced as a child to the local authorities, and she developed a strategy for organizing her siblings and their spouses. The family reunion turned into a confrontation of her father when at least six of the grandchildren were discovered to have been violated. The siblings and spouses were able to convince him to go into sexual offender treatment after assuring him that their children would all know what he had done and would never be left alone with him again. The local reporting agency provided the legal muscle to effect the family's plan.

Occasionally a woman will ask if anything can be done to punish the perpetrator, even if years have passed since the abuse stopped. Statute of limitations provisions do apply, and they differ from state to state. It may be possible to press charges, depending on when the abuse last occurred. Recently, victims in some jurisdictions have sued for damages resulting from abuse that occurred in childhood. An added dimension to some of these suits has been that the statue of limitations clock was regarded as beginning to run when the repressed memories surfaced. Public sentiment seems to have swung back regarding repressed memories, as the result of several well publicized cases; the willingness of juries to accept repressed memory evidence is currently not great. You may want to recommend that your patient receive local legal advice. (See chapter 23 for a further discussion of forensic implications of abuse.)

THE ADULT SURVIVOR MOVEMENT

In addition to group therapy, peer support groups have evolved to respond to the needs of people victimized in childhood. Several of the more prominent organizations include Survivors of Incest Anonymous,[41] Parents United, and VOICES in Action.[45] Incest Survivors Anonymous is a twelve-step program that has more than 300 groups meeting around the country. Following the model of Alcoholics Anonymous, accurate records are not kept of membership. Parents United has a base in California and is an outgrowth of the work of Giarretto. VOICES in Action is based in Chicago but has a national agenda; it sponsors meetings for professionals and survivors. These organizations have in common an ability to respond to individuals needing confirmation from others with shared experiences.

The unofficial bible of the adult survivor self-help movement remains *The Courage to Heal*.[3] This best-selling book offers advice and suggestions for numerous life situations in a format that many patients find helpful.

CONCLUSION

Adults sexually victimized as children appear in the primary care physician's office frequently and for many different reasons. The individual may have unexplained physical symptoms, atypical exam behavior, or a history of emotional problems. The primary tool of the physician is the ability to communicate and make the patient feel comfortable when revealing the pertinent history and when undergoing necessary medical procedures. The fundamental treatment strategy for these patients should be to facilitate the construction of a supportive network of professionals, friends, and family within which the person can make sense of the childhood experience, and get on with his or her life.

REFERENCES

1. Alexander PC, Neimeyer RA, Follette VM, Moore MK, Harter SA. A comparison of group treatments of women sexually abused as children. *J Consult Clin Psychol* 1989;57:479–483.

2. American Psychiatric Association. *Diagnostic and statistical manual of mental disorders*, 3rd ed., rev'd. Washington DC: American Psychiatric Press. 1987.

3. Bass E, Davis L. *The courage to heal: A guide for women survivors of child sexual abuse*. New York: Harper and Row. 1988.

4. Beitchman JH, Zucker KJ, Hood JE, et al. A review of the long-term effects of child sexual abuse. *Child Abuse Negl* 1992;16:101–118.

5. Briere J. *Therapy for adults molested as children*. New York: Springer. 1989.

6. Briere J, Zaidi LY. Sexual abuse histories and sequelae in female psychiatric emergency room patients. *Am J Psychiatry* 1989;146:1602–1606.

7. Brown GR, Anderson B. Psychiatric morbidity in adult inpatients with childhood histories of sexual and physical abuse. *Am J Psychiatry* 1991;148:55–61.

8. Bryer JB, Nelson BA, Miller JB, Krol PA. Childhood sexual and physical abuse as factors in adult psychiatric illness. *Am J Psychiatry* 1987;144:1426–1430.

9. Burnam MA, Stein JA, Golding JM, et al. Sexual assault and mental disorders in a community population. *J Consult Clin Psychol* 1988;56:843–850.

10. Conte JR. The effects of sexual abuse on children: Results of a research project. *Ann N Y Acad Sci* 1989;326–330.

11. Courtois CA. *Healing the incest wound: Adult survivors in therapy*. New York: W. W. Norton. 1985.

12. Courtois CA. The memory retrieval process in incest survivor therapy. *J Child Sexual Abuse* 1992;1:15–31.

13. Denbo R, Berry E, William L, et al. The relationship between physical and sexual abuse and illicit drug use: A replication among a new sample of youths entering a juvenile detention center. *Int J Addictions* 1988;23:1101–1123.

14. Domino JV, Haber JD. Prior physical and sexual abuse in women with chronic headache: Clinical correlates. *Headache* 1987;27:310–314.

15. Finkelhor D. Early and long-term effects of child sexual abuse: An update. *Professional Psychology: Research and Practice* 1990;21:325–330.

16. Finkelhor D. *Sexually victimized children.* New York: Free Press, 1979.

17. Friedman LS, Samet JH, Roberts MS, Hudlin M, Hans P. Inquiry about victimization experiences: A survey of patient preferences and physician practices. *Arch Intern Med* 1992;152:1186–1190.

18. Fromuth ME, Burkhart BR. Long-term psychological correlates of childhood sexual abuse in two samples of college men. *Child Abuse Negl* 1989;13:533–542.

19. Giarretto H, Giarretto A, Sgroi SM. Coordinated community treatment of incest. In Burgess AW, Groth AN, Holmstrom LL, and Sgroi SM (eds.), *Sexual assault of children and adolescents,* 231–240. Lexington, MA: Lexington Books. 1978.

20. Herman JL, Schatzow E. Recovery and verification of memories of childhood sexual trauma. *Psychoanal Psychol* 1987;4:1–14.

21. Herman JL, Schatzow E. Time-limited group therapy for women with a history of incest. *Int J Group Psychother* 1984;34:605–616.

22. Hooper PD. Psychological sequelae of sexual abuse in childhood. *Br J Gen Pract* 1990; 40:29–31.

23. Jones DPH, McGraw JM. Reliable and fictitious accounts of sexual abuse to children. *J Interpers Viol* 1987;2:27–45.

24. Lanktree C, Briere J, Zaidi L. Incidence and impact of sexual abuse in a child outpatient sample: The role of direct inquiry. *Child Abuse Negl* 1991;15:447–453.

25. Lindberg FH, Distad LJ. Post-traumatic stress disorders in women who experienced childhood incest. *Child Abuse Negl* 1985;9:329–334.

26. Maltzman I, Schweiger A. Individual and family characteristics of middle-class adolescents hospitalized for alcohol and other drug abuse. *Br J Addict* 1991;86:1435–1447.

27. Moran MA. Conversion disorders in 1991: Diagnosis and treatment. Paper presented November 1991, Denver, CO.

28. Morgan E, Froning ML. Child sexual abuse sequelae and body-image surgery. *Plast Reconstr Surg* 1990;86:475–480.

29. Ogata SN, Silk KR, Goodrich S, et al. Childhood sexual and physical abuse in adult patients with borderline personality disorder. *Am J Psychiatry* 1990;147:1008–1013.

30. Pope HG, Hudson JI. Is childhood sexual abuse a risk factor of bulimia nervosa? *Am J Psychiatry* 1992;149:455–463.

31. Putnam F. *Diagnosis and treatment of multiple personality disorder.* New York: Guilford Press. 1989.

32. Roesler TA. The effect on adult psychological functioning of reactions to disclosure of childhood sexual abuse. Unpublished manuscript.

33. Roesler TA. Unpublished data.

34. Roesler TA, Daffler CE. Chemical dissociation in adults sexually victimized as children: Alcohol and drug use in adult survivors. Unpublished manuscript.

35. Roesler TA, Wise TW. Telling the secret: Disclosure of incest by adult women. Unpublished manuscript.

36. Roesler TA, Czech N, Camp W, Jenny C. Network therapy using videotape disclosures for adult sexual abuse survivors. *Child Abuse Negl* 1992;16:575–583.

37. Rohsenow DJ, Corbett R, Devine D. Molested as children: A hidden contribution to substance abuse? *J Subst Abuse Treat* 1988;5:13–18.

38. Russell DEH. The incidence and prevalence of intrafamilial and extrafamilial sexual abuse of female children. *Child Abuse and Negl* 1983;7:133–146.

39. Saunders BE, Villeponteaux LA, Liipovsky JA, Kilpatrick DG, Veronen LF. Child sexual assault as a risk factor for mental disorders among women. *J Interpers Viol* 1992;7:189–204.

40. Schatzow E, Herman JL. Breaking secrecy: Adult survivors disclose to their families. *Psychiatr Clin North Am* 1989;12:337–349.

41. Survivors of Incest Anonymous, PO Box 21817, Baltimore, MD 21222.

42. Survivors United Network, 3607 Martin Luther King Blvd., Denver, CO 80205.

43. Terr LC. Childhood traumas: An outline and overview. *Am J Psychiatry* 1991;148:10–20.

44. Terr LC. Terror writing by the formerly terrified. *Psychoanal Study Child* 1989;44:369–390.

45. VOICES in Action, PO Box 148309, Chicago, IL 60614.

46. Walker E, Katon W, Harrop-Griffiths J, et al. Relationship of chronic pelvic pain to psychiatric diagnoses and childhood sexual abuse. *Am J Psychiatry* 1988;145:75–80.

47. Williams LM. Adult memories of childhood abuse: Preliminary findings from a longitudinal study. *APSAC Advisor* 1992;5:19–21.

PART II

Physical Abuse

Chapter 6

Initial Medical Treatment of the Physically Abused Child

Lawrence R. Ricci, M.D.

The medical practitioner plays a critical role in the diagnosis and initial treatment of physical child abuse, with a function that ultimately will be tightly linked to forensic aspects of the case. The goals of initial medical intervention are twofold—treating physical injury and setting the stage for later psychosocial and legal action. The health care provider can offer support to families, but his or her primary obligation is to ensure the safety of the child. Child abuse management considerations require a clear understanding of the complexity of decision making and an appreciation of the benefits of multidisciplinary collaboration. Sometimes hospitalization is indicated, not only for the injury but also for the purpose of assessing the safety of the home and the advisability of returning the child to a potentially abusive family environment. The medical practitioner may be in an excellent position to stay involved in the treatment process after diagnosis and medical stabilization, and to support the child and family through the treatment process.

GENERAL CONSIDERATIONS

Physical abuse of a child can be conceptualized along a spectrum of nonaccidental injury. At one end lie inflicted minor bruises and lacerations, at the other end severe multisystem trauma and death.[20] It has been estimated that 1.4 million children in the United States are abused in some manner each year—between 2 percent and 3 percent of the population under 18 years of age.[82] Of these children, 160,000 are thought to suffer from serious or life-threatening injuries.

The present medical interest in physical child abuse began in 1962 when C. Henry Kempe introduced the term *battered child syndrome.*[37] Dr. Kempe and colleagues found 302 cases of the battered child ("serious physical abuse generally from a parent or foster parent") in their nationwide survey of 71 responding hospitals. Of those 302 children, 33 died, and 85 of the survivors suffered permanent brain injury.

Some of the initial treatment considerations of the physically abused child are similar to those discussed for the sexually abused child (see chapter 1). As in the case of sexual abuse, the treatment of the physically abused child requires that the medical practitioner understand not only the multiple psychosocial and biomechanical causes of abusive injuries but also the physical, psychosocial, and legal sequelae as well.[30] Physical child abuse is a complex phenomenon resulting from a combination of individual, family, and societal factors.[29,45] Newberger has suggested that physical abuse results from the interaction of three types of stressors:

- child-produced stressors (physically, mentally, temperamentally, or behaviorally different children)
- social situational stressors (poverty, unemployment, excessive mobility, isolation, domestic violence, attachment problems, punitive child-rearing styles)
- parent-produced stressors (low self-esteem, abused as children themselves, depression, substance abuse, character disordered, unrealistic expectations of the child)

These stressors usually result in physical abuse in the context of a triggering situation, for example, discipline, argument or family conflict, substance abuse, or any acute problem in the family environment.[8]

In this model, the injury is the visible expression of a more pervasive family problem and represents, from an optimistic view, a gateway into analysis and treatment of family dysfunction, the issue of ultimate import for the child.[78] With this model in mind, the goals of initial medical intervention become twofold: not only treating physical injury but also setting the stage for later psychosocial and legal action.

The general principles of medical intervention with the physically abused child can be viewed as a series of diagnostic and therapeutic steps:

1. suspecting abuse
2. establishing the diagnosis
3. treating injuries
4. addressing safety issues
5. reporting to child protective agencies and law enforcement
6. documenting findings
7. recommending follow-up treatment

In addition, the practitioner might be involved in continued work with the child and family, expert testimony when required, and referral, when available, to a child abuse medical specialist for definitive medical forensic assessment. This chapter reviews the unique medical intervention needs of the physically abused child during the critical period immediately following diagnosis.

TREATMENT PRINCIPLES

The management issues requiring medical decision making include

- what immediate medical intervention is indicated,
- whether the child is at ongoing risk,
- what protective steps should be taken, and
- what follow-up should occur.[20,59]

Such management considerations require a clear understanding of the complexity of child abuse decision making and an appreciation of the benefits of multidisciplinary collaboration.[29]

History taking is the first step in decision making. It requires a compassionate yet objective approach. History obtained from the child and the parents can be critically important in assessing the cause of an inflicted injury. The medical provider plays a vital role in the preservation of this verbally relayed evidence.[56,59] Good interviewing technique is important, not only for later criminal and child protective intervention, but for treatment as well. It is essential to carefully and completely gather as much detailed information as possible, while avoiding interrogating or alienating the family.[82] Remember, though, that the information offered is subject to interpretation. Whereas in most other clinical encounters, the medical provider can expect the proffered history to be truthful, it is not uncommon for an abusive caretaker to either fabricate an explanation or offer no explanation at all for the injuries.[55] Important concepts to keep in mind while interviewing include: interviewing everyone alone, using open ended, nonleading questions particularly with younger children, and inquiring about not only physical abuse but sexual abuse, domestic violence, and witnessed abuse as well.[20,68,82] For more information about the forensic implications of history taking, see chapter 23.

In closing out interviews with parents and children, it is important to answer their questions and thank them for their participation. However, the provider should not offer specific information as to the believed etiology of the injuries—for example shaking as an etiology for subdural hematoma and retinal hemorrhage—before careful forensic assessment has been completed.[44] Such prematurely released information about the mechanism of a possible criminal act could seriously impede later law enforcement interrogation.

It is appropriate to be supportive and interested, but it is not appropriate to make promises to children and families that are beyond the provider's ability to keep. It is likewise best for the interviewer not to interrupt history taking by expressing a critical opinion, for example, about the inappropriateness of parental behavior. Such an interruption may only serve to limit the honesty of the historian. These discussions should be saved until the assessment has been completed. Important historical red flags for abuse, apart from an inconsistent history of the injury, include domestic violence, substance abuse, and child abuse in the caretaker's own history.[8,50,60,76,82] The classic physical indicators of nonaccidental trauma include multiplanar injuries, injuries in various stages of healing, and injuries in an assaultive pattern.[20,55,62,82]

The physical examination offers an opportunity not only to assess the child for the classic injuries of physical abuse such as burns, bruises, fractures, and head trauma but also to observe the child's behavior and parent-child interaction. A sensitive and gentle approach to the child and family during the examination can avoid retraumatizing the child and establish the seeds for a later trusting relationship.

The single most important treatment priority for the medical provider is to insure the safety of the child.[20] No child should be sent unprotected back to an abusive environment. However, it is also important that the provider act in a nonjudgmental and compassionate manner, as an advocate for both the child and the family, while collecting information critical to the well-being of the child. Nurturing this relationship from the outset allows the physician to function as a positive support and a bridge between the family and the many other professionals who will later become involved. Balancing the need of the child for protection with the need of the family for preservation and the need for complete and critical data collection with the need for a sensitive, supportive approach to children and adults, remains the most difficult yet critical task for the medical provider working with families where abuse has occurred.

OUTPATIENT TREATMENT

Physical child abuse may present to the private office or emergency department in one of two ways: the child may present accompanied by a parent or child protective authority with the primary complaint of abuse, or the child may present accompanied by a caretaker with injuries that the practitioner subsequently determines to be abuse. Whatever the presentation, proceeding with a sensitive nonjudgmental manner yet critical eye will go a long way to defusing a potentially tense situation and setting the stage for later intervention.[20] One helpful approach in working with a parent or caretaker is simply not to assume during data collection that the caretaker giving the history is the person who abused or failed to protect the child.

The presentation of the abused child to the private office presents both opportunity and challenge. Usually the practitioner knows the family well and can continue to use that knowledge and rapport as the investigation evolves and in follow-up treatment. The challenge is that such a prior relationship sometimes can bias the practitioner to underreport or even misidentify clear-cut abuse.[35,53,74]

Not infrequently, the physically abused child is first transported to the hospital by ambulance. The prehospital emergency medical provider is in an ideal position to observe and document the initial appearance of the child and family in their home environment.[61,75] In doing so, the prehospital provider must, like other medical professionals, suspect abuse yet not act suspicious, while at the same time treating injuries according to local and national treatment protocols. The initial statement of how the injury occurred, taken before the family has an opportunity to devise a more complete story, should be carefully documented. This can be important for comparison, should the story later change. Observations and concerns of the prehospital medical provider should be conveyed to hospital personnel. A detailed descriptive report should be written. Most importantly, the provider must report to, or see that a report is made to, the appropriate authorities. This is legally mandated in all jurisdictions in the United States whenever child abuse is suspected (see chapter 8).

The emergency department, where many physical abuse cases first present, has the advantage of immediate social service consultation and multidisciplinary collaboration.[34,45,54] The initial medical treatment of the physically abused child in the emergency department should proceed no differently from that for the accidentally injured child, except that forensic data collection and analysis takes on a particular and pressing importance. Multidisciplinary collaboration in the emergency department should involve a hospital social worker who can interview families and children and coordinate reporting to appropriate authorities. Such reporting is often traumatic to families, yet, if handled sensitively, can be accomplished in such a way as to continue to support the family. The family should be informed that such reporting will occur and is required by law unless the professional feels that notification will pose a risk to the child, such as by causing the parents to flee with the child.[63] Concern for the child should be emphasized, rather than accusation. But more than this, the family should also be told that the clinical circumstances of the case demand a report, that the practitioner is not only required to report but believes that a report is indicated by the clinical circumstances.

It is helpful to establish an institutional protocol for the treatment of abuse cases. Such a protocol should state what diagnostic and therapeutic steps are to be taken, who should be consulted (for example, institutional social services) and how to notify state agencies.

INPATIENT TREATMENT

Severity of injuries should not be the sole determining factor for hospitalization. Because the safety of the child is all important, strong consideration should be given to hospitalizing an abused child if safety cannot otherwise be guaranteed. Hospitalization may be indicated as the best immediate recourse for protecting the child while further investigation is in process.[5] In addition to providing immediate protection and a place for medical treatment of injuries, hospitalization may offer time to sort out difficult diagnostic decisions (whether the injury is abusive or not) and therapeutic decisions (whether it is safe for the child to return home). Another advantage of hospitalization is the opportunity to observe parental behavior and parent-child interaction in a controlled setting.

Child abuse cases particularly benefit from multidisciplinary collaboration in the hospital. Many hospitals have so-called Trauma X or suspected child abuse and neglect (SCAN) teams made up of medical providers (physicians, nurses), mental health providers (social workers, psychologists), and sometimes legal, child protective, and community health providers.[78] Such teams are invaluable in addressing the needs of the individual case as well as in addressing the institutional needs for identification of and appropriate intervention in all child abuse cases. An important immediate function for such teams is to assure that all professionals in the institution convey the same message to the family. In the heated atmosphere of a child abuse evaluation, parents will often compare and contrast differing messages from professionals. Such apparent lack of concurrence can seriously disrupt later attempts at coordinated intervention.

The nurse, both outpatient and inpatient, plays a critical role as a team member in identifying and treating the physically abused child.[13,57,73] Nursing history should be carefully documented and include direct quotes of questions and answers.[52] Such nursing history can later be compared to other histories for inconsistencies. Parental reactions, child behavior, and parent-child interaction should also be noted. In the hospital, the nurse should attempt to establish a therapeutic relationship with both the child and the parents. It is vitally important for the nurse to stay neutral in encounters with the family, not try to prove abuse by accusations, not display horror or anger, not make judgmental statements, yet be factual and honest in discussions with parents. Therapeutically, the nurse can model appropriate adult-child behavior for the parents by recognizing and appropriately responding to the needs of the child. In this way the nurse can promote parental adequacy and support the parent-child relationship. The nurse can play a vital role in child abuse prevention through preventive health care, child behavior management instructions, encouraging the use of community resources, and educating families about risk factors for abuse and shaken baby syndrome.

The child life specialist, trained to understand all phases of hospital activity and child development, can greatly assist the children in acclimatizing to the hospital environment and beginning the process of recovering from abuse.[4,22,33] Such specialists can educate children about the hospital environment, prepare them for hospital procedures, organize diagnostic and therapeutic play, help children work through their feelings about the abuse and hospitalization, and assure that the hospital environment is conducive to the psychological well-being of the child. Child life specialists may also work with parents to provide children with appropriate emotional support, observe and document parent-child interaction and child behavior, and administer developmental screening tests to children.

One particular institutional intervention—attention to staff reaction—is important.[45] Perhaps in no other field of medicine can staff emotions be so strong and potentially so damaging to the professional and the family alike. There is no place in the treatment of the abused child for the medical provider who openly attacks the family or who is blatantly accusatory. Meetings among staff to discuss personal reactions and inservice education can be particularly helpful, both to minimize bias and to prevent adverse staff reactions to frequently troubling case material.[49,65,69] Somewhere between denial and outrage lies the most appropriate and most useful professional response.

TRAUMA MANAGEMENT

Initial assessment and treatment of the seriously physically abused child should proceed according to established guidelines such as those contained in the *Advanced Trauma Life Support Course for Physicians*[17] or in the *Textbook of Pediatric Advanced Life Support.*[1] Priorities include recognition of airway, breathing, and circulatory problems; instituting airway and ventilatory management; and establishing vascular access for fluid resuscitation and medication administration.[83] The medical care of the seriously injured abused child should be team based and include a physician experienced in the treatment of pediatric emergencies, a surgeon experienced in managing childhood trauma, and a physician experienced in the management of the abused child. The team may require the services of specialists in pediatric radiology, neurology, neurosurgery, and ophthalmology.

Treatment of the child with serious injuries, whether inflicted or otherwise, must focus simultaneously on diagnosis and treatment. Most seriously injured children are best monitored in an intensive care setting.[1] Depending on the complexity of services needed, the clinician should consider transferring the child to a specialized pediatric center. Not uncommonly, the child will present in extremis from circulatory or central nervous system compromise, without any history of trauma.[2] Thus, a high index of suspicion for occult head, chest, and abdominal trauma is important, as is a physiologic approach to resuscitation. In the abused child, particular attention should be placed on a search for head trauma as well as serious blunt abdominal and chest trauma. Most often, shock in these children is due to occult blood loss, but it may also result from dehydration, toxins, central nervous system dysfunction, external loss from lacerations or burns, or in rare cases infection (e.g., ruptured small bowel with resulting peritonitis).[18,19]

Head Injuries

Head injury is the most common cause of death in the abused child. The critically head-injured child is best treated aggressively in a specialized intensive care center.[28] Classic inflicted serious head traumas include subgaleal hematomas, skull fractures, subarachnoid hemorrhages, subdural hematomas, and parenchymal brain injuries.[11] Epidural hematomas may be inflicted but are more likely to be accidental.[72]

The abused head-injured child is often acutely critically ill at the time of presentation, although not uncommonly the child will present with subtle subacute or chronic symptoms such as vomiting, lethargy, irritability, or increasing head circumference, all without visible head trauma or a history of head injury.[7] The child who is apneic, convulsing, or comatose requires airway support. In the face of cerebral edema, fluid restriction, steroids, hyperventilation, and osmolar drugs may be of benefit.[2,11] A subdural anterior fontanel tap may be indicated both diagnostically and therapeutically.[11] A spinal or subdural tap may be diagnostic if blood is present. Xanthochromia should be noted, particularly if the differential is between traumatic tap and old subarachnoid blood. However, careful thought should be given before performing lumbar puncture, because of the possibility of causing cerebellar herniation. Seizures, if present, should be treated according to standard guidelines. Intracranial lesions requiring surgical treatment are not common in the abused head-injured child. Such treatment should be guided by the results of a computerized tomography scan and clinical examination.[11,28] Cervical spine injuries, uncommon in child abuse, still require consideration, particularly in the unresponsive or seriously head-injured child.[48]

Abdominal Injuries

The second leading cause of death in the abused child is abdominal trauma. Death usually occurs either from a direct blow that causes blood loss, such as from a ruptured solid viscus (liver, spleen) or a lacerated vessel (mesenteric), or from infection, such as from a perforated hollow viscus.[43] Duodenal or jejunal obstruction from intramural hematoma secondary to blunt trauma can also occur.[12,18] Blunt trauma to the abdomen can also result in pancreatic trauma.[12,18]

The nature of the injury may provide clues to its cause. In one analysis comparing children with accidental versus inflicted blunt abdominal trauma, most inflicted injuries were hollow viscera while most accidental injuries were to single solid organs, with the former more likely requiring surgical intervention.[43]

Symptoms of abdominal trauma secondary to perforation, obstruction, or bleeding include vomiting, pain, tenderness, shock, and sepsis. Life-threatening abdominal trauma, like head trauma, may present without visible external signs or history to suggest such an injury.[18,34] Computerized tomography scanning of the abdomen may be useful in the child who is unconscious or when abdominal trauma is suspected, particularly if a bleeding source cannot be identified.[18] Blunt abdominal trauma from child abuse, because of its attendant high mortality, should be identified quickly and treated aggressively.[19]

Bruises, Burns, and Fractures

Though unlikely to require aggressive resuscitative treatment, serious cutaneous bruising has been described as leading to hypovolemic shock from subcutaneous blood loss or renal failure from rhabdomyolysis.[25,39,46] Documentation of such findings can have importance not only medically but legally, in later assessing a risk of serious harm. Inflicted burns, whether by contact or immersion, require careful attention to fluid resuscitation and wound care.[26,70] Photographs should be taken of all visible cutaneous injuries before treatment.[65]

Kleinman divides fractures into three categories depending on their specificity for abuse:[38]

1. Highly specific fractures: e.g., posterior rib, scapular, spinous process, sternal, and metaphyseal lesions
2. Moderately specific fractures: e.g., multiple especially if bilateral, those of different ages, epiphyseal separations, vertebral body, digital, complex skull
3. Common but low specificity fractures: e.g., clavicle, long bone shaft, linear skull

He further indicates that moderate and low specificity fractures become highly specific when a credible history of accidental trauma is absent.

The treatment of abuse-related skeletal injury differs little from the treatment of accidental fractures.[51] Many injuries, particularly older ones, require no treatment at all. When treatment is indicated, simple casting is usually satisfactory. Closed reduction and cast immobilization are required for displaced fractures, to restore length as well as rotational and angular alignment. Operative treatment, either open or closed, is rarely necessary.

Death

The infant who is brought to the hospital dead or who dies shortly after admission often presents a particular diagnostic and therapeutic dilemma. In this situation, the central differential diagnosis is between sudden infant death syndrome and child abuse.[3,14,64] In such circumstances families should be managed supportively while appropriate investigative information is gathered. Such a process often involves expeditious consultation with child protective services and law enforcement. Though it may be appropriate to discuss with the family the possible differential diagnosis, such as sudden infant death syndrome, it is equally important to remember that sudden infant death syndrome is a diagnosis of exclusion requiring a complete autopsy and death scene investigation. However, there is little to gain from an accusatory, inconsiderate approach to families and much to gain by attempting to engage the family in the assessment process. Many families, particularly those who truly don't know why their child died, welcome appropriate investigation if they are approached with compassion and care. The involvement of a child abuse medical specialist early in the investigation of a suspicious death can be of benefit, particularly in gathering history and interpreting the history in comparison to the findings at autopsy.

IMPORTANCE OF MULTIDISCIPLINARY TEAMS AND ROLE OF THE CHILD ABUSE SPECIALIST

The child abuse field has been a model for multidisciplinary collaboration.[10,32,40,42,77,79,81] Such collaboration is useful for joint decision making, planning, and mutual support. Teams may be hospital or community based, state or local. Many teams include medical providers, social services agency personnel, mental health providers, and law enforcement professionals. Hospital-based suspected abuse and neglect (SCAN) teams function to collect data, encourage appropriate reporting, and convene multidisciplinary case discussion.[81] State and local multidisciplinary child death review teams have proliferated throughout the United States and offer an excellent modality for death assessment as well as case-specific and communitywide treatment and prevention.[24]

The philosophy of the diagnostic multidisciplinary team is that having multiple professionals evaluate multiple aspects of a case offers the best chance for accurate diagnosis and effective treatment planning. A logical extension of this has been the development of community- or hospital-based child abuse diagnostic centers. The functions of many such case-specific diagnostic teams include substantiation of child abuse, development of a case plan, and, in some centers, monitoring of the implementation of the plan. A child abuse specialist who understands the forensic implications of child abuse diagnosis and treatment can be invaluable, if involved early in the diagnostic assessment and care of the physically abused child. Such consultation can be particularly beneficial in initial forensic data collection and interpretation and later, when court appearance is requested.[41] In 1988, the American Academy of Pediatrics formed the Section on Child Abuse. Currently the section has more than 500 members, pediatricians throughout the United States and Canada who have a special interest or expertise in child abuse diagnosis and treatment. In 1990, the Section on Child Abuse performed a national survey throughout the United States and Canada and found more than 100 child abuse diagnostic teams that had a medical component.[71]

LEGAL CONSIDERATIONS

Reporting issues for the medical provider include reporting to the department of human services and, when indicated, to law enforcement.[67] Child protective services and police investigators should be involved expeditiously when suspicions arise that an injury is non-accidental. Crime scene information fades rapidly. Medical providers should never assume that abusive injuries are a one-time event that will not reoccur, nor that they alone can intervene to protect children without other agency assistance.

There has been concern expressed about the so-called criminalization of child abuse. It has been suggested that movement has been away from a helping approach and toward a prosecutorial approach to abusive parents.[76] It is true that the legal system has increasingly served to drive child welfare and medical professionals together to gather evidence for prosecution. This may, at times, seem to conflict with the offering of services to promote family welfare; however, the determination of precisely what happened and who did it is as important to the ultimate welfare of the child as the family dynamics and treatment needs. Such determination, particularly in the case of the physically abused child, relies heavily on the clarity and specificity of the medical findings. Not infrequently, "what happened and when" can be converted by law enforcement and child protective professionals into "who did it and why."

For both medical and legal purposes, accurate written documentation is important.[56] Such documentation should include a history that is as factual and as detailed as possible. Written documentation of verbal evidence should be accomplished immediately. The source of information should be clearly noted. A recent study found that details of the history and the consistency or lack thereof of the history of the presenting injury was addressed or implied in only 59 percent of clinical records in suspected abuse cases.[15]

For a more detailed discussion of legal intervention with the physically abused child, see chapters 8 and 23.

EFFECTS OF PHYSICAL ABUSE
AND HOW TO FOLLOW UP

The physically abused child requires immediate medical, psychological, and protective attention. Later, more detailed assessment and treatment in each area is required. Surgical follow-up may be indicated for head trauma or other evidence of serious multisystem trauma. Orthopedic follow-up may be indicated for serious skeletal injuries. Ophthalmologic follow-up may be indicated for retinal and other eye injuries. The details of these treatments are discussed in chapter 9.

The physically abused child will also likely have psychosocial and developmental follow-up needs. Many physically abused children also suffer from neglect[82] and may have developmental delays requiring assessment and intervention. Long-term developmental follow-up is also critical for the neurologically injured abused child, who often suffers from significant developmental delays.[9] All this may best be coordinated by a committed and knowledgeable pediatrician who can integrate the myriad specialists, both medical and mental health, involved with the child and family. Developmental consequences for physically abused children are discussed in full in chapter 10.

Although the medical practitioner's main responsibility in child abuse management is initially diagnostic, he or she may also play a significant role in intervention, both short and long term. In the highly charged emotional atmosphere of child abuse assessment and intervention, treatment begins at first contact. In no other area of medical practice does diagnostic assessment and treatment proceed in such a linked fashion. How families are managed during the assessment period often sets the stage for later intervention. The practitioner should stay involved in the treatment process after diagnosis and medical stabilization. In many circumstances, the practitioner may be in an excellent position to participate in case management and to support the child and family through the treatment process.

Child abuse and neglect frequently occur in concert with other forms of family violence, including spousal abuse and violence between siblings.[80] In one study of the hospital records of mothers of 32 abused children, the records of 60 percent of the mothers were diagnostic or highly suggestive of previous maternal spousal victimization.[50] This study suggests that abused children are at high risk for exposure to violence against their mothers. The possibility of such violence should be actively investigated and, if found, aggressively treated in collaboration with community-based domestic violence programs.[23,58]

Long-term mental health consequences of physical abuse include violent and criminal behavior, substance abuse, self-injurious and suicidal behavior, depression, anxiety, and dissociation.[47] Many abused children–although not the majority–later abuse their own children.[36] Moderating influences do exist and include the characteristics of the maltreatment (who abused, how much, whether concurrent neglect is present), of the individual (e.g., men may become violent while women may become self-injurious), of the family (family violence, substance abuse), and of the environment (supportive relationships, therapy).[47]

Treatment frequently involves working with the family and working separately with individual members, particularly the child victim.[27,66,82] Positive results have been reported in some education programs for physically abusive and neglectful parents and in preventive home visits to young mothers at high risk for abusing their children.[16] Family preservation programs, designed to stabilize families and allow children to remain at home, are currently popular alternatives to foster care. Such programs, however, have not been demonstrated to be superior to treatment that separates the child from the family, nor have they been shown to reduce the number of children placed out of the home.[6,31]

CONCLUSION

In the care of the physically abused child, medical and forensic diagnosis and treatment are tightly linked. Accurate diagnosis must precede and inform any attempt at effective treatment. The forensic purpose of the evaluation is to collect evidence, through history, physical examination, and laboratory data, and to provide expert interpretation of this evidence. The traditional medical role of suspicion of abuse, diagnosis, medical treatment, and referral has recently expanded to include serving on hospital and community teams, directing specialized diagnostic and treatment centers, participating in community case and advisory review boards, and general advocacy.

A new subspecialist pediatrician, the forensic pediatrician or child abuse specialist, now exists in many locales around the United States. Though not yet pediatric board recognized, such specialists complement the role of the generalist medical provider in clearly establishing a legally defensible diagnosis of abuse and in providing specialized treatment services for abused children. The emergence during the past ten years of this cadre of forensically skilled pediatricians specializing in the diagnosis and treatment of the abused child, and the development of regional centers for such evaluations and treatment mirrors the parallel evolution of pediatric emergency medicine specialists and pediatric trauma centers. The latter developments have clearly had a significant and positive impact on the outcome for the seriously injured child.[83]

Of paramount importance in the treatment of the physically abused child is a supportive approach to families, yet a comprehensive and cautious approach to the protection of children. Indeed, if any treatment option is unacceptable, it is that an abused child be sent back unprotected to a potentially abusive environment.

REFERENCES

1. American Academy of Pediatrics. *Textbook of pediatric advanced life support,* Chameides L, Hazinski MF (eds.). American Heart Association. 1994.

2. American Academy of Pediatrics, Committee on Child Abuse and Neglect. Inflicted cerebral trauma. *Pediatrics* 1993;92:872–875.

3. American Academy of Pediatrics, Committee on Child Abuse and Neglect and Committee on Community Health. Investigation and review of unexpected infant and child deaths. *Pediatrics* 1993;92:88–89.

4. American Academy of Pediatrics, Committee on Hospital Care. Child life programs. *Pediatrics* 1993;91:671–673.

5. American Academy of Pediatrics, Committee on Hospital Care. Medical necessity for the hospitalization of the abused and neglected child. *Pediatrics* 1987;79:90.

6. Bath HI, Haapula DA. Intensive family preservation services with abused and neglected children: An examination of group differences. *Child Abuse Negl* 1993;17:213–215.

7. Berkowitz CD. Pediatric abuse: New patterns of injury. *Emerg Med Clin North Am* 1995; 13:321–341.

8. Bittner S, Newberger EH. Pediatric understanding of child abuse and neglect. *Pediatr Rev* 1981;2:197–207.

9. Bonnier C, Nassagne MC, Evrard P. Outcome and prognosis of whiplash shaken infant syndrome: Late consequences after a symptom-free interval. *Dev Med Child Neurol* 1995;37:943–956.

10. Bourne R, Newberger EH. Interdisciplinary group process in the hospital management of child abuse and neglect. *Child Abuse Negl* 1980;4:137–144.

11. Bruce DA. Neurosurgical aspects of child abuse. In Ludwig S, Kornberg AE (eds.), *Child abuse: A medical reference,* 2nd ed., 117–130. New York: Churchill Livingston. 1992.

12. Chadwick DL, Merten DF, Reece RM. Thoracic and abdominal injuries associated with child abuse. In Reece RM (ed.), *Child abuse: Medical diagnosis and treatment,* 54–69. Philadelphia: Lea and Febiger. 1994.

13. Chiocca EM. Shaken baby syndrome: A nursing perspective. *Pediatr Nursing* 1995;21:33–38.

14. Christoffel KK, Zieserl EJ, Chiaramonte J. Should child abuse and neglect be considered when a child dies unexpectedly? *Am J Dis Child* 1985;139:876–880.

15. Christopher NC, Anderson D, Gaertner L, et al. Childhood injuries and the importance of documentation in the emergency department. *Pediatr Emerg Care* 1995;11:52–57.

16. Cohn AH, Daro D. Is treatment too late: What 10 years of evaluation research tells us. *Child Abuse Negl* 1987;11:433–442.

17. Committee on Trauma. *Advanced trauma life support course for physicians,* 5th ed. Alexander RH, Proctor HJ (eds.). American College of Surgeons. 1994.

18. Cooper A: Thoracoabdominal trauma. In Ludwig S, Kornberg AE (eds.), *Child abuse: A medical reference,* 2nd ed., 131–150. New York: Churchill Livingston. 1992.

19. Cooper A, Floyd T, Barlow B, et al. Major blunt abdominal trauma due to child abuse. *J Trauma* 1988;28:1483–1487.

20. Council on Scientific Affairs. AMA diagnostic and treatment guidelines concerning child abuse and neglect. *JAMA* 1985;254:796–800.

21. Crothers D. Vicarious traumatization in the work with survivors of childhood trauma. *J Psychosoc Nurs Ment Health Serv* 1995;33:9–13.

22. Dolan A. A day in the life of a hospital play therapist. *Br J Theatre Nurs* 1993;3:31–32.

23. Dubowitz H, King H. Family violence: A child-centered, family-focused approach. *Pediatr Clin North Am* 1995;42:153–166.

24. Durfee MJ, Gellert PA, Tilton-Durfee D. Origins and clinical relevance of child death review teams. *JAMA* 1992;267:3172–3175.

25. Eichelberger SP, Beal DW, May RB. Hypovolemic shock in a child as a consequence of corporal punishment. *Pediatrics* 1991;87:570–571.

26. Finkelstein JL, Schwartz, Madden MR, et al. Pediatric burns: An overview. *Pediatr Clin North Am* 1992;39:1145–1163.

27. Fontana VJ. The maltreatment syndrome in children. *Pediatr Ann* 1994;13:736–744.

28. Ghajar J, Hariri RJ. Management of pediatric head injury. *Pediatr Clin North Am* 1992;39:1093–1125.

29. Green FC. Child abuse and neglect: A priority problem for the private physician. *Pediatr Clin North Am* 1975;22:329–339.

30. Halverson KC, Elliott BA, Rappley M, et al. Treatment of child abuse. *Prim Care* 1993;20:355–357.

31. Heneghan AM, Horwitz SM, Leventhal JM. Evaluating intensive family preservation programs: A methodological review. *Pediatrics* 1996;97:535–542.

32. Hochstadt NJ, Harwicke NJ. How effective is the multidisciplinary approach? A follow-up study. *Child Abuse Negl* 198 5;9:365–372.

33. Hughes M. Child life specialist: A new profession. *J Nurs Care* 1979;12:14.

34. Hyden PW, Gallagher PW. Child abuse intervention in the emergency room. *Pediatr Clin North Am* 1992;39:1053–1081.

35. James J, Womack WM, Stauss F. Physician reporting of sexual abuse of children. *JAMA* 1978;240:1145–1146.

36. Kaufman J, Zigler E. Do abused children become abusive parents? *Am J Orthopsychiatry* 1987;57:186–192.

37. Kempe CH, Silverman FN, Steele BF, et al. The battered-child syndrome. *JAMA* 1962; 181:17–24.

38. Kleinman PK: Skeletal trauma: General considerations. In Kleinman PK (ed.), *Diagnostic imaging of child abuse,* 5–28. Baltimore: Williams and Wilkins. 1987.

39. Knottenbelt JD. Traumatic rhabdomyolysis from severe beating: Experience of volume diuresis of 200 patients. *J Trauma* 1994;37:214–219.

40. Kovitz JE, Gougan P, Reinhold R, et al. Multidisciplinary team functioning. *Child Abuse Negl* 1984;8:353–360.

41. Krugman RD. Future role of the pediatrician in child abuse and neglect. *Pediatr Clin North Am* 1990;37:1003–1011.

42. Krugman RD. The multidisciplinary treatment of abusive and neglectful families. *Pediatr Ann* 1994;13:761–764.

43. Ledbetter DJ, Hatch EI, Feldman KW, et al. Diagnostic and surgical implications of child abuse. *Arch Surg* 1988;123:1101–1105.

44. Levitt CJ, Smith WL, Alexander RC. Abusive head trauma. In Reece RM (ed.), *Child abuse: Medical diagnosis and treatment,* 1–22. Philadelphia: Lea and Febiger. 1994.

45. Ludwig S. Child abuse. In Fleisher GR, Ludwig S (eds.), *Textbook of pediatric emergency medicine,* 2nd ed., 1127–1163. Baltimore: Williams and Wilkins. 1988.

46. Malik GH, Sirwal IA, Reshi AR, et al. Acute renal failure following physical torture. *Nephron* 1993;63:434–437.

47. Malinosky-Rummell R, Hansen DJ. Long-term consequences of childhood physical abuse. *Psychol Bull* 1993;114:68–79.

48. Manary MJ, Jaffee DM. Cervical spine injury in children. *Pediatr Ann* 1996;25:423–428.

49. McCann L, Pearlman LA. Vicarious traumatization: A framework for understanding the psychological effects of working with victims. *J Trauma Stress* 1990;3:131–149.

50. McKibben L, DeVos E, Newberger EH. Victimization of mothers of abused children: A controlled study. *Pediatrics* 1989;84:531–535.

51. Merten DF, Cooperman DR, Thompson GH. Skeletal manifestations of child abuse. In Reece RM (ed.), *Child abuse: Medical diagnosis and treatment,* 23–53. Philadelphia: Lea and Febiger. 1994.

52. Michalek JB. Nursing and child protection. In Newberger EH (ed.), *Child abuse,* 217–234. Boston: Little, Brown. 1982.

53. Morris JL, Johnson CF, Clasen M. To report or not to report: Physicians' attitudes toward discipline and child abuse. *Am J Dis Child* 1985;139:194–197.

54. Mundie PE. Team management of the maltreated child in the emergency room. *Pediatr Ann* 1994;13:771–776.

55. Myers JEB. Proof of physical child abuse. *Missouri Law Rev* 1988;53:189–225.

56. Myers JEB. Role of the physician in preserving verbal evidence of child abuse. *J Pediatr* 1986;109:409–411.

57. Neill K, Kauffman C. Care of the hospitalized abused child and his family: Nursing implications. *Matern Child Nurs J* 1976;1:117–123.

58. Newberger EH. Child physical abuse. *Prim Care* 1993;20:317–327.

59. Newberger EH. Pediatric interview assessment of child abuse: Challenges and opportunities. *Pediatr Clin North Am* 1990;37:943–954.

60. Newberger EH, Hyde JN. Child abuse: Principles and implications of current pediatric practice. *Pediatr Clin North Am* 1975;22:695–715.

61. Nordberg M. When parents kill. How do you deal with the unthinkable? *Emerg Med Serv* 1995;24:22–25.

62. Pascoe JM, Hildebrandt HM, Tarrier A, et al. Patterns of skin injuries in non-accidental and accidental injury. *Pediatrics* 1979;64:245–247.

63. Racusin RJ, Felsman JK. Reporting child abuse: The ethical obligation to inform parents. *J Am Acad Child Adolesc Psychiatry* 1986;25:485–489.

64. Reece RM. Fatal child abuse and sudden infant death syndrome: A critical diagnostic decision. *Pediatrics* 1993;91:423–429.

65. Ricci LR: Photodocumentation of the abused child. In Reece RM (ed.), *Child abuse: Medical diagnosis and treatment,* 248–266. Philadelphia: Lea and Febiger. 1994.

66. Rivara FP. Physical abuse in children under two: A study of therapeutic outcomes. *Child Abuse Negl* 1985;9:81–87.

67. Rose M, Schwartz R. Civil and criminal judicial intervention. In Ludwig S, Kornberg AE (eds.), *Child abuse: A medical reference,* 2nd ed., 423–441. New York: Churchill Livingston. 1992.

68. Saywitz KJ, Geiselman RE, Bornstein GK. Effects of cognitive interviewing and practice on children's recall performance. *J Appl Psychol* 1992;77:744–756.

69. Schetky DH, Devoe L. Countertransference issues in forensic child psychiatry. In Schetky DH, Benedek EP (eds.), *Clinical handbook of child psychiatry and the law,* 230–245. Baltimore: Williams and Wilkins. 1992.

70. Schiller WR. Burn management in children. *Pediatr Ann* 1996;25:431–439.

71. Section on Child Abuse and Neglect. *A guide to references and resources in child abuse and neglect,* 107–137. Elk Grove Village, IL: American Academy of Pediatrics. 1994.

72. Shugerman RP, Paez A, Grossman DC, et al. Epidural hemorrhage: Is it abuse? *Pediatrics* 1996;97:664–668.

73. Smith JB. Care of the hospitalized abused child and family: A framework for nursing intervention. *Nurs Clin North Am* 1981;16:127–137.

74. Ten Bensel RW, Wilcox M. Facilitating physician reporting of child abuse. *Minn Med* 1986;69:651–653.

75. Thomas JL, Towberman DB. Responding to the child within: Child abuse and the EMS provider. *J Emerg Med Serv* 1992;17:98–99,101–106,108.

76. Vandeven AM, Newberger EH. Child abuse. *Annu Rev Public Health* 1994;15:367–379.

77. Weimer CL, Goldfarb W, Slater H. Multidisciplinary approach to working with burn victims of child abuse. *J Burn Care Rehabil* 1988;9:79–82.

78. White KM, Snyder J, Bourne R, Newberger E. *Treating child abuse and family violence in hospitals: A program for training and service.* Lexington, MA: Lexington Books. 1989.

79. Whitworth JM, Lanier MW, Skinner RG, et al. A multidisciplinary hospital-based team for child abuse cases: A hands-on approach. *Child Welfare* 1981;60:233–243.

80. Widom CS. The cycle of violence. *Science* 1989;244:160–166.

81. Wilson EP. Multidisciplinary approach to child protection. In Ludwig S, Kornberg AE (eds.), *Child abuse: A medical reference,* 2nd ed., 79–84. New York: Churchill Livingston. 1992.

82. Wissow LS. Child abuse and neglect. *N Engl J Med* 1995;33:1425–1431.

83. Yurt RW. Triage, initial assessment and early treatment of the pediatric trauma patient. *Pediatr Clin North Am* 1992;39:1083–1091.

Initial Psychosocial Treatment of the Physically Abused Child: The Issue of Removal

Kerry M. Drach, Psy.D., and
Lesley Devoe, M.S.W.

The initial psychosocial treatment of the physically abused child revolves around the issue of removal from the home. While preliminary assessments will not provide the detailed informa-tion of later family analysis, attention to three key considerations can inform the process and benefit early decision making. These considerations are: parenting characteristics that may predict the risk of physical abuse; attachment difficulties between parent and child; and trau-matic response of the child, including risk of further trauma. While the safety of the child is the primary concern, removal of a child from the home, even a physically abusive home, also puts a child at risk for negative psychosocial consequences.

GENERAL CONSIDERATIONS

When a child is diagnosed as physically abused, child protective caseworkers, mental health providers, and other community professionals are called upon to make critical deci-sions that are likely to change significantly the child's psychosocial adjustment and devel-opment. It must be determined quickly whether it is possible for the child to remain safely in the home or whether removal into protective custody is necessary in order to keep the child safe. If placement is judged necessary, case managers are pressed to make decisions early in the placement about whether to allow and how to regulate the child's contact with the family. Case planners must also begin to consider how quickly the child may be returned to the home in order to minimize potential negative consequences of placement itself.

Much is known about physical child abuse as a risk factor for many types of psychoso-cial problems in children. For example, controlled empirical research studies have found that child victims of physical abuse exhibit increased risk for anxiety-related problems, depression, and posttraumatic stress disorder.[17,29,36,39,40,62] Studies likewise document in-creased risk for the development of conduct disorder, physical aggression, peer relationship disturbances, academic performance problems, and decreased cognitive functioning in children who have experienced physical abuse.[38,39,50,52,71]

Studies of long-term consequences of physical maltreatment indicate that the behavioral and emotional problems found among abused children often persist well into adulthood. Such problems include violent behavior, criminality, and psychiatric disorder.[47,56,69] Findings like these lend strong support to the intervention strategy of removing the physically abused child from the home in order to minimize the likelihood of such short-term and long-term psychosocial sequelae.

However, placement of children outside the home may in itself pose a risk factor for negative psychosocial consequences, because of the radical disruption children may experience in their primary emotional attachments and routines. Children frequently experience intense reactions of anxiety, loss, grief, and depression when precipitously separated from their family, even an abusive family, and placed in foster care.[5–7,20] Such intense emotional experiences may interfere significantly with the child's ability to negotiate critical "stage salient" developmental tasks[11] and thereby disrupt or distort the child's psychosocial development.

Physical abuse often occurs along with other forms of child maltreatment, including verbal abuse, physical or emotional neglect, and sexual abuse.[51] Some degree of emotional abuse is, by definition, present in most cases of physical abuse. When children are injured physically by primary caretakers, their emotional well-being, especially self-esteem and self-concept, is likely to be damaged.[25] In addition, witnessing acts of physical violence—for example, domestic violence between parents, physical abuse of siblings, rape, murder, and suicide attempts—is known to have negative psychosocial sequelae for children.[34,53,59]

The initial treatment program focuses on the weeks following the diagnosis of physical child abuse. During this time, the results from comprehensive and formal psychological, psychiatric, or infant mental health evaluations are usually not yet available. This chapter looks at the types of information that medical staff, child protective caseworkers, and other early intervenors may collect on their own to help determine whether or not to remove the child from the home.

Three specific psychosocial dimensions should be considered when deciding between placement and family preservation strategies:

- parental characteristics that predict risk of further physical abuse of the child
- indicators of attachment difficulties in the parent-child relationship that would predict risk either of future abusive treatment or of future psychosocial problems in the child
- indicators of traumatic response by the child, as well as the risk for further traumatization if the child remains in the home

Case examples presented at the end of the chapter illustrate how these concepts inform practice.

PARENTAL CHARACTERISTICS AS INDICATORS OF RISK

Reviews of the empirical research on characteristics of child-abusive parents[48,49,70] generally agree on a number of parental characteristics that predict increased risk of physically abusive behavior. Some of these characteristics are

- a history of unresolved child abuse in the parent's own childhood
- social isolation and lack of adequate social and emotional support
- inability or unwillingness to recognize and utilize social supports that are available
- a pattern of negatively toned interpersonal interactions between the parent and the child
- high levels of distress experienced by the parent combined with absent or ineffectual stress management strategies
- limited ability to respond empathically to the needs of the child
- limited child developmental knowledge
- developmentally inappropriate perceptions and unrealistic expectations of the child's behavior
- incorrect attributions about causes of the child's behavior
- reliance on authoritarian and other coercive discipline strategies
- limited problem-solving, abstract-reasoning, and other cognitive abilities

In the past, the mere presence of mental illness (major depression, schizophrenia, etc.), alcoholism, or other psychiatric or substance abuse disorder in a parent or caretaker was considered adequate grounds for removing a child from an abusive situation, for it was believed that such disorders more or less directly *caused* child abuse.[58] Now, however, it is recognized that child protective personnel and other intervenors must document specifically *if* and *how* a particular parent's psychiatric condition or problem drinking pattern is likely to increase the risk of child abuse.[32] Similarly, mentally retarded individuals have in the past been considered unfit as parents simply because of their cognitive limitations.[63] Again, it is now understood to be necessary to identify whether and in what specific respects a particular cognitively limited parent is likely to be at risk of physically abusive behavior.

In the immediate postdiagnostic period it will generally not be possible to complete formal, comprehensive evaluations of parenting strengths and weaknesses, including the risk factors for physically abusive behavior listed above. However, child protective workers and other professionals involved with the family should be alert to the presence of such risk factors. For example, when a single parent enjoys strong emotional support from relatives willing to help in times of stress, acknowledges full responsibility for the abusive behavior, and appears genuinely motivated to learn more positive parenting skills, the risk for further physical abuse may be judged to be reasonably low. However, it is reasonable to be concerned about the potential for further physically abusive behavior if a single, cognitively limited parent attributes full responsibility for the abusive behavior to the child, has no circle of social supports, routinely uses coercive, negative, authoritarian parenting methods, systematically misinterprets normal childish energy as opposition and defiance, and is unable to empathize with the child's obvious fear of being hurt. Where multiple indicators surface about the parent's potential for physically abusive behavior, intervenors may be well advised to request formal evaluation of the parent's ability to provide at least minimally adequate, safe parenting.

ATTACHMENT-BASED INDICATORS OF RISK

Attachment has become a central consideration in child development research,[28,31] especially in the field of developmental psychopathology.[10–12,45,46] The idea of attachment was initially conceptualized in the seminal works of Bowlby[4–7] and operationalized in terms of a reliable empirical research methodology by Ainsworth and her colleagues.[2,3] Bowlby[5] describes the attachment of human and other primate infants to their primary caretakers as an evolutionarily based behavioral system that functions to keep the vulnerable infant and later the young child physically close to the caretaker, thereby decreasing the risk of predation and other life-threatening environmental dangers. Attachment difficulties are linked to the development of human psychopathology, first through the feelings of anxiety and anger incurred when the child is separated from the attachment figure,[6] and second through the grief, depression, and psychological defenses that result when the child is cut off from access to the attachment figure.[7]

Through the development of a standardized laboratory methodology for observing and classifying attachment patterns in young children, Ainsworth and her colleagues[2,3] were originally able to identify three primary patterns of attachment among middle-class 12–18-month-old babies observed with their mothers. These patterns are

- secure attachments
- insecure/avoidant attachments
- insecure/ambivalent attachments

Continued research examining attachment behaviors in children from more diverse socio-economic backgrounds has resulted in the identification of additional insecure attachment patterns—a mixed pattern with both avoidant and ambivalent qualities[14] and a disor-ganized/disoriented pattern.[46] More recent work has extended the classification of at-tachment patterns to later age groups, including older children, adolescents, and adults.[1,12,28,41,43,55] The development of the Adult Attachment Interview (AAI) by Main and her colleagues[44] has spawned a large body of empirical research into the relationship between adult attachment patterns and the presence of insecure versus secure attachment patterns in their children.

In cases of physical abuse, early attention to attachment issues is a necessary compo-nent of risk assessment during the immediate postdiagnostic period. Two types of attachment-related research findings are particularly relevant. The first is the finding that insecure attachment status is a significant risk factor in the development of behavioral and emotional problems, including psychiatric disorder, in children,[42] adolescents,[54] and adults.[23,67] The second is that insecure attachment status in itself is a significant risk factor for child maltreatment, in that insecure attachment patterns are found to be especially predominant in samples of maltreated children.[9,15,71] In addition, abusive mothers and fathers are much more likely than nonabusive parents to exhibit insecure attachment pat-terns in their own histories and current relationships.[16] It is not reasonable to expect child protective caseworkers and other community professionals to complete a comprehensive assessment of a child's security of attachment in the few weeks following diagnosis of physical child abuse. However, a number of attachment-related indicators can be noted without a formal assessment. For example, several types of child behavior directed toward the caregiver may indicate attachment difficulties.[72,73] In extreme forms, such behaviors exhibited in the child-caretaker relationship may be viewed as indicators of attachment disorder and thus indicators of significant long-term risk for negative psychosocial prob-lems for the child. Child behaviors indicative of attachment difficulties include

- absence of or promiscuous affection-based behavior
- absent, peculiar, or ambivalent comfort seeking by the child
- developmentally excessive dependence on the caregiver or failure to turn to the caregiver for support when needed

- chronically noncompliant or overly compliant behavior
- inhibition of exploratory behavior, especially in younger children, or failure to check back with the caregiver while exploring
- oversolicitous attempts by the child to function as caretaker to the adult or excessively bossy and controlling behavior
- avoidance of, anger at, or lack of affection toward the caregiver after separations

In cases of physical maltreatment, it is unlikely that a child will be removed into protective custody solely on the basis of attachment concerns. However, heightened awareness of and sensitivity to the quality of the child's attachment to adult caregivers will help shape case management decisions in the immediate postdiagnostic period. For example, it is perhaps best that the child be removed from the home in situations where the child appears to enjoy no secure attachments within the family, where extreme and long-term disturbances in the child-caregiver relationship are clearly evident, and where the primary attachment figure either is the abuser or is unable to protect the child from abuse. However, in other situations, even when the child may have suffered a fairly severe injury, the decision might be made to keep the child in the home or to return the child to the home as soon as possible if the abuser was not the child's primary attachment figure or if the abuse was clearly precipitated by transient stressors in an otherwise healthy attachment environment. Such a decision organized around a family preservation strategy is especially likely to serve the best interests of the child if the child has enjoyed a reasonably secure attachment to the primary caretaker prior to the current stressful conditions, and if the caretaker is willing to accept assistance.

TRAUMA-BASED INDICATORS OF RISK

The concept of psychic trauma may also be useful in helping to guide decision making during the immediate postdiagnostic period in physical child abuse cases. Psychic trauma occurs when an external event is so threatening that the emotional and physical coping mechanisms of the victim are overwhelmed.[24,33] The response is psychobiological in nature. It has both cognitive and physiological components, and it may present in two different forms. The traumatized individual either relives the trauma, having constant, unbidden images of the events and exhibiting hypervigilance, startle responses, and autonomic arousal; or he or she endeavors to avoid all memory or risk of recurrence, appears numb and dazed, and avoids normal life activities.[18,35,57,64,65] Some individuals typically display behaviors consistent with one or the other form, while others alternate between the two forms. Research suggests that central nervous system functioning may be altered either temporarily or permanently in response to trauma.[26,65,66,68]

Traumatic experiences are known to shape children's development.[19] The impact of trauma may be *localized,* meaning more or less immediate and time-limited, or *developmental,* meaning that it interferes with the completion of stage-salient developmental tasks or distorts the child's progress.[21] Traumatic experiences may occur in isolated acute episodes or in multiple chronic episodes experienced over time, or as a combination of both.[30,60,61] The developmental effects are generally considered more severe when the abuse is repetitive, when it alters the child's relationship with his or her primary social support network, when it occurs in the context of other significant life stressors, or when it interrupts an important developmental transition.[21]

It has long been recognized that trauma-based emotional difficulties, especially posttraumatic stress disorder, are a frequent outcome of childhood sexual abuse.[8,21,22,37,38] (See chapter 2 for further discussion of posttraumatic stress disorder in children who have been sexually abused.) Less has been written about the traumatic impact of physical child abuse. Kolko,[39] however, discusses posttraumatic stress disorder and other indicators of psychological trauma as sequelae of physical abuse and, relying on behavioral descriptions provided by Terr,[60] lists the following signs of abuse-related traumatization in the child:

- strongly visualized or repeatedly perceived traumatic memories
- posttraumatic behavior, often observed in play and artwork, that appears to repeat or replay the abuse experience (reenactment)
- personality changes organized around feelings of grief and loss
- trauma-specific fears, such as fear of individuals who resemble the abuser, cringing when an adult raises a hand or speaks loudly, and fear of entering a room where abuse has taken place

Children respond to longstanding, repeated exposure to extreme events through a variety of trauma-related coping strategies, all of which appear motivated by a need on the part of the child to manage the intense, dysphoric effects associated with the abusive experience and the abuser. These coping strategies include

- denial, dissociation, withdrawal, or identification with the aggressor
- emotional numbing or indifference to pain
- reactions of rage, including self-injurious behaviors
- unremitting depression and sadness[39,60]

One extreme coping strategy described in the literature is traumatic bonding, in which, like a hostage, the child comes to view the abuser (captor) as a savior and to fear and hate rescuers, that is, child protective caseworkers and other community professionals.[27,33]

Core trauma-related questions focus on the extent to which the child is exhibiting behavioral or emotional signs of traumatization, the ability of the family to protect the child from further traumatization, and the willingness of the abuser to acknowledge responsibility and accept helping resources in order to prevent future traumatization. Circumstances that would suggest removal from the home are when the physically abused child is exhibiting multiple signs of traumatic response—frequent aggressive play, self-abusive behaviors, clear-cut reactions of acute fears when approached by strange adults—and the primary caretaker does not appear to be able or willing to guarantee the child's safety in the future. It is likely in this case that a plan will be developed to remove the child from the abuser's care in order to prevent further traumatization.

Similarly, in the case of a child who has undergone repeated, severe physical maltreatment and who appears detached, socially distant, emotionally indifferent, and depressed, it may also be decided to remove the child into protective custody. In this case, it is reasonable to interpret the child's psychosocial symptoms as efforts to cope psychologically with the cumulative effects of repeated abuse, especially if it appears likely that the symptoms represent an abuse-related change in the child's behavior from an earlier time when such abuse was not occurring.

ILLUSTRATIVE CASES

With the above principles in mind, a look at the cases of Susan, Johnny, and Marion illustrates how simultaneous attention to parental characteristics, attachment problems, and trauma indicators may guide early case management decisions when physical abuse has been diagnosed.

FOUR-YEAR-OLD Susan was seen in the emergency room for second degree burns on her leg and abdomen that had become infected. She was hospitalized and a child protective referral was made, because staff were concerned that Susan's parents had sought medical care only after the burns became infected. They were also concerned that Susan appeared poorly attached to her parents. She expressed a desire to be adopted by everyone on the unit, and nursing staff noted that she typically seemed withdrawn and emotionally "absent" when her mother visited her. At night, staff frequently had to stay by her side because of frightening dreams.

Child protective social workers investigated the referral by interviewing Susan's parents and the neighbors in the family's apartment building. It was found that Susan was often left unsupervised by her parents for extended periods of time, that both parents were unemployed and evasive about their personal histories, and that the father was an active, untreated alcoholic. Neighbors reported hearing sounds of Susan being hit by both parents, but much more by her father. The couple was isolated from family and friends, and they had little social contact with neighbors in the building. The mother appeared to have limited intellectual ability.

Susan stayed in the hospital a full week. On day five, her father announced that he was leaving town. Her mother expressed a desire to go with him, but she decided to stay so that she could continue her daily visits with Susan. Observation of the mother indicated that she had negative expectations of Susan and was uneven and inconsistent in her responses to her daughter. She blamed Susan for causing the accident that had led to her burn, claiming that the girl had bumped into her mother when she was holding a cup of hot coffee in her hand. She was openly hostile toward child protective staff and toward her neighbors for reporting her. As time progressed, she visited her daughter less frequently and for shorter periods of time. Meanwhile, Susan appeared to attach too easily to hospital staff. She blamed herself for the burn and for the times her parents "have to hit me."

This is a case in which risk factors for further abuse predominated, and it was judged that keeping Susan in the home would place her at risk for abusive treatment. The decision was appropriately made to remove Susan from her mother's custody. The initial assessment led to the conclusion that she was at high risk of continued physical abuse by her parents and that her parents had exhibited poor protective judgment around her safety and well-being. In addition, it was clear that Susan's attachment to her parents was insecure and that she was exhibiting signs of traumatization by her contacts with her mother. Because the father moved out of town and was expressing no interest in continued contact with his daughter, reunification efforts were planned to focus solely on the mother, who stated that she wanted Susan returned to her care. The mother was referred for more complete assessment of her capacity to provide appropriate parenting, her capacity to function as a consistent attachment figure, and her ability to respond to intervention.

FOUR-YEAR-OLD Johnny is a child with attention deficit hyperactivity disorder (ADHD) who was taken into emergency foster care because of multiple bruises identified by his pediatrician, inflicted in the name of discipline. Once confronted with the question of abuse, Johnny's parents, Mike and Sonya, both full-time accountants, were fully cooperative with child protective investigators and forthcoming about their problems. Financial difficulties, Mike's drinking, and the parents' decreasing ability to cope with Johnny's attentional problems and associated behavioral difficulties were all identified as situational factors leading to overly harsh physical discipline, especially by Mike. Johnny, however, was clearly traumatized by being removed from his family. His foster mother reported that he cried inconsolably for hours every day, that he isolated himself from the rest of the foster family, and that he frequently awoke from sleep crying for his mother or father.

Early evaluation of the family indicated that Johnny enjoyed reasonably healthy attachments to his parents and that both Mike and Sonya had been reasonably successful in learning to understand and manage their son's ADHD-related behavioral problems. They participated in educational programming for parents of ADHD children. The use of overly harsh physical punishment had emerged only in recent months in the context of other family stresses.

The occasion of removal of Johnny from the home proved to be a wake-up call for both parents. Mike recognized that he should not drink and agreed to undergo substance abuse counseling and attend Alcoholics Anonymous. Sonya agreed to attend Alanon. Both cooperated fully with child protective staff at all times, through which they demonstrated their primary motive: that Johnny be returned to their home as soon as possible.

Because of the level of cooperation and follow-through demonstrated by the parents, because the precipitating stressors on the family were primarily situational (with the exception of Johnny's ADHD-related problems), because of the degree of warmth and nurturance observed in parent-child interactions during early visits, and because placement itself proved psychologically traumatic for Johnny, child protective staff decided to pursue a family reunification plan after only a few weeks of foster care. In this case, protective factors appeared to predominate over risk factors, and it was possible to achieve a successful reunification of the family.

FOUR-YEAR-OLD Marion was placed in emergency foster care after the police found her wandering alone in the streets at 11:30 P.M. Her three siblings, aged 2 to 8, were also placed in emergency foster care. The family was well-known to the police because of multiple domestic violence complaints involving Marion's mother, Judy, and her many boyfriends. When the police took Marion back to her home, they found Judy passed out drunk on the living room floor. The other children had gone to sleep in their clothes in their mother's bed. Police contacted child protective services, and immediate arrangements were made to remove all four children from the home.

Once sober, Judy was furious about the removal of her children, and her interactions with child protective staff investigating the case were extremely hostile. She was found to be a harsh disciplinarian who valued unquestioning obedience and became enraged when the children did not provide it. She boasted about how she "had" to spank her children on a regular basis, because "that's all they'll listen to." She was spanked as a child, she added, and it did not hurt her. Her manner of talking about her children demonstrated an extreme lack of empathy for their feelings. She admitted openly to shooting the children's puppy in front of them "to teach them a lesson," and she spoke in an extremely critical manner about the children, about their multiple fathers, none of whom were marital partners, and about "the system."

In the foster home, Marion was abusive to pets, experienced frequent nightmares, and engaged in a variety of self-injurious behaviors, such as biting her arm until it bled and head-banging. She became extremely upset by visits with her mother. According to the foster mother, the visits appeared to trigger memories of past traumas while in Judy's care.

After the visits, Marion evidenced periods of apparent dissociation ("as though she's not there," said the foster mother) alternating with periods of hypervigilance and aggressive behavior. At such hypervigilant times she was likely to cry and scream, and she was extremely difficult to soothe. She often cried, "My mommy is bad!" The foster mother reported that such difficulties persisted for two or three days after contacts with Judy. Marion's softest feelings, however, seemed to be reserved for her siblings, who were placed in different foster homes.

Marion was clearly an extremely traumatized child who exhibited severe attachment difficulties and who was already showing signs of significant emotional and behavioral disorder related to her history of abusive and neglectful care. Her mother was impulsive and appeared completely lacking in empathy. She openly blamed the children for her use of abusive disciplinary methods. Her drinking and resultant unconscious states placed the children at immediate risk of serious harm, and she demonstrated no motivation to engage in any type of recovery programming. She clearly did not accept responsibility for her problems. Based on such considerations, it was most appropriate for Marion to remain in protective custody for a long period of time.

CONCLUSION

The primary issue in the initial psychosocial treatment of the physically abused child is whether it is safe for the child to remain with the family. There are three key psychosocial dimensions critical to risk assessment in the time period immediately following the diagnosis of physical child abuse—parenting characteristics that predict risk of physical abuse, attachment-related indicators of psychosocial risk, and trauma-based indicators of psychosocial risk. Careful attention to these dimensions will greatly benefit the early case planning and decision making, especially decisions about whether to pursue strategies of family preservation or removal of the child into protective custody, as well as early planning of contact with the family if the child is removed.

Although the same emotional and behavioral indicators may be used to guide longer-term treatment planning—for example, helping the parent change those personal characteristics that increase risk of abuse; resolving the child's trauma issues through play therapy; improving the security of the child's attachment to the parent through treatment of the parent-child dyad—it is unlikely that such detailed treatment planning will be completed in the immediate postdiagnostic period. Rather, such comprehensive treatment and intervention planning will more likely be addressed only after formal psychological, psychiatric, infant mental health, or family systems evaluations are scheduled and completed.

REFERENCES

1. Aber JL, Baker AJL. Security of attachment in toddlerhood: Modifying assessment procedures for joint clinical and research purposes. In Greenberg MT, Cicchetti D, Cummings EM (eds.), *Attachment in the preschool years: Theory, research and intervention,* 427–460. Chicago: University of Chicago Press. 1990.

2. Ainsworth MDS, Wittig BA. Attachment and exploratory behavior of one-year-olds in a strange situation. In Foss BM (ed.), *Determinants of infant behavior.* London: Methuen. 1969.

3. Ainsworth MDS, Blehar MC, Waters E, Wall S. *Patterns of attachment: A psychological study of the strange situation.* Hillsdale, NJ: Erlbaum, 1978.

4. Bowlby J. The nature of the child's tie to his mother. *Int J Psychoanal* 1958;39:250–373.

5. Bowlby J. *Attachment and loss,* vol. 1, *Attachment.* New York: Basic Books. 1969 [1982].

6. Bowlby J. *Attachment and loss,* vol. 2, *Separation: Anxiety and anger.* New York: Basic Books. 1973.

7. Bowlby J. *Attachment and loss,* vol. 3, *Loss: Sadness and depression.* New York: Basic Books. 1980.

8. Briere JN, Elliot DM. Immediate and long-term impacts of child sexual abuse. *Future Child* 1994;4:54–69.

9. Carlson V, Cicchetti D, Barnett D, Braunwald KG. Finding order in disorganization: Lessons from research on maltreated infants' attachments to their caregivers. In Cicchetti D, Carlson V (eds.), *Child maltreatment: Theory and research on the causes and consequences of child abuse and neglect,* 494–528. London: Cambridge University Press. 1989.

10. Cicchetti D. Developmental psychopathology in infancy: Illustration from the study of maltreated youngsters. *J Consult Clin Psychol* 1987;55:837–845.

11. Cicchetti, D. How research on child maltreatment has informed the study of child development: Perspectives from developmental psychopathology. In Cicchetti D, Carlson V (eds.), *Child maltreatment: Theory and research on the causes and consequences of child abuse and neglect,* 377–431. London: Cambridge University Press. 1989.

12. Cicchetti D, Toth SL. Child maltreatment and attachment organization. In Goldberg S, Muir R, Kerr J (eds.), *Attachment theory: Social, developmental, and clinical perspectives,* 279–308. Hillsdale, NJ: Analytic Press. 1995.

13. Cicchetti D, Toth SL., Lynch M. Bowlby's dream comes full circle: The application of attachment theory to risk and psychopathology. *Adv Clin Child Psychol* 1995;17:1–75.

14. Crittenden PM. Maltreated infants: Vulnerability and resilience. *J Child Psychol Psychiatry* 1985;26:85–96.

15. Crittenden PM, Ainsworth MDS. Child maltreatment and attachment theory. In Cicchetti D, Carlson V (eds.), *Child maltreatment: Theory and research on the causes and consequences of child abuse and neglect,* 432–463. London: Cambridge University Press. 1989.

16. Crittenden, PM, Partridge MF, Claussen AH. Family patterns of relationship in normative and dysfunctional families. *Dev Psychopathol* 1991;3:491–449.

17. DePaul J, Arruabarrena MI. Behavior problems in school-aged physically abused and neglected children in Spain. *Child Abuse Negl* 1995;19:409–418.

18. Dorsey J. Dynamics of post-traumatic symptomatology and character changes. In Krystal H (ed.), *Massive psychic trauma.* New York: International Universities Press. 1968.

19. Eth S, Pynoos R. Developmental perspective on psychic trauma in childhood. In Figley C (ed.), *Trauma and its wake.* New York: Brunner/Mazel. 1985.

20. Fahlberg VI. *A child's journey through placement.* Indianapolis: Perspectives Press. 1991.

21. Finkelhor D. The victimization of children: A developmental perspective. *Am J Orthopsychiatry* 1995;65:177–193.

22. Finkelhor D, Browne A. The traumatic impact of child sexual abuse: A conceptualization. *Am J Orthopsychiatry* 1985;55:530–541.

23. Fonagy P, Leigh T, Steele M, Steele H, Kennedy R, Mattoon G, Target M, Gerber A. The relations of attachment status, psychiatric classification, and response to psychotherapy. *J Consult Clin Psychol* 1996;64:22–31.

24. Furst S. *Psychic trauma.* New York: Basic Books. 1967.

25. Garbarino J. Psychological child maltreatment: A developmental view. *Family Violence and Abusive Relationships* 1993;20:307–315.

26. Giller, E (ed.). *Biological assessment and treatment of post-traumatic stress disorder.* Washington, DC: American Psychiatric Press. 1990.

27. Goddard CR, Stanley JR. Viewing the abusive parent and the abused child as captor and

hostage: The application of hostage theory to the effects of child abuse. *J Interpers Viol* 1994; 9:258–269.

28. Goldberg S. Recent developments in attachment theory and research. *Can J Psychiatry* 1991;6:393–400.

29. Graham-Bermann, SA, Cutler, SE, Litzsenberger, BW, Schwartz, WE. Perceived conflict and violence in childhood sibling relationships and later emotional adjustment. *J Fam Psychol* 1994;8:85–97.

30. Green AH. Dimensions of psychological trauma in abused children. *J Am Acad Child Adolesc Psychiatry* 1983;22:231–237.

31. Greenberg MT, Cicchetti D, Cummings EM (eds.). *Attachment in the preschool years: Theory, research and intervention.* Chicago: University of Chicago Press. 1990.

32. Grisso, T. *Evaluating competencies: Forensic assessments and instruments.* New York: Plenum Press. 1986, pp. 187–267.

33. Hermann J. *Trauma and recovery.* New York: Basic Books. 1992.

34. Jaffe P, Wolfe D, Wilson S, Zak L. Similarities in behavioral and social maladjustment among child victims and witnesses to family violence. *Am J Orthopsychiatry* 1986;56:142–146.

35. Kardiner A. The traumatic neuroses of war. In Arieti S, *American handbook of psychiatry.* New York: Basic Books. 1941.

36. Kaufman J. Depressive disorders in maltreated children. *J Am Acad Child Adolesc Psychiatry* 1991;30:257–265.

37. Kendall-Tackett KA, Williams L, Finkelhor D. Impact of sexual abuse in children: A review and synthesis of recent empirical studies. *Psychol Bull* 1993;113:164–180.

38. Knutsen JJ. Psychological characteristics of maltreated children: Putative risk factors and consequences. *Annu Rev Psychol* 1995;46:401–31.

39. Kolko, DJ. Characteristics of child victims of physical violence: Research findings and clinical implications. *J Interpers Viol* 1992;7:244–276.

40. Lizardi H, Klein DN, Ouimette PC, Riso LP, Anderson RL, Donaldson SK. Reports of childhood home environment in early-onset dysthymia and episodic major depression. *J Abnorm Psychol* 1995;104:132–139.

41. Lynch M, Cicchetti D. Patterns of relatedness in maltreated and nonmaltreated children: Connections among multiple representational models. *Dev Psychopathol* 1991;3:207–226.

42. Lyons-Ruth K. Attachment relationships among children with aggressive behavior problems: The role of disorganized early attachment patterns. *J Consult Clin Psychol* 1996;64:64–73.

43. Main M, Cassidy J. Categories of response to reunion with a parent at age 6: Predictable from infant attachment classifications and stable over a one-month period. *Dev Psychol* 1988;24:415–426.

44. Main M, Goldwyn R. Adult attachment classification system, version 5. Unpublished manuscript, University of California, Berkeley, 1991.

45. Main M, Hesse E. Parents' unresolved traumatic experiences are related to infant disorganized attachment status: Is frightened and/or frightening parental behavior the linking mechanism? In Greenberg MT, Cicchetti D, Cummings EM (eds.), *Attachment in the preschool years: Theory, research and intervention,* 161–182. Chicago: University of Chicago Press. 1990.

46. Main M, Solomon J. Procedures for identifying infants as disorganized/disoriented during the Ainsworth Strange Situation. In Greenberg MT, Cicchetti D, Cummings EM (eds.), *Attachment in the preschool years: Theory, research and intervention,* 121–160. Chicago: University of Chicago Press. 1990.

47. Malinosky-Rummell R, Hansen D. Long-term consequences of childhood physical abuse. *Psychol Bull* 1993;114:68–79.

48. Milner J. Assessing physical child abuse risk: The Child Abuse Potential Inventory. *Clin Psychol Rev* 1994;14:547–583.

49. Milner J, Dopke CA. Child physical abuse: Review of offender characteristics. Unpublished manuscript. 1995.

50. Mueller E, Silverman N. Peer relations in maltreated children. In Cicchetti D, Carlson V

(eds.), *Child maltreatment: Theory and research on the causes and consequences of child abuse and neglect,* 529–578. London: Cambridge University Press. 1989.

51. Ney PG, Fung T, Wickett AR. The worst combinations of child abuse and neglect. *Child Abuse Negl* 1994;1:705–714.

52. Perez CM, Widom CS. Childhood victimization and long-term intellectual and academic outcomes. *Child Abuse Negl* 1994;18:617–633.

53. Pynoos R, Eth S. Children traumatized by witnessing acts of personal violence: Homicide, rape, or suicide behavior. In Eth S, Pynoos R (eds.), *Post-traumatic stress disorder in children.* American Psychiatric Association, 1985.

54. Rosenstein DS, Horowitz HA. Adolescent attachment and psychopathology. *J Consult Clin Psychol* 1996;64:244–253.

55. Schneider-Rosen K. The developmental reorganization of attachment relationships: Guidelines for classification beyond infancy. In Greenberg MT, Cicchetti D, Cummings EM (eds.), *Attachment in the preschool years: Theory, research and intervention,* 185–220. Chicago: University of Chicago Press. 1990.

56. Schwartz IM, Rendon J, Hsieh C-M. Is child maltreatment a leading cause of delinquency? *Child Welfare* 1994;73:639–655.

57. Scrignar, CB. *Post-traumatic stress disorder,* 2nd ed. New Orleans: Bruno Press. 1988.

58. Steele BF, Pollock CB. A psychiatric study of parents who abuse infants and small children. In Helfer RE, Kempe CH (eds.), *The battered child,* 2nd ed., 103–147. Chicago: University of Chicago Press. 1974.

59. Sternberg KJ, Lamb ME, Greenbaum C, Cicchetti D, Dawud S, Cortes, RM, Krispin O, Lorey F. Effects of domestic violence on children's behavior problems and depression. *Dev Psychol* 1993;29:44–52.

60. Terr LC. Childhood traumas: An outline and overview. *Am J Psychiatry* 1991;148:10–20.

61. Terr LC. *Unchained memories.* New York: Basic Books. 1994.

62. Toth SL, Manly JT, Cicchetti D. Child maltreatment and vulnerability to depression. *Dev Psychopathol* 1992;4:97–112.

63. Tymchuk AJ. Predicting adequacy of parenting by people with mental retardation. *Child Abuse Negl* 1992;16:165–178.

64. Van der Kolk BA (ed.). *Post-traumatic stress disorder: Psychological and biological sequelae.* Washington, DC: American Psychiatric Press. 1984.

65. Van der Kolk BA. *Psychological Trauma.* Washington, DC: American Psychiatric Press. 1987.

66. Van der Kolk BA, Fisler RE. Childhood abuse and neglect and lost of self-regulation. *Bull Menninger Clin* 1994;58:135–168.

67. Van I, Jzendoorn MH, Bakermans-Kranenburg MJ. Attachment representations in mothers, fathers, adolescents, and clinical groups: A meta-analytic search for normative data. *J Consult Clin Psychol* 1996;64:8–21.

68. Walker A. The psychobiology of trauma. In Wilson JP (ed.), *Trauma, transformation, and healing.* New York: Brunner/Mazel. 1989.

69. Widom CS. Does violence beget violence? A critical examination of the literature. *Psychol Bull* 1989;106:3–28.

70. Wolfe D. Child-abusive parents: An empirical review and analysis. *Psychol Bull* 1985; 97:462–482.

71. Youngblade LM, Belsky J. Child maltreatment, infant-parent attachment security, and dysfunctional peer relationships in toddlerhood. *Topics in Early Childhood Special Education* 1989;9:1–15.

72. Zeanah C. Beyond insecurity: A reconceptualization of attachment disorders in infancy. *J Consult Clin Psychol* 1996;64:42–52.

73. Zeanah CH, Mammen OK, Lieberman AF. Disorders of attachment. In Zeanah CH (ed.), *Handbook of infant mental health,* 332–349. New York: Guilford Press. 1993.

Chapter 8

Legal Intervention for the Physically Abused Child

Anita M. St. Onge, J.D., and
Megan L. Elam, J.D.

Legal intervention is a potential outcome of any allegation of physical child abuse, and medical, mental health, child protective, and law enforcement agencies must work cooperatively for effective legal intervention. There are two types of legal intervention: civil and criminal. Civil action focuses on the safety of the child and may involve removal from the home. Criminal action focuses on identification and prosecution of the perpetrator. Each type of proceeding has three phases: investigation, case assessment, and trial. Different evidentiary rules often apply to civil and criminal proceedings, but case workers and law enforcers can work together to minimize further trauma for the abused child in either setting.

GENERAL CONSIDERATIONS

Discovering an inflicted physical injury in a child is one of the most difficult dilemmas faced by medical and mental health professionals, social workers, educators, and others concerned with the well-being of children. Allegations of physical abuse are commonly reviewed by both the police and a child protective agency, and all professionals serving the needs of abused children must realize the potential for legal intervention as a result of this discovery. It is critical from a legal standpoint that these diverse systems—medical, mental health, child protective, and law enforcement—work together and with a common understanding of each other's roles in investigating and pursuing prosecution. In many jurisdictions, criminal prosecutors, police departments, and child protective agencies have memoranda of understanding about how to proceed with their investigations in a mutually agreeable fashion. Many medical and mental health systems have protocols outlining how a case of suspected child abuse will be handled. This chapter examines the legal considerations in managing child physical abuse in the immediate postdiagnostic period. For a more general discussion of the specific forensic issues involved in child abuse cases, see chapter 23.

SAFETY OF THE CHILD

The most urgent concern following a diagnosis of child physical abuse is the safety of the child. An appropriate investigation must determine who committed the abuse, the extent of injuries, and to what extent the child is in danger of further harm. Two separate investigations will take place with two separate legal interventions occurring. Understanding the proceedings of each is essential for a fuller understanding of the consequences of a referral. One investigation is conducted by the governmental agency mandated to protect children, known generically as child protective services (CPS). That agency's goal is to identify the source of the abuse, provide service to the family, and, in some cases, remove the child to a safer home by means of a civil court process. The second investigation is done by a law enforcement agency whose primary mandate is to investigate the circumstances of the case, apprehend the alleged abuser, and refer the matter to the state or county prosecutor for possible criminal action. Professionals may be required by law to report suspected cases of inflicted physical abuse to both types of agencies.[1]

CIVIL VERSUS CRIMINAL PROCEEDINGS

The purpose of the child protective service agency's civil investigation is to protect the child from further harm. The agency, however, has a further mandate to prevent removal of the child from his or her home if appropriate safeguards can be applied. The purpose of the initial investigation is to gather sufficient information to determine if child maltreatment occurred, if there is a risk of future maltreatment, and the level of that risk.

If it is decided that the child is safe in the home, CPS must determine what interventions will ensure the child's protection and maintain the family unit. They should also determine if continuing agency services are needed to reduce the risk of future maltreatment.[2] For example, if a child has been physically assaulted by one parent and the other parent has taken steps to have the assaultive parent removed from the home through a protection from abuse order, CPS will not generally pursue independent civil proceedings for custody, because the home should have been rendered safe for the child. In this same case, the criminal system may pursue a criminal prosecution of the assaultive parent, however. In a case where the primary caretaker is suspected of assaulting a child and claims that he or she was not present or that the injury was accidental, both the criminal and child protective systems will be investigating to determine whether a nonaccidental injury occurred and whether the child is in danger.

Criminal proceedings differ from civil proceedings in several important ways. First, the goal of a criminal proceeding is primarily to identify the abuser, gather sufficient evidence to successfully prosecute the abuser, and, after conviction, to fashion a sentence that punishes the crime, reflects the particular vulnerability of the child victim, reflects the particular circumstances of the abuser, and provides for rehabilitation of the offender and safety for the child. Additionally, the criminal process is designed to serve as a deterrent to others.

Although both the civil and the criminal processes strive ultimately to ensure safety for the child, the criminal process focuses more on the offender than the victim. Both the civil process and the criminal process ultimately may result in court proceedings. In a criminal case, the burden of proof is on the state, and it must prove its case beyond a reasonable doubt. The burden of proof in a civil proceeding is generally by a preponderance of evidence, a substantially lower standard. Additionally, the rules regarding the admissibility of certain kinds of evidence differ between the two types of proceedings and among jurisdictions. One key difference is that most child protection proceedings allow child hearsay evidence to be admitted. The child hearsay rule allows the child's statements to be considered by the court without requiring the child to appear as a witness. The use of this exception is severely limited in criminal proceedings.[3] (Hearsay rules are explained in greater detail in chapter 23.) Furthermore, the defendant's right to confront accusatory witnesses limits the use of measures such as videotaped testimony or one-way screens designed to shield young witnesses.[4] Finally, the criminal process is almost always public, while the civil child protection hearing is most often confidential. (Again, see chapter 23 for further discussion.)

In the criminal process, the abuse allegation is generally investigated by a law enforcement official, from the state police, the county sheriff's office, a local police department, or the office of the prosecuting attorney. A prosecutor may become involved during the course of the investigation or after the investigation is completed. The prosecutor's role is to ensure that the investigation is sufficient to determine how the injury was inflicted and who inflicted it. The prosecutor must also be able to prove to a jury of average citizens at trial or to a judge that the evidence is of sufficient quality to prove, beyond a reasonable doubt, that the person or persons charged inflicted the injuries in a nonaccidental manner.

Both civil and criminal proceedings for cases involving physical abuse of a child have three major components: investigation, case assessment, and trial.

INVESTIGATION

It is important for both police and social workers to employ proper investigative techniques, even in situations that may warrant sympathy for the parents. For example, in a case that appears to be a death resulting from sudden infant death syndrome, it is crucial to separate the parents or other family members who had access to the child and to get each of their accounts of events recorded separately, to rule out the possibility of an act of physical abuse. When the parties are interviewed jointly, it is impossible to conduct a proper interview subsequently, because all parties now know one another's version of events.

Treating all potential physical abuse cases as possible crimes, the investigation should include photographs and interviews of all potential witnesses. Police officers and social workers should coordinate their investigations when possible to avoid duplicating efforts or potentially damaging the other agency's case.

The child protective investigation will focus on the nature of the injury and the risk of further harm to the child. Considerations will include the family structure and past history of abuse as well as the family's willingness to accept necessary services to ameliorate the circumstances of jeopardy in the home.

In the case of inflicted physical injury, criminal proceedings are generally instituted in one of two ways: direct report to a law enforcement agency or referral by another agency. It is not common for a report of inflicted physical injury to be made directly by a victim or a victim's family. In a child abuse case the victims themselves are often not equipped to make a direct report, because of their age and lack of experience and because the families of child victims are often the source of the injury.

If the child is old enough to describe how he or she got hurt, it is critical to attempt to interview the child. The earlier this interview can be done the better. This is especially true in the case of a child who may have been assaulted by a loved one. The child may feel conflict and confusion in implicating such a person. Pressure may be brought to bear—either intentionally or unwittingly—to convince the child that the injury was an accident or was prompted by the child's own misbehavior. While the child's medical needs must be addressed first, an interview at the medical facility can be very productive. The child may perceive this setting as free of consequences for his or her abuser, thinking, for example, "They're asking these questions to help me get better, not to get Mommy in trouble."

Whatever the location of the interview, the setting must be quiet, unhurried, and non-threatening to the child. Confusion and interruption make it difficult for a child to remain focused on the task at hand. Impatience on the part of the interviewer may be perceived by the child as disinterest or disbelief and may result in an unwillingness by the child to tell the full story.

The question of who should participate in the interview with the child requires collaborative decision making. Often civil and criminal investigations proceed on parallel but separate tracks. In the past, criminal investigators and social service caseworkers have done their interviews independently. Recently, however, many agencies have begun to conduct joint interviews, with both investigators present. However, the differing natures of their respective objectives should be recognized as a source for potential conflict. The criminal investigator's goal is to put together a case in which the abuser can be successfully prosecuted. The social service caseworker's goal is to protect the child, offer the opportunity for treatment to both victim and offender and, if possible, reunify a family separated by abuse. It is important for law enforcement officers and child protective caseworkers to communicate with one another prior to the interview, to clarify how the interview will be conducted and to assure that both investigators' responsibilities are carried out.[5]

Whether the interviews are done by teams of investigators or a single investigator, several questions need to be answered:

- What happened?
- Who did it?
- When did it happen?
- How often did it happen?
- Who knows it happened (either because they witnessed it or because the child told them about it)?

Determining what happened from the child's account is sometimes the only way to distinguish between an accidental injury and an inflicted injury. Who inflicted the injuries is valuable information, because in cases of physical abuse there are often multiple caretakers and therefore multiple suspects. The date of the injury can be an important support to medical opinions as to time of injury. It is important, however, to take into account the child's developmental age and understanding of time. In far too many cases, initial interviews of very young children ruled out a particular suspect or circumstance because the child told an investigator that the injury occurred "yesterday." It might later be learned that, to this child, any past event, whether last week or last month, occurred "yesterday."[6]

If repetitive injury can be established, it is potentially powerful evidence that these injuries are not recurring accidents but instead purposely inflicted injuries. If the child reports that others, such as siblings or the other parent, witnessed the abuse, the investigator can interview those people in an effort to corroborate the child's statement. In addition, knowledge of the infliction of an injury by a caretaker who is not directly responsible for the injury is important information. In civil cases it can help determine whether the nonabusive parent can adequately protect the child from further harm. From the criminal aspect, although it is rare, a person may be charged with a crime for failure to protect the child.[7]

While a child is often physically battered without other witnesses being present, there is a host of people who can provide essential information to an investigator. All members of the household should be interviewed. Their first reaction may be to deny that they have anything valuable to offer. Sometimes siblings may have seen the abuse and are reluctant to say so out of fear of or loyalty to the abuser. However, sometimes siblings are hoping someone will give them the opportunity to tell what they know. Siblings should be interviewed with the same sensitivity to the difficulty of their situation as the victim. Adults in the household must also be interviewed. Adults may be hostile if the investigator is perceived as trying to "pin the blame" for the child's injuries on a family member they love. They may refuse to consider that the child was hurt purposely. They may be suspicious, but hopeful that it was really an accident, or they may be firmly convinced that abuse occurred and may cooperate with the investigation. Whatever their posture, an interview with adults should focus on the surrounding circumstances of the injury. The following information needs to be obtained:

- where everyone was when the injury occurred;
- where objects were in the area in which the child was hurt;
- most importantly, what explanation was offered by the adult who was with the child at the time of the injury.

Family members are often the first to respond to the injured child. Consequently, they may hear an explanation from the abuser before the abuser has a chance to concoct a plausible story that is in accord with subsequent medical findings. For this reason investigators should consult with medical experts in the early stages of the investigation to compare historical information to medical findings. Anyone with whom the victim or suspect discussed the circumstances of the injury should be interviewed. When the victim's or the suspect's account remains consistent, it is likely to be reliable. However, inconsistencies in their reports raise questions about the veracity of their stories.

Finally, the suspect should be interviewed, if possible. If the suspect speaks of the details surrounding the injury, the investigator should record as much detail as possible, for it is in the detail that the truth may be found. If possible, the suspect should be asked to reenact the circumstances of the injury at the location of the injury, using furniture or other items that were present at the time. The investigator should consider videotaping the reenactment for review by medical experts to determine if the mechanism demonstrated is consistent or inconsistent with the medical findings. Investigators may offer potential suspects the opportunity to take a polygraph. While the results of a polygraph are not admissible in court proceedings, pre- and postpolygraph interviews may be admissible and may present an opportunity to test the consistency of the suspect's story and to confront a deceptive person with an inconsistency.

Sometimes the child victim is too young, too badly injured, or too traumatized to be a useful witness. Even in these cases, though, an investigation may lead to a legal intervention, if there is compelling medical and physical evidence to establish that the child's injury was nonaccidental and to identify the person responsible for it. In a child protection proceeding, the identity of the perpetrator may not even be required, if it can be proven that the child was intentionally injured while in the care of the parent or parents.

Of primary importance is a thorough medical evaluation by medical personnel specially trained in the indicators of inflicted trauma in children. A thorough medical evaluation can help establish abuse or clear an unfounded suspicion of abuse. The nature of the injury must be diagnosed accurately. Testing must be done to rule out organic causes for the injuries or illness. To the extent possible, testing should be undertaken to determine if this is a single episode or a chronic problem. Medical personnel should take careful note of the history provided about the injury. It is especially important to record statements by the child and parents given to medical personnel—these statements may later be admitted at a trial as a statement made for purposes of diagnosis and treatment, an exception to the hearsay rule.[8] Additionally, medical personnel should note the behavior of the parents of an injured child: if the parent refuses to discuss the circumstances of the injury with medical personnel; if the parent only comes to see the child when the parent thinks he or she will not be confronted by staff; or if the parent is available but fails to visit the child altogether. All these behaviors can suggest an attempt to cover up abuse.

Investigators should obtain search warrants to gather evidence when probable cause exists to believe that a crime has been committed. Careful evaluation of the locale in which the injury took place can establish the placement of objects which suspects or witnesses say caused the injury, for example, coffee tables on which the child is claimed to have struck his head, bureaus from which the child is said to have fallen. Measurements, photographs, videotapes, and diagrams of these scenes may have future evidentiary value that is not immediately apparent. If the child has been burned by immersion in water, checking the water temperature of tub water can help an expert to estimate how long a child's feet or hands were immersed to cause the burn. In cases of neglect, determining the status of the household in terms of food, state of habitability, and child safety can provide evidence of disregard for the well-being of the children living there. Video documentation of a scene of chronic neglect can be powerful evidence.

CASE ASSESSMENT AND LEGAL INTERVENTION

Once an investigation is complete, the criminal prosecutor and child protective agency must decide whether or not to proceed with legal intervention. Determining whether to pursue criminal prosecution essentially involves two considerations: Did a crime occur? Can it be proven beyond a reasonable doubt? Determining whether a crime occurred is largely based on a review of

- the statement of the victim if such statement is available
- statements by other witnesses
- the suspect's version of the injury-producing event
- the physical evidence gathered from the scene
- the medical evaluation of the victim's injuries

To the extent that these factors reinforce or corroborate each other, the prosecutor may gain confidence that this is a case of child abuse. However, it is a rare case which has all of these elements. If prosecutors required total corroboration or consistency before undertaking a criminal prosecution for child abuse, few cases would be pursued. Sometimes it is clear that only one person had access to the child at the time of the injury but unclear that the injury was inflicted, rather than accidental or organic. In other cases it is clear that a child has suffered inflicted injury but unclear who inflicted the injury.

When it is clear that the child suffered an inflicted injury but not clear who the perpetrator was, it is instructive to consider the motive or lack of motive for the child or caretakers to accuse one another falsely. Is there an ongoing custody battle? Is there a longstanding animosity between the accuser and the accused? Have other injuries occurred when the child has been in the care of others, or only when the child has been with the accused? When a motive to fabricate or exaggerate exists, prosecution becomes much more difficult.

When it is unclear whether the injury is inflicted or accidental, even if someone is strongly suspected to be an abuser, the prosecutor must be sure that the medical assessment was done or reviewed by a person with sufficient expertise to make the necessary judgments. The close-call case is not one for medical personnel who only occasionally evaluate child abuse. It is important to both not miss a child abuse diagnosis and not make an incorrect child abuse diagnosis.

Once it is decided that a crime has occurred and the perpetrator has been identified, the prosecutor must assess the likelihood of a conviction. Where the prosecutor has a conscientious belief, based on credible evidence, that a crime has been committed and the criminal identified but believes that conviction is unlikely, plea negotiation can provide a measure of justice. This assessment must be made in a detached, professional manner based on the best instincts of an experienced prosecutor. Just as the medical personnel who review these matters must have sufficient experience, so too must the prosecutors who handle these cases. The effects on a child of the rigors of a trial should not be underestimated.[9] Basing a charging decision on emotion or sympathy can result in increased hardship for the child the prosecutor seeks to help. A negotiated plea can offer a resolution that can mean protection for the child and a decrease in guilt for the child, because the abuser admits wrongdoing. A negotiated plea can offer the opportunity for treatment for the truly remorseful defendant and the chance for reunification of the family. It can provide punishment for the unrepentant abuser.

In a civil case, the decision to pursue a child protection action is most often made by the child protective agency. The agency may decide to proceed without legal intervention if the child's caretaker is willing and able to take steps to protect the child. If the agency has determined that the child has been physically abused, that the parent either caused the abuse or failed to protect from abuse, and that there are no services that can be put in place to allow the child to safely remain in the home, the agency will make a determination of whether the child is in immediate danger requiring protective custody. Some state statutes allow the agency to take the child into custody for a limited period of time without a court order.[10] Most states provide that the social service agency may petition the court for an *ex parte* (without other parties) hearing when a child is in immediate danger.[11] The parent is then entitled to an emergency hearing, usually within 24 hours to 10 days.[12] At that hearing, the court will determine whether the circumstances warrant emergency detention and whether the child should remain in the temporary custody of the agency. A finding against the agency at the emergency detention hearing does not preclude the agency from pursuing its underlying petition alleging that the parent has either physically abused or failed to protect the child from abuse.

Between the time the agency files a petition for a child protection order and the time the matter is scheduled to be heard by the court, the process of discovery and negotiation occurs. All involved parties—the parents, the child,[13] the agency and any other parties, such as grandparents, foster parents, or other relatives—will engage in "discovery," the process of reviewing records and reports, talking to witnesses, and conducting an independent investigation into the circumstances of the case. The parties will discuss the likelihood of resolution without a hearing, establishment of court findings, and expectations of the parties, with the goal of safely returning the child home.

TRIAL

In both the civil and criminal arenas, if a case cannot be resolved by negotiation it will proceed to trial. In a criminal trial before a jury, in order for the defendant to be convicted, each member of the jury must be convinced beyond a reasonable doubt that the victim suffered a nonaccidental injury and that the defendant is the person criminally responsible for the injury.

If the child is able to testify, he or she will likely be the most important witness in the case. When children are able to describe the injuries they suffered and who caused them in a consistent, credible way, the chances of conviction are greatly improved. In order for the child to do well at trial, it is imperative that the child be prepared for the process. Steps as simple as showing the child the courtroom and where everyone will be sitting can ease anxiety. Telling children who they will be seeing in court and explaining what each person does may demystify the courtroom experience. Honestly describing the procedure for the child without exaggerating or minimizing the difficulty of it can provide the child with a sense of confidence. Prosecutors should ask the child questions in anticipation of trial, including questions expected from the defense attorney. This will provide the child with the opportunity to process the question and not be taken by surprise. While most defense attorneys will not be overtly hostile to a child for fear of alienating the jury, the defense attorney will be skeptical and attempt to show inconsistencies in the child's testimony and any prior statements the child may have made.

In some instances, most notably child homicides and cases of injuries to preverbal children, the child cannot be called to testify. Other witnesses to the surrounding circumstances of the assault may testify to establish that abuse occurred. The investigator may testify and the medical experts will certainly be asked to testify to establish what the injuries were, whether the injuries were inflicted or accidental, and whether an injury is or is not consistent with the defendant's version of the circumstances surrounding it. Witnesses will also be subject to cross-examination by the defense.

The defendant may choose to offer a defense, though a defendant cannot be compelled to testify in a criminal case. Possible defenses include claiming that the injury was inflicted but not by the defendant or that the injury occurred while the child was in the defendant's care but it was accidental. It is at this point that the time and effort put into the investigation will bear fruit. If the surrounding circumstances indicate that the defendant's version of the injury is inconsistent with the true nature of the injury, such an inconsistency suggests that the defendant is less than truthful.

Criminal convictions in child abuse cases are difficult to obtain for a number of reasons. Often the victim is unable or unwilling to testify against his or her abuser. Also, few episodes of child abuse occur in the presence of neutral third-party witnesses. Lastly, the myth lives on that physical abuse of children happens only in impoverished families and is done only by obviously depraved, vicious people. Such beliefs make it difficult for jurors to convict seemingly loving, otherwise affectionate caretakers.

A civil trial will focus on two separate issues: whether the child was physically abused and whether the circumstances existing within the home are such that another injury or other harm will be likely without legal intervention. In considering the first issue, evidence will be presented at trial about the nature and cause of the child's injury: Was it inflicted or accidental? Was it the result of some disease or other organic cause? With regard to the latter issue, the court will consider: (a) whether the parents breached a responsibility to protect the child from the injury, regardless of who inflicted it, (b) the physical and psychological effects of the injury, and (c) the parents' response to the injury. Finally, the court will ask whether the parents have ameliorated the circumstances that caused the child to be injured.

Testimony will often be given by experts such as physicians or psychologists, as well as by investigators and social workers. Child protection cases usually proceed without requiring the child to testify, but there are circumstances when the child will be required to present information. Often, special protections for the child will be allowed.[14] These protections might include having the child testify over closed-circuit television, in the judge's chambers or, in civil cases, outside of the presence of the alleged abusers. Once abuse and responsibility have been established, the court will then focus on the needs of the child and on the plan to rehabilitate the family in order for the child to be able to return home safely. In those circumstances where the parents cannot or will not be able to change the circumstances within the home, the court must determine as soon as possible what alternative disposition will ensure the child a permanent and stable living arrangement.

CONCLUSION

Legal intervention is needed in the case of physically abused children, not only for the immediate safety of those children, but also to help stop the cycle of violence which begins in childhood for too many children. It is critical that those involved in this intervention coordinate their response to make the legal system more responsive to the needs of victims of abuse and their families and in a manner that does not revictimize the child abuse victim.

N O T E S

1. Most state child abuse statutes mandate a wide range of professionals—medical and osteopathic physicians, dentists, podiatrists, fire inspectors, school officials, and code enforcement officers, among others—to report child abuse or neglect when they have reasonable cause to suspect it.

2. D DePanfilis and M Salus, *Child protective services: A guide for caseworkers,* The User Manual Series, National Center on Child Abuse and Neglect, 1992, p. 5.

3. Most state statutes require a finding that the child's statement is reliable and that the child either testifies or is unavailable as a witness. When the child is unavailable, many states require additional corroborative evidence before admitting the hearsay statements. See JEB Myers, *Evidence in child abuse and neglect cases,* 2nd ed. (Somerset, NJ: Wiley Law Publications, 1992), vol. 1, pp. 266–273.

4. See *Maryland v. Craig,* 110 S. Ct. 3157 (1990); *Coy v. Illinois,* 487 U.S. 1012 (1988).

5. For a discussion of team investigation and some of the problems and recommendations for resolving these conflicts, see D Pence and C Wilson, *The role of law enforcement in the response to child abuse and neglect,* The User Manual Series, National Center on Child Abuse and Neglect, 1992, pp. 8–11.

6. For a discussion of children's reality and how to integrate developmental psychology into the legal system, see BW Dziech and CB Schudson, *On trial* (Boston: Beacon Press, 1989), pp. 41–72.

7. See, e.g., *People v. District Court,* 803 P.2d 193 (Colo. 1990); Myers, *Evidence in child abuse and neglect,* vol. 1, p. 198.

8. *White v. Illinois,* 112 S. Ct. 736 (1992). This exception includes statements by a parent describing the child's medical history or symptoms. *State v. Hebert,* 480 A.2d 742 (Me. 1984).

9. Although the impact of court involvement is still not entirely clear, studies suggest that certain

court practices, including long delays and requirements to testify on multiple occasions, pose risks to a child's recovery from sexual abuse. C Kendall-Tackett and D Finkelhor, Impact of sexual abuse on children: A review and synthesis of recent empirical studies, *Psychol Bull* 1993;113, no. 1:164–180.

10. See, e.g., Connecticut statutes CGS § 17a-101(e), 96-hour hold by DCF; Maine, 16 M.R.S.A. § 3501, a law enforcement officer may take a juvenile into interim care (up to 6 hours) if the officer has reasonable grounds to believe that the juvenile is abandoned, lost, or seriously endangered in his surroundings and that immediate removal is necessary for his protection.

11. Maine, 22 M.R.S.A. § 4036 (immediate risk of serious harm).

12. Michigan Court Rule 5.965 provides that a preliminary hearing must commence no later than 24 hours after the child has been taken into court custody, excluding Sundays and holidays. Illinois, California, and Colorado provide for hearings within 48 hours of removal: Ill. Ch. 37 § 802-9; Cal. Welf. & Inst. Code §§ 313 and 315; Colo. 19-3-43 . Maine, Connecticut, and New Mexico provide for 10-day hearings, although New Mexico law allows an earlier hearing upon written request of the respondent: 22 M.R.S.A § 4036; CGS 46b-129; N. M. Stat. Ann. § 32-4-16.

13. Under federal law, 42 U.S.C. § 5106a(b)(6) states must provide a guardian ad litem for all children in the child protective court system, in order to receive federal funds. States will either appoint a volunteer advocate, usually associated with the court appointed special advocate (CASA) program, or an attorney, or both to represent the child's interests in court. For a discussion of the attorney's role in advocating for a child, see N Haralambie, *The child's attorney: Representing children in domestic relations and civil juvenile cases,* American Bar Association, Section on Family Law, 1993.

14. See Dziech and Shudson, *On trial,* pp. 163–181.

Chapter 9

Long-term Medical Consequences of Physical Abuse

Robert H. Wharton, M.D.,
Suzanne Rosenberg, M.D.,
Robert L. Sheridan, M.D., and
Daniel P. Ryan, M.D.

Injuries that are most likely to cause lingering medical problems for the physically abused child are in three categories: traumatic brain injuries, burns, and abdominal injuries. All three present significant risk of morbidity, and abused children suffer more severe traumatic brain injuries and burns than children whose injuries are accidental. Traumatic brain injury presents the greatest risk of mortality. Appropriate specialty care and an integrated team approach are necessary to treat the physical injuries of abuse. Traumatic brain injuries can result in a range of consequences, including paralysis, blindness, cognitive impairment, neurobehavioral disorders, seizures, psychomotor impairment, and attention deficit. There is no single best protocol for these children and an individualized treatment plan is necessary. While modern technology and techniques mean significantly improved outcomes for burn patients compared to two decades ago, these are also complex cases requiring a team approach, and attention must be paid to all phases of treatment: initial evaluation and resuscitation, initial wound excision and biologic closure, definitive wound closure, and rehabilitation. Abdominal injuries from abuse are usually blunt rather than penetrating and can damage a number of organs, including the liver, pancreas, kidneys, bladder, spleen, stomach, and intestines. Patients who survive these injuries generally do well, but they are at risk for a number of complications, depending on the severity of the injury.

GENERAL CONSIDERATIONS

Children who sustain severe physical abuse will often have persisting medical consequences in addition to long-term emotional sequelae. While physical abuse affecting any part of the body may result in long-term medical complications, there is an extraordinarily high incidence of morbidity and mortality among young victims of shaking.[9,27] In addition to these often catastrophic injuries, children who have been burned or who have been the victims of abdominal trauma will also have long-lasting medical complications.

While initial efforts must be directed at management of life-threatening medical concerns, early and aggressive attention to such issues as increased intracranial pressure, abnormal tone, and spasticity will help markedly reduce or avoid many potential long-term physical and musculoskeletal complications. As detailed in previous chapters, in the immediate evaluation and treatment of nonaccidental trauma, efforts are directed primarily at resuscitation and stabilization of the child and, secondarily, on investigation and accumulation of data for diagnostic and forensic purposes. Orthopedic and surgical injuries are identified and treated. In the case of traumatic brain injury, the primary lesions such as depressed skull fractures, contusions, and diffuse axonal injuries require expedient recognition and treatment where possible. Secondary injury occurs as a result of increased intracranial pressure, decreased perfusion pressure, and ischemia. This may be caused by both intracranial factors, such as hematomas, swelling, hemorrhage, and hydrocephalus, and by extracranial systemic factors, such as hypotension and hypoxia. Neurosurgical and intensive care interventions are targeted at these pathological processes.

The impairments and resultant disabilities faced by victims of child abuse are far ranging. A team of caregivers with diverse skills most effectively addresses the needs of these children and their family. An interdisciplinary team assures appropriate specialty care and diverse therapeutic input. This interdisciplinary model lends itself to the acute management period, during which a physician or other health care provider assumes the role of team leader and facilitates communication. This inpatient rehabilitation model can be continued after a child is discharged, ensuring that the multiple needs of each child are addressed without omission of key elements of care. A follow-up program might have input available from physicians; nurses; physical, occupational, speech, and recreational therapists; as well as psychologists, psychiatrists, and social workers.

TRAUMATIC BRAIN INJURY

Mechanism of Injury

The precise mechanism of the injury to the brain in abused children remains controversial. The principal uncertainty is whether shaking itself can be sufficient to cause the severe injuries seen or whether a forceful impact is required.

Traumatic brain injury in children leading to severe permanent sequelae is generally caused by such events as being an unrestrained passenger in a high-speed motor vehicle crash, being struck by a car as either a pedestrian or an unhelmeted bicycle rider, or other such high-velocity, high-impact events. The mechanism of injury in crashes such as these is rotation of the brain around its center of gravity, causing diffuse axonal injuries and less frequently, subdural hematomas.[27]

On the other hand, common and more typical minor falls of childhood have a significantly different mechanism of injury. Here, the problem is one of translation of forces in which the brain moves with the center of gravity. These insults do not often result in severe injuries to the brain, and the sequelae from the injury are determined by the amount of force and the specific point of contact of the brain against the skull wall.

The first speculation that whiplash forces cause subdural hematomas by tearing cortical bridging veins occurred in 1971,[41] one year before the term *whiplash shaken baby syndrome* was used to describe a constellation of findings in infants including retinal hemorrhages, subdural and/or subarachnoid hemorrhages.[4,16,41] While it is now accepted that minor whiplash or shaking injuries cannot cause significant brain damage, disagreement persists whether violent shaking alone can cause significant neurologic sequelae.

Duhaime, using infant models, found that the magnitude of deceleration is 50 times as great when an infant held by the trunk forcefully strikes a surface as when shaking alone occurs, and that the brain only reaches thresholds necessary for injury at the moment of impact.[25] Concluding that the sudden angular deceleration experienced by the brain and cerebral vessels causes intracranial injury and that the majority of abused infants have some form of evidence of blunt impact to the head,[25] she and her colleagues suggested that the term *shaken-impact syndrome* be used to describe the syndrome, as it may more accurately reflect the mechanism of injuries.[27]

General Sequelae

This subgroup of children with traumatic brain injury who have been abused demonstrates a particularly high degree of morbidity and mortality.[45] Interhemispheric falx hemorrhage, subdural hematomas, large extradural fluid collections, and basal ganglia edema were found to be significantly more prevalent in nonaccidental head injury than in head injury occurring in the general pediatric population.[55] In survivors of the shaken baby/shaken impact syndrome, the most common motor sequelae include tetraplegia, hemiplegia, blindness, cognitive impairment, neurobehavioral disorders, hemiparesis, and psychomotor delay. Spasticity, lack of coordination, and ataxia are the most common types of psychomotor impairments.[73] However, it may take several years for the full consequence of the injury to appear, a situation that leads to the description of a "symptom-free interval."[12]

Deficits in attention with and without hyperactivity are commonly seen after traumatic brain injury. Impulsivity and disinhibition are associated with frontal lobe injury, although clinically these patients may also develop inanition and an apathetic affect. Neuropsychological testing frequently demonstrates decreased scores on performance IQ and memory deficits. Visual motor and visual spatial skills are also found to be relatively compromised.[56]

Prognosis

Investigators have tried to establish parameters for prognostication after pediatric traumatic brain injury. In 1992 Jaffe summarized the literature of mostly accidental injuries and identified several favorable prognosticators:

- absence of hypoxemia
- absence of prolonged periods of increased intracranial pressure
- Glasgow Coma Scale score of 4 to 6 at 72 hours
- coma of less than 24 hours
- posttraumatic amnesia period of less than two weeks

Defining coma as ending when the patient can follow commands or imitate gestures, Brink found that 94 percent of children and adolescents were independent in all activities of daily living and mobility if their duration of coma was less than 6 weeks. After 12 weeks of coma, however, 38 percent of children were completely dependent for all activities of daily living.[15]

In infants, the deceleration of brain growth, retinal hemorrhages, and the presence of intracranial lesion on CT scan have been associated with poorer prognosis.[12] Epidural hematomas carry a generally good prognosis, while subdurals are associated with a poorer outcome.[80] Ophthalmologists may have input into assessing the degree of neurologic injury, as the severity of retinal hemorrhage has been shown to correlate with acute injury with vitreous hemorrhage and subhyaloid hemorrhage, both of which are associated with more severe injury in the acute period.[115] Nonaccidental trauma in general carries a worse prognosis than other traumatic brain injury diagnoses.[15] The Glasgow Coma Scale has only limited value as a predictor of functional outcome,[120] although a GCS of 3 was associated with 100 percent mortality in one study.[7]

Specific Sequelae

Neurobehavioral Concerns

The type of injury seen in shaken-impact syndrome generally results in severe global neurobehavioral sequelae. However, less severe insults can lead to sequelae similar to those generally seen in traumatic brain injuries.

Neuropsychological testing has identified disorders of learning and memory as the most common weakness after traumatic brain injury. Reflecting the more serious nature of intentional injury, a study by Ewing-Cobbs and her colleagues on developmental findings after inflicted and noninflicted traumatic brain injury in young children noted that 45 percent of children with inflicted injury had cognitive test scores in the mentally deficient range, compared to only 5 percent of children with noninflicted traumatic brain injury.[31]

Additional studies consistently reveal this disparity in developmental outcome between inflicted and noninflicted injuries.[29,30] Key to the analysis are the ages of the abused children, as well as their environmental and socioeconomic backgrounds. There is some disagreement about the relationship between age at injury and cognitive outcome. While one study reported that age at injury was not predictive of long-term outcome following severe traumatic brain injury, others identified worse outcomes in children whose injuries occurred when they were less than 6 years of age.[22,61] However, the fact that children under 2 years of age are more vulnerable to violent shaking injuries may be a sufficient explanation for their worse cognitive outcome, compared to older children. There are no data to support the suggestion that the disparity in sequelae in physically abused children is based on premorbid socioeconomic and family factors.[61]

Posttraumatic personality change and slowness in rate of information processing are also commonly seen in abused children who have suffered traumatic brain injury.[104] Deficit in attention; memory problems, including visual memory and visual and verbal recognition memory; and deficits in short-term or working memory have commonly been seen after traumatic brain injury.[64] In addition, neurobehavioral changes seen after brain injury include hyperactivity, impulsivity, and aggressive behavior, as well as poor adaptive functioning, social judgment, and attention.

Unfortunately, the severity of the neurobehavioral sequelae does not dissipate with time. Disinhibition, impulsivity, and aggression have been found to increase in adulthood after childhood traumatic brain injury.[19] However, Glasgow Outcome Scores and the Barthel Index tend to improve with time, reflecting increased independence in activities of daily living. Scales of social adjustment and community integration reveal the greatest deficiencies, suggesting that more attention should be paid to emotional, behavioral, social, and family issues throughout the rehabilitative process.

Pharmacological treatment should be directed at an individual's symptoms, rather than trying to choose a medication that will consistently help traumatic brain injury itself. In other words, treatment decisions should be individualized for specific symptoms. The validity of this approach is supported by the disparity reflected in the studies of stimulant medication for pediatric brain injury. Whereas some authors state that children with brain injury respond to neurostimulants such as methylphenidate, with improvements noted in cognition, behavior, and arousal similar to improvements noted in children with attention deficit/hyperactivity disorder,[53] other studies have found no benefit in methylphenidate in a brain-injured population, compared to controls.[116] In addition to the stimulant medications, several other classes of medications may play a role when appropriately employed. These include

- medications such as carbamazepine and valproic acid, which often successfully control disordered regulation of behavior
- medications such as clonidine and quanfacine, which help control children with excessive arousal
- antidepressant medications such as the SSRIs, which manage mood disturbances

Sensory Impairments

Visual disturbance is a frequent complication of traumatic brain injury. Acute loss of vision may be due to retinal or vitreous hemorrhage or may be cortical in nature. Cortical blindness is more commonly seen when there is associated hypoxic injury and tends to be transient.[78] Field defects may be permanent, requiring compensatory techniques and adaptation within the child's classroom.[78] Cranial nerve injuries may cause double vision, which will resolve with time.[56]

Audiological and vestibular disturbances may lead to significant functional morbidity. Longitudinal temporal bone fractures can lead to hearing loss through disruption of middle ear structures, the tympanic membranes, or the external auditory canal.[46] Transverse temporal bone fractures and sensorineural hearing loss may also present as a complication. Evaluation of hearing may include brainstem auditory evoked responses to help clarify the nature of the child's problems.

Seizures

The incidence of posttraumatic seizures is reported to be between 1 and 8 percent.[78] The risk for early posttraumatic seizures increases for children, however, in the presence of low Glascow Coma Scale scores, cerebral edema, acute subdural hematomas, and open, depressed skull fractures with parenchymal damage.[112] In these cases prophylactic neuroleptic treatment is generally initiated. Although phenytoin is often the initial treatment, carbamazepine may be better tolerated for long-term use and may avoid the concern of delayed development associated with use of phenobarbital and phenytoin in young children. Anticonvulsants have not been shown to be effective in preventing late traumatic seizures.[56]

Spasticity

Spasticity, the velocity-dependent increase in tonic stretch reflexes with exaggerated tendon jerks, is a frequent sequela of severe traumatic brain injury. The upper motor neuron syndrome more broadly includes exaggerated cutaneous reflexes, dystonia, and muscle spasms.[119] Spasticity and abnormal tone, present in the upper and lower extremities, the trunk, the jaw, and the oropharynx, interfere with activities of daily living, mobility, hygiene and, if severe, respiratory effort. Consequences of inadequately treated spasticity and hypertonicity include soft tissue contractures with resultant loss of range of motion and pain.

Spasticity and abnormal tone often can be controlled to some degree by decreasing nociceptive stimulation. In fact, a change in a patient's tone may herald a urinary tract infection or a decubitus ulcer. Therefore, much like treatment for insomnia, diagnostic investigation should be the primary effort of the clinician. In children with traumatic brain injury, overstimulation, an ineffective seating system, or metabolic or musculoskeletal pathology may cause the problem. If the stretch reflex results in gross clonus or spasticity, these reactions can often be prevented by an appropriately set footrest or lateral support on a wheelchair. As synergy is seen in association with certain patterns of abnormal tone— such as decerebrate or decorticate posturing—the disruption of the pattern at one end may be reflected throughout the kinetic chain. For example, flexion of the neck or dorsiflexion of the ankle may help break up the extensor tone in the trunk or extremities.

Proper positioning can also help to minimize noxious stimulation and prevent contractures. Sustained stretches can reduce spasticity and retard contracture formation. The use of splints and inhibitive or serial casting also allows for sustained stretch and appropriate positioning.

When nonpharmacological strategies alone are ineffective at managing tone, systemic and locally acting pharmaceutical agents should be considered as additional therapy. The primary antispastic medications are divided into centrally and peripherally acting agents. Baclofen and diazepam fall into the former category. Baclofen is a chemical analogue of the inhibitory neurotransmitter gamma aminobutyric acid (GABA). It acts presynaptically to diminish transmission within the spinal cord. It has no peripheral muscle relaxant activity. Diazepam enhances the effects of GABA, increasing presynaptic inhibition. Tizanidine is a relatively selective alpha 2 adrenergic receptor agonist which reduces synaptic transmission of nociceptive stimuli in the spinal pathways and causes postsynaptic reduction in excitatory transmitter activity.[119] Dantrolene acts peripherally on skeletal muscle by reducing calcium release from the sarcoplasmic reticulum, thereby interfering with excitation-contraction coupling.

Treatment of spasticity through local injection of neurolytic agents is indicated when oral agents are either ineffective or cause intolerable side effects. Phenol can be injected into the motor points of selected muscles by using a neurostimulator.[117] Both the nerve stimulation and the injection can be painful and this procedure will require sedation or general anesthesia, depending on the age of the patient and length and invasiveness of the procedure. Phenol is nonselective and may result in paresthesias in mixed nerves or sensory branches. For this reason, its use is often limited to the branches of the obturator nerve and the tibial portion of the sciatic nerve, which serve the hip adductors and hamstrings, respectively. Injection into the dermis could cause sloughing. Its immediate effect, long duration, availability for repetitive use, and low cost, however, make it the procedure of choice in many circumstances.

Botulinin toxin A is one of seven toxins produced by *Clostridium botulinum.*[20] It is selective for the neuromuscular junction, where it inhibits acetylcholine release, thereby weakening muscle. While initially used ophthalmologically to treat strabismus and blepharospasm, its beneficial effect on reducing spasticity has been well described.[18,38] Its selectivity for the neuromuscular junction allows it to be used in small muscles of the upper extremity as well as any lower extremity muscle without risk of sensory paresthesias. Its effect becomes apparent two to seven days post injection. Neurostimulation may be used to isolate muscles when necessary. Topical cream anesthetic may be used with or without conscious sedation. The duration of effect of an injection of botulinin toxin A is three to six months. While the frequency of antibody formation is reported to be below 5 percent,[121] repetitive use and more frequent administration does carry this associated risk. The procedure itself is generally free from adverse effects except for mild pain at the injection site.

The next available treatment modality for spasticity is orthopedic intervention. Tenotomy or myotomy are generally considered when spasticity has progressed to the point of disabling soft tissue contracture or when the degree of spasticity has plateaued and it is anticipated that muscle lengthening will bring about improved function. Heel cord lengthening may be achieved percutaneously. Tendon transfers can manipulate muscle balance for more efficient upper extremity function or correction of gait abnormalities. Surgical intervention is often scheduled to follow a growth spurt, to minimize the need to repeat lengthening procedures. Communication between orthopedic surgeons and physiatrists allows for effective utilization of pharmacological management so that surgery can be appropriately timed and, in ideal situations, exposure to anesthesia may be used for both surgical procedures and injections.

Baclofen may be administered intrathecally via a "pump" reservoir maintained under the skin. While this does allow lower doses to be administered locally at the target organ system, the procedure carries the risks of surgery, anesthesia, and foreign body insertion. Usually the placement of the intrathecal device is preceded by administration of a trial dose of baclofen via lumbar puncture. Patients must be carefully monitored for respiratory depression. Ideally, the lower dosages achieve improved tone management with minimal side effects. Dosage flow rates are titrated based on clinical effect using computerized telemetry, and the reservoirs are easily refilled as needed. Unfortunately, the size of the reservoir prohibits use in small children.

Finally, selective dorsal rhizotomy (SDR) is a neurosurgical procedure in which posterior lumbar rootlets are selected for irreversible resection using electrophysiologic criteria. The procedure is thought to reduce spasticity by diminishing excitatory input to the anterior horn. While studies have rather consistently reported a reduction in spasticity after this procedure, its functional relevance has been questioned. As use of physical therapy postoperatively has intensified, the contribution of surgery versus therapy has also been called into question. Recently, two investigations were published attempting to answer this question. Interestingly, one study concluded that SDR does lead to statistically significant improvement in gross motor function compared to children who receive therapy alone,[118] while the other demonstrated no relative improvement in function despite a strong effect on spasticity.[70] The authors of the latter study theorized that their inclusion of a strengthening program might be partially responsible for the similarity in gains made by the group who received physical therapy alone. There were no serious or persistent adverse events noted in either study series.

BURNS

Admission of young children to burn centers is frequently a result of child abuse. Nearly 20 percent of children referred to burn centers are considered victims of child abuse, and of these, 20 percent are subsequently discharged into foster care.[92] The range of injury severity among these patients is enormous. Unfortunately, victims with burns from abuse commonly suffer extensive injuries with significant long-term morbidity.[54]

Like any subtle diagnosis in medicine, the diagnosis of abuse by burning is often not immediately obvious. It is therefore important to consider the possibility of abuse when evaluating any burn patient. There are three components to making the diagnosis: history, examination, and investigation.

First, when evaluating a burn, as with taking a history for any situation when child abuse is being considered, several important points of history should alert the clinician to a possible diagnosis of abuse.[49,67,83] These include delayed presentations for care and conflicting or confusing stories.

Second, suspicious patterns in burns caused by abuse include

- deep contact burns, particularly on the dorsal surface of the hand or foot;
- immersion stocking or glove pattern scalds, particularly if there are no splash burns and the injury is of uniform depth;
- tub immersion injuries, particularly if there is flexor sparing in the popliteal fossa or porcelain contact sparing of the perianal skin.[33,57,63]

An accurate burn diagram should be drawn and the injury photographed promptly from several angles and with proper lighting, as splash marks and other superficial injury components are often evanescent. The patient should be thoroughly examined for other injuries and healed burns.[6]

Investigation of child abuse by burning begins with a proper and well-documented initial evaluation.[95,100] State authorities should perform prompt home inspections of tap water temperature before any charges are made. Knowing the depth of the burns and the water temperature will help investigators determine the duration of exposure to hot liquids and thereby clarify the actual mechanism of injury.[75]

Treatment

Management of the child with acute burn injuries has improved dramatically over the past two decades. Children now routinely survive, with high quality outcomes, injuries that were uniformly lethal a few years ago.[47,83,106] However, achieving these outcomes requires a focused multidisciplinary effort by an experienced team.[91] These are complex hospitalizations and should be structured to organize the efforts of the many parties involved. An optimal structure includes four phases:

1. initial evaluation and resuscitation
2. initial wound excision and biologic closure
3. definitive wound closure
4. rehabilitation

Initial Evaluation and Resuscitation

During the first 24 to 72 hours after injury, patients suffering serious burns develop an enormous capillary leak, the extent of which is seen in no other disease or injury process. To support continued perfusion of the viscera and soft tissues requires that a careful resuscitative effort be promptly initiated, monitored, and titrated to the individual patient's physiology. While this fluid resuscitation is under way, a careful evaluation must be performed to thoroughly exclude other injuries.

Initial Wound Excision and Biologic Closure

The central event in modern burn care, the key to modifying the natural history of the disease, is the surgical maneuver of initial wound excision and immediate biologic closure. This surgery requires that full-thickness burns be identified and excised and that the wounds thus generated undergo immediate biologic closure. If adequate autograft is not available for wound closure, temporary wound closure materials should be used, such as human allograft skin. These operations can be physiologically stressful events and must be conducted with proper attention to body temperature, blood loss, and hemodynamic stability. When properly performed, this strategy can have a dramatic effect on patient survival and length and number of hospital stays. This process should be completed before the otherwise inevitable development of wound colonization and infection, ideally within the first seven days after injury.

Definitive Wound Closure

This phase of care typically begins at the end of the first week after the burns were suffered and continues through six or more weeks post-injury, depending on the availability of autograft. It is here that temporary wound closure materials are replaced with autograft and wounds of high complexity but small anatomic size, like those on the face and hands, are addressed.

Rehabilitation

Although rehabilitation efforts begin during resuscitation, they increase in intensity throughout the hospital stay. At the end of the acute hospitalization, rehabilitation efforts will involve many hours a day; after discharge, rehabilitation continues as a major component of burn aftercare programs. After surviving a serious burn, optimal long-term outcomes are difficult to attain without participation in a coordinated burn aftercare program, the central components of which are rehabilitation, reconstruction, and reintegration.

Rehabilitation during the critical phase of illness begins with ranging, splinting, and antideformity positioning. Subsequently, passive and active motion, ambulation, self-care activities, and strengthening become rehabilitation priorities. Aggressive rehabilitation efforts begun early will greatly enhance the patient's subsequent efforts to develop independence.

Reconstruction

Seriously burned patients usually need reconstructive surgery to achieve optimal functional and cosmetic outcomes. Timing of these operations must balance the immediate needs of the patient with the physical and psychological trauma of repeated hospitalization and surgery. However, many of these operations are not extensive and can be performed with short-stay hospitalization. Pressing functional and cosmetic needs should be promptly addressed.

Reintegration

The objective of burn care is to return patients to their pre-injury state as much as possible—back to community, school, work, and family. To enhance patient reintegration, it is helpful to address the common psychological sequelae of serious burns. Posttraumatic stress disorder is reported to occur in up to 30 percent of those surviving serious burns;[33] to address this problem can significantly improve all aspects of recovery. Support of the patient's family is also important, as family dysfunction will render the child's recovery far more problematic.[5,17,113]

Long-term Outcomes

The few long-term outcome studies of seriously burned children have focused on psychological adjustment, although none has specifically addressed outcomes of children suffering burns of abuse. Posttraumatic stress disorder,[79] depression,[99] and low self-esteem are unfortunately common.[1] Despite these difficulties, most children will have surprisingly good long-term psychological outcomes.[10,74,97,98] Two important findings are the often devastating effect of the injuries on families[69,81] and the favorable influence of a healthy family on the patient's recovery.[11,72] These data underscore the importance of family evaluation and support to achieve optimal outcomes.

Unfortunately, methodological problems abound in the evaluation of long-term outcomes after burns,[32] and this is particularly true of functional and cosmetic results. There are no widely accepted tools to measure these important endpoints. Without such data, we must use other measures as a proxy for functional and cosmetic outcome, such as frequency and type of reconstructive surgery, social relationships, and employment. However, the majority of children surviving serious burns can achieve satisfying long-term outcomes.[87,102,103] Available data suggest that if seriously injured children participate in a burn aftercare program, if they endure the essential serial reconstructive surgical procedures and participate in rehabilitation efforts, most will achieve functional and cosmetic long-term outcomes they consider satisfactory.

This is even true of those suffering massive burns. However, clearly there is a knowledge gap here that should be addressed in a prospective fashion using objective outcome measures. On the whole, children suffering burns of abuse will do well in the long term if they are managed in an organized fashion by a committed team. However, they will require prolonged and often painful therapies to reach this result, and they will carry physical and psychological scars for the rest of their lives.

ABDOMINAL TRAUMA

Most abdominal injuries from child abuse are secondary to blunt force trauma. Penetrating injuries are much less common. The injury patterns are similar to other cases of blunt abdominal trauma and include

- solid organ injury to the liver or spleen and to retroperitoneal organs like the kidneys or pancreas
- hollow viscus injuries to the bladder or bowel
- injuries to the abdominal wall or diaphragm

The treatment protocols and procedures are the same for abused children as they are for other patients with blunt trauma to the abdomen, regardless of the injuring agent. The evaluation for intra-abdominal injuries must be tailored to the patient. Before the abdomen can be evaluated with a proper CT scan, hemodynamic stability must be achieved and other severe injuries that require immediate operation must be treated.[77,85] Institutions with appropriate resources may be able to treat many solid organ injuries with nonoperative protocols in selected patients.[42]

Long-term medical complications are related to the specific organ injured and the methods of treatment used. Most patients who survive severe abdominal injuries do well in the long term. Those who have been able to avoid open surgical intervention have fewer problems than ones who have had a laparotomy.[109] After discharge from the hospital, patients who have lost their spleens or had a major bowel injury are the most likely to go on to develop later problems.

Patients who have had liver injuries are at risk for three significant problems, not necessarily related to whether they were treated operatively.[51,82] First, bile leaks can require surgical drainage, either percutaneous or operative; the resulting fistula will close without further surgery in nearly all patients. Some may need other therapies, like endoscopic papillotomy and biliary drainage, although the success of these techniques is anecdotal. If a major bile duct has been injured and the leak persists, internal drainage to the jejunum will be needed.[96]

A second potential complication is hemobilia. This will often occur within five to ten days after the injury and present with pain, bleeding, hemetemesis, and occasionally fever. Angiography can both define the source of the bleeding and treat the problem by occluding the distal vessel that is the bleeding source.

The third problem is infection and liver abscess. Large hematomas seldom become infected. Patients with injuries that leave significant segments of the liver devascularized have a higher likelihood of developing abscesses. This complication will often present within two weeks of the injury, usually before the patient has been discharged from the hospital.

Injuries to the spleen are common from blunt forces to the abdomen. Many of these will not need surgical intervention and will eventually heal completely.[3,68] Delayed rupture of the spleen is not unusual in the adult population but seems to be rare in children.[14,88] This occurs 5 to 14 days after the injury and presents with acute onset of left upper quadrant pain and hypotension. Most cases of delayed rupture will require splenectomy to control the bleeding.

The long-term problems associated with splenectomy are well documented.[23,52,66,90] The most feared is the overwhelming postsplenectomy infection. This is associated with the encapsulated organisms, such as pneumococcus, H. flu, and meningococcus. The incidence of this problem seems variable in the trauma population and is more frequent in patients who have had splenectomies for hematological conditions. The incidence is quoted at anywhere from below 1 percent to 13.5 percent in various studies.[28,40,111] One difficulty with calculating the true incidence is that an overwhelming infection can occur up to 50 years after the splenectomy.

Currently, all patients who have had a splenectomy should be vaccinated against the encapsulated organisms listed above and their antibody response should be monitored. The effectiveness of the vaccines is reduced when given following the splenectomy, especially if they are given during the period of postsurgical and postinjury stress. None of the vaccines provides complete immunity to all possible strains of the organisms, however. The role of prophylactic antibiotics is not clear. Many physicians recommend using oral penicillin daily for at least two years after a splenectomy, the time period in which infections seem to be most likely.[39,96,110] Unfortunately, the infections often present with very nonspecific symptoms, similar to the beginnings of a cold or viral syndrome. The rapid, fulminant course and high mortality rates (30%–50%) have led to the movement to save as many spleens after trauma as possible, either with nonoperative management or by surgical repair of the injured spleen.[8]

Injuries to the pancreas from blunt trauma occur when the organ is crushed against the vertebral bodies. This can result in various degrees of injury from contusions to transection. Pancreatitis or ductal disruption may then lead to problems with pancreatic necrosis, infection, or late pseudocyst formation. The most common late problem is with pseudocysts, although these are often present and detected prior to discharge. Posttraumatic strictures of the pancreatic duct may lead to either recurrent pancreatitis or chronic pancreatitis.[89,94]

Renal injuries most often become manifest by hematuria. Injuries to the collecting systems may lead to retroperitoneal urine leaks that will often resolve but may require a late repair or drainage. A more subtle problem, although perhaps more serious in the long term, is the development of hypertension following renal trauma. Segmental areas of injury to the kidney may lead to significant hypertension many weeks after the injury. Therefore, all patients with renal trauma need close follow-up and documentation of their blood pressure for a minimum of six months to detect if there is a problem. Some patients who have hypertension early due to a hematoma contained within Gerota's fascia will have it resolve over a few months. Those with persistent hypertension should be evaluated for a potentially correctable lesion, either a renal artery stenosis, segmental ischemia, or compressive lesion on the kidney.

Hollow viscus injuries occur in about 1 percent of all patients with blunt abdominal trauma.[62,76,86] The areas injured may be anywhere from the esophagus to the rectum and result in free rupture, intramural hematoma, or a mesenteric injury that may have acute bleeding or late stenosis from ischemia. Duodenal hematomas often occur in conjunction with pancreatic injuries and often by the same mechanism. These present with gastric outlet obstruction and may resolve with conservative treatment, but the patient will usually benefit from early surgery to evacuate the hematoma and relieve the obstruction. Late stenosis of an injured area of intestine, at the duodenum or elsewhere, will present with signs of partial or complete bowel obstruction.

Traumatic bladder rupture from blunt abdominal trauma is usually recognized soon after the injury, because of anuria and hematuria. These injuries tend to do well following repair, with few long-term problems. A rupture of the diaphragm may not be recognized in the acute setting and may present late with chest or abdominal pain, inability to swallow, and perhaps a bowel obstruction.[21,24,44,65] Acute dilatation of the stomach within the left chest may lead to respiratory symptoms as well. The diagnosis is often evident on a chest x-ray, but confirming it may require an upper GI series. If the patient has a dilated stomach and it cannot be decompressed by a nasogastric tube, urgent surgical evaluation is necessary, because the stomach may be developing vascular compromise.[35,60,107]

CONCLUSION

Continuing and long-term health consequences of physical abuse necessitate continuing medical follow-up, especially since these consequences sometimes do not present symptoms until long after the abuse has occurred. Because of the complexity of injuries and the psychological and social as well as medical damage that is often suffered by physically abused children, an integrated team approach is the best way to ensure that these children have the best possible chance for optimal outcomes in all areas.

REFERENCES

1. Abdullah A, Blakeney P, Hunt R, et al. Visible scars and self-esteem in pediatric patients with burns. *J Burn Care Rehabil* 1994;15:164–168.
2. Alexander R, Sato Y, Smith W, Bennett T. Incidence of impact trauma with cranial injuries ascribed to shaking. *Am J Dis Child* 1990;144:724–726.
3. Allins A, Ho T, Nguyen TH, Cohen M, et al. Limited value of routine follow-up CT scans in nonoperative management of blunt liver and splenic injuries. *Am Surg* 1996;62:883–886.
4. Anonymous. Shaken baby syndrome: Inflicted cerebral trauma. *Pediatrics* 1993;92:872–875.
5. Ayoub C, Jacewitz MM. Families at risk of poor parenting: A descriptive study of sixty at-risk families in a model prevention program. *Child Abuse Negl* 1982;6:413–422.
6. Ayoub C, Pfeifer D. Burns as a manifestation of child abuse and neglect. *Am J Dis Child* 1979;133:910–914.
7. Barzilay Z, et al. Variables affecting outcome from severe brain injury in children. *Intensive Care Med* 1988;14:417–421.
8. Benya EC, Bulas DI, Eichellberger MR, Sivit CJ. Splenic injury from blunt abdominal trauma in children: Follow-up evaluation with CAT. *Radiology* 1995;195:685–688.
9. Billmire ME, Myers PA. Serious head injury in infants: Accident or abuse. *Pediatrics* 1985;75:340–342.
10. Blakeney P, Herndon DN, Desai MH, Beard S, Wales-Seale P. Long-term psychosocial adjustment following burn injury. *J Burn Care Rehabil* 1988;9:661–665.
11. Blakeney P, Portman S, Rutan R. Familial values as factors influencing long-term psychological adjustment of children after severe burn injury. *J Burn Care Rehabil* 1990;11:472–475.
12. Bonnier C, et al. Outcome and prognosis of whiplash shaken infant syndrome: Late consequences after a symptom-free interval. *Dev Med Child Neurol* 1995;37:943–956.
13. Bontke CF, et al. Principles of brain injury rehabilitation. In Braddom RL, *Physical medicine and rehabilitation.* Philadelphia: W. B. Saunders. 1996.
14. Brasel KJ, DeLisle CM, Olson CJ, Borgstrom DC. Splenic injury: Trends in evaluation and management. *J Trauma* 1998;44:283–286.
15. Brink JD, et al. Physical recovery after severe closed head trauma in children and adolescents. *J Pediatr* 1980;97:721–727.

16. Caffey J. Brain damage from whiplash-shaking of infants. *Am J Dis Child* 1972:161–169.

17. Cahners SS, Bernstein NR. Rehabilitating families with burned children. *Scand J Plast Reconstr Surg* 1979;13:173–175.

18. Calderon-Gonzalez R, et al. Botulinum toxin A in management of cerebral palsy. *Pediatr Neurol* 1994;10:284–288.

19. Cattelani R, et al. Traumatic brain injury in childhood: Intellectual, behavioral and social outcome into adulthood. *Brain Injury* 1998;12:283–296.

20. Chutorian AM, et al. Management of spasticity in children with botulinum A toxin. *Int Pediatr* 1994;9:35–43.

21. Cifti AO, Tanyel FC, Salman AB, Buyukpamukcu N, Hicsonmez A. Gastrointestinal tract perforation due to blunt abdominal trauma. *Pediatr Surg Int* 1998;13:259–264.

22. Costeff H, Grosswasser Z, Goldstein R. Long-term follow-up review of 31 children with severe closed head trauma. *J Neurosurg* 1990;73:684–687.

23. Cullingford GL, Watkins DN, Watts AD, Mallon DF. Severe late postsplenectomy infection. *Br J Surg* 1991;78:716–721.

24. Czyrko C, Weltz CR, Markowitz RI, O'Neil JA. Blunt abdominal trauma resulting in intestinal obstruction: When to operate? *J Trauma* 1990;30:1567–1571.

25. Duhaime AC, Gennarelli TA, Thibault LE, Bruce DA, Margulies SS, Wiser R. The shaken baby syndrome: A clinical, pathological, and biomechanical study. *J Neurosurg* 1987;66:409–415.

26. Duhaime AC, et al. Head injury in very young children: Mechanisms, injury types, and ophthalmologic findings in 100 hospitalized patients younger than 2 years of age. *Pediatrics* 1992:179–185.

27. Duhaime AC, Christian CW, Rorke LB, Zimmerman RA. Nonaccidental head injury in infants: The "shaken-baby syndrome." *N Engl J Med* 1998;338:1822–1829.

28. Ein SH, Shandling B, Stephens CA, Bandi SK, Biggar WD, Freedman MH. The morbidity and mortality of splenectomy in childhood. *Ann Surg* 1977;185:307–310.

29. Ewing-Cobbs L, Miner ME, Fletcher JM, Levin HS. Intellectual, motor, and language sequelae following closed head injury in infants and preschoolers. *J Pediatr Psychol* 1989;14:531–547.

30. Ewing-Cobbs L, Duhaime A, Fletcher JM. Inflicted and noninflicted traumatic brain injury in infants and preschoolers. *J Head Trauma Rehabil* 1995;10(5):13–24.

31. Ewing-Cobbs L, Kramer L, Prasad M, Canales DN, Louis PT, et al. Neuroimaging, physical, and developmental findings after inflicted and noninflicted traumatic brain injury in young children. *Pediatrics* 1998;102:300–307.

32. Eyles P, Browne G, Byrne C, et al. Methodological problems in studies of burn survivors and their psychosocial prognosis. *Burns* 1984;10:427–433.

33. Fauerbach JA, Lawrence J, Haythornthwaite J, McGuire M, Munster A. Preinjury psychiatric illness and postinjury adjustment in adult burn survivors. *Psychosomatics* 1996;37:547–555.

34. Feldman KW, et al. Cervical spine MRI in abused infants. *Child Abuse Negl* 1997;21:199–205.

35. Frykberg ER, Phillips JW. Obstruction of the small bowel in the early postoperative period. *South Med J* 1989;82:169–173.

36. Glod C, et al. Increased nocturnal activity and impaired sleep maintenance in abused children. *J Am Acad Child Adolesc Psychiatry* 1997;36:1236–1243.

37. Golson E. The affective and cognitive sequelae of child maltreatment. *Pediatr Clin North Am* 1991:1481–1496.

38. Gooch JL, et al. Botulinum toxin for spasticity and athetosis in children with cerebral palsy. *Arch Phys Med Rehabil* 1996;77:508–511.

39. Green JB, Shackford SP, Sise MJ, Fridlund P. Late septic complications in adults following splenectomy for trauma: A prospective analysis in 144 patients. *J Trauma* 1986;26:999–1004.

40. Green JB, Shackford SP, Sise MJ, Powell RW. Postsplenectomy sepsis in pediatric patients following splenectomy for trauma: A proposal for a multi-institutional study. *J Pediatr Surg* 1986;21:1084–1086.

41. Guthkelch AN. Infantile subdural hematoma and its relationship to whiplash injury. *Br Med J* 1971;2:430–431.

42. Haller JA Jr, Papa P, Drugas G, Colombani P. Nonoperative management of solid organ injuries in children: Is it safe? *Ann Surg* 1994;219:625–628.

43. Hammond J, Perez-Stable A, Ward CG. Predictive value of historical and physical characteristics for the diagnosis of child abuse. *South Med J* 1991;84:166–168.

44. Hardacre JM, West KW, Rescorla FR, Vane DW, Growfield JL. Delayed onset of intestinal obstruction in children after unrecognized seat belt injury. *J Pediatr Surg* 1990;25:967–968.

45. Haviland J, et al. Outcome after severe non-accidental head injury. *Arch Dis Child* 1997;77:504–507.

46. Healy GB. Hearing loss and vertigo secondary to head injury. *N Engl J Med* 1982;306:1029–1031.

47. Herndon DN, LeMaster J, Beard S, et al. The quality of life after major thermal injury in children: An analysis of 12 survivors with greater than or equal to 80% total body, 70% third-degree burns. *J Trauma* 1986;26:609–619.

48. Hight DW, Bakalar HR, Lloyd JR. Inflicted burns in children: Recognition and treatment. *JAMA* 1979;242:517–520.

49. Hobson MI, Evans J, Stewart IP. An audit of non-accidental injury in burned children. *Burns* 1994;20:442–445.

50. Holdsworth RJ, Irving AD, Cuschieri A. Postsplenectomy sepsis and its mortality rate: Actual versus perceived risks. *Br J Surg* 1991;78:1031–1038.

51. Hollands MJ, Little JM. Post-traumatic bile fistula. *J Trauma* 1991;31:117–120.

52. Hollands MJ, Little JM. Nonoperative management of blunt liver trauma. *J Trauma* 1991;78:968–972.

53. Hornyak J, et al. The use of methylphenidate in pediatric traumatic brain injury. *Pediatr Rehabil* 1997;1:15–17.

54. Hummel RP 3d, Greenhalgh DG, Barthel PP, et al. Outcome and socioeconomic aspects of suspected child abuse scald burns. *J Burn Care Rehabil* 1993;14:121–126.

55. Hymel KP, et al. Comparison of intracranial computed tomographic (CT) findings in pediatric abusive and accidental head trauma. *Pediatr Radiol* 1997;27:743–747.

56. Jaffe KM, et al. Rehabilitation following childhood injury. *Pediatr Ann* 1992;21:438–447.

57. Keen JH, Lendrum J, Wolman B. Inflicted burns and scalds in children. *Br Med J* 1975;4:268–269.

58. Keller MS, Stafford PW, Vane DW. Conservative management of pancreatic trauma in children. *J Trauma* 1997;42:1097–1100.

59. Kempe CH, Silverman FN, Steele BF, Droegemueller W, Silver HK. The battered-child syndrome. *JAMA* 1962;181:17–24.

60. Klausner JM, Rozin RR. Late abdominal complications in war wounded. *J Trauma* 1995;38:313–317.

61. Kriel RI, Krach LE, Panser LA. Closed head injury: Comparison of children younger and older than 6 years of age. *Pediatr Neurol* 1989;5:296–300.

62. Kurkchubasche AG, Fendya DG, Tracy TF Jr, Silen MK, Weber TR. Blunt intestinal injury in children: Diagnostic and therapeutic considerations. *Arch Surg* 1997;132:652–657.

63. Lenoski EF, Hunter KA. Specific patterns of inflicted burn injuries. *J Trauma* 1977; 17:842–846.

64. Levin HS, Eisenberg HM, Wigg NR, Kobayashi K. Memory and intellectual ability after head injury in children and adolescents. *Neurosurgery* 1982;11:668–673.

65. Lien GS, Mori M, Enjoji M. Delayed posttraumatic ischemic stricture of the small intestine: A clinicopathologic study of four cases. *Acta Pathol Jpn* 1987;37:1367–1374.

66. Linet MS, Nyren O, Gridley G, Adami HO, Buckland JD, McLaughlin JK, Fraumeni JF Jr. Causes of death among patients surviving at least one year following splenectomy. *Am J Surg* 1996;172:320–323.

67. Lung RJ, Miller SH, Davis TS, Graham WP 3d. Recognizing burn injuries as child abuse. *Am Fam Physician* 1977;15:134–135.

68. Lynch JM, Meza MP, Newman B, Gardner MJ, Albanese CT. Computed tomography grade

of splenic injury is predictive of the time required for radiographic healing. *J Pediatr Surg* 1997;32:1093–1095.

69. Mason S, Hillier VF. Young, scarred children and their mothers: A short-term investigation into the practical, psychological and social implications of thermal injury to the preschool child. Part 3: Factors influencing outcome responses. *Burns* 1993;19:507–510.

70. McLaughlin J. Selective dorsal rhizotomy: Efficacy and safety on an investigator-masked randomized clinical trial. *Dev Med Child Neurol* 1998:226–232.

71. Meekes I, van der Staak F, van Oostrom C. Results of splenectomy performed on a group of 91 children. *Eur J Pediatr Surg* 1995;5:19–22.

72. Meyer WJ, Blakeney P, Moore P, Murphy L, Robson M, Herndon D. Parental well-being and behavioral adjustment of pediatric survivors of burns. *J Burn Care Rehabil* 1994;15:62–68.

73. Michaud LJ, et al. Traumatic Brain Injury in Children. *Pediatr Clin North Am* 1993;40:553–565.

74. Moore P, Blakeney P, Broemeling L, Portman S, Herndon DN, Robson M. Psychologic adjustment after childhood burn injuries as predicted by personality traits. *J Burn Care Rehabil* 1993;14:80–82.

75. Moritz AR, Henriques FC. Study of thermal injury: The relative importance of time and surface temperature in the causation of cutaneous burns. *Am J Pathol* 1947;23:695–720.

76. Nance ML, Peden GW, Shapiro MB, Kauder DR, Rotondo MF, Schwab CW. Solid viscus injury predicts major hollow viscus injury in blunt abdominal trauma. *J Trauma* 1997;43:628–632.

77. Neish AS, Taylor GA, Lund DP, Atkinson CC. Effect of CT information on the diagnosis and management of acute abdominal injury in children. *Radiology* 1998;206:327–331.

78. Nelson SV. Pediatric head injury. *Phys Med Rehabil Clin North Am* 1992;3:461–478.

79. Powers PS, Cruse CW, Daniels S, Stevens B. Post-traumatic stress disorder in patients with burns. *J Burn Care Rehabil* 1994;15:147–153.

80. Raimondi A, et al. Head injury in the infant and toddler: Coma scoring and outcome scale. *Childs Brain* 1984:12–35.

81. Rizzone LP, Stoddard FJ, Murphy JM, Kruger LJ. Posttraumatic stress disorder in mothers of children and adolescents with burns. *J Burn Care Rehabil* 1994;15:158–163.

82. Roche B, Mentha G, Bugmann P, LaScala G, LeCoultre C. Intrahepatic biliary lesions following blunt liver trauma in children: Is nonoperative management or conservative treatment always safe? *Eur J Pediatr Surg* 1993;3:209–212.

83. Rosenberg NM, Marino D. Frequency of suspected abuse/neglect in burn patients. *Pediatr Emerg Care* 1989;5:219–221.

84. Rosenberg NM, Meyers S, Shackleton N. Prediction of child abuse in an ambulatory setting. *Pediatrics* 1982;70:879–882.

85. Ruess L, Sivit CJ, Eichelberger MR, Gotschall CS, Taylor GA. Blunt abdominal trauma in children: Impact of CT on operative and nonoperative management. *Am J Roentgenol* 1997;169:1011–1014.

86. Sarna S, Kivioia A. Blunt rupture of the diaphragm: A retrospective analysis of 41 patients. *Ann Chir Gynaecol* 1995;84:261–265.

87. Sawyer MG, Minde K, Zuker R. The burned child—scarred for life? A study of the psychosocial impact of a burn injury at different developmental stages. *Burns* 1983;9:205–213.

88. Shafi S, Gilbert JC, Carden S, Allen JE, Glick PL, Caty MG, Azizkhan RG. Risk of hemorrhage and appropriate use of blood transfusions in pediatric blunt splenic injuries. *J Trauma* 1997;42:1029–1032.

89. Shah P, Applegate KE, Buonomo C. Stricture of the duodenum and jejunum in an abused child. *Pediatr Radiol* 1997;27:281–283.

90. Shatney CH. Complications of splenectomy. *Acta Anaesthesiol Belg* 1987;38:333–339.

91. Sheridan RL. The acutely burned child: Resuscitation through reintegration. *Curr Probl Pediatr* 1998;28:101–132.

92. Sheridan RL, Ryan CM, Petras LM, Lydon MK, Weber JM, Tompkins RG. Burns in chil-

dren younger than two years of age: An experience with 200 consecutive admissions. *Pediatrics* 1997;100:721–723.

93. Sheridan RL, Tompkins RG, Burke JF. Management of burn wounds with prompt excision and immediate closure. *Intensive Care Med* 1994;9:6–19.

94. Shilyansky J, Sena LM, Kreller M, Chait P, et al. Nonoperative management of pancreatic injuries in children. *J Pediatr Surg* 1998;33:343–349.

95. Showers J, Garrison KM. Burn abuse: A four-year study. *J Trauma* 1988;28:1581–1583.

96. Steiner Z, Brown RA, Jamieson DH, Millar AJ, Cywes S. Management of hemobilia and persistent biliary fistula after blunt liver trauma. *J Pediatr Surg* 1994;29:1575–1577.

97. Stoddard FJ, Norman DK, Murphy JM. A diagnostic outcome study of children and adolescents with severe burns. *J Trauma* 1989;29:471–477.

98. Stoddard FJ, Norman DK, Murphy JM, Beardslee WR. Psychiatric outcome of burned children and adolescents. *J Am Acad Child Adolesc Psychiatry* 1989;28:589–595.

99. Stoddard FJ, Stroud L, Murphy JM. Depression in children after recovery from severe burns. *J Burn Care Rehabil* 1992;13:340–347.

100. Stone NH, Rinaldo L, Humphrey CR, Brown RH. Child abuse by burning. [Review]. *Surg Clin North Am* 1970;50:1419–1424.

101. Styrt B. Infection associated with asplenia: Risks, management and prevention. *Am J Med* 1990;88:(network 5N) 33N–42N.

102. Tarnowski KJ, Rasnake LK, Linscheid TR, Mulick JA. Behavioral adjustment of pediatric burn victims. *J Pediatr Psychol* 1989;14:607–615.

103. Tarnowski KJ, Rasnake LK. Long-term psychosocial sequelae. In Tarnowski KJ, ed. *Behavioral aspects of pediatric burns,* 81–118. New York: Plenum Press. 1994.

104. Tate RL, et al. Patterns of neuropsychological impairment after severe blunt head injury. *J Nerv Ment Dis* 1991;179:117–126.

105. Telzrow CF. Management of academic and educational problems in head injury. *J Learn Disabil* 1987;20:536–545.

106. Tompkins RG, Remensnyder JP, Burke JF, et al. Significant reductions in mortality for children with burn injuries through the use of prompt eschar excision. *Ann Surg* 1988;208:577–585.

107. Tortella BJ, Lavery RF, Chandrakantan A, Medina D. Incidence and risk factors for early small bowel obstruction after celiotomy for penetrating abdominal trauma. *Am Surg* 1995; 61:956–958.

108. U.S. Department of Health and Human Resources. *Child maltreatment, 1995: Reports from the states to the National Child Abuse and Neglect Data File.* Washington, D.C.: U.S. Government. 1997.

109. Velanovich VD. Decision analysis in children with blunt splenic trauma: The effects of observations, splenorrhaphy, or splenectomy on quality-adjusted life expectancy. *J Pediatr Surg* 1993; 28:179–185.

110. Waghorn DJ, Mayon-While RT. A study of 42 episodes of overwhelming post-splenectomy infection: Is current guidance for asplenic individuals being followed? *J Infect* 1997;35:289–294.

111. Walker W. Splenectomy in childhood: A review of England and Wales, 1960–1964. *Br J Surg* 1976;63:36–43.

112. Ward J. Pediatric issues in head trauma. *New Horiz* 1995;3:539–545.

113. Weimer CL, Goldfarb IW, Slater H. Multidisciplinary approach to working with burn victims of child abuse. *J Burn Care Rehabil* 1988;9:79–82.

114. Wescott H. The abuse of disabled children: A review of the literature. *Child Care Health Dev* 1991:243–258.

115. Wilkinson WS, et al. Retinal hemorrhage predicts neurologic injury in the shaken baby syndrome. *Arch Ophthalmol* 1989;107:1472–1474.

116. Williams SE, Ris MD, Ayyangar R, Schefft, Berch D. Recovery in pediatric brain injury: Is psychostimulant medication beneficial? *J Head Trauma Rehabil* 198:13(3):73–81.

117. Wood K. The use of phenol as a neurolytic agent: A review. *Pain* 1978;5:205–229.

118. Wright F. Evaluation of selective dorsal rhizotomy for the reduction of spasticity in cerebral palsy: A randomized controlled trial. *Dev Med Child Neurol* 1998:239–247.

119. Young RR, et al. Current issues in spasticity management. *Neurologist* 1997;3:261–275.

120. Zafonte RD, et al. Relationship between Glasgow Coma Scale and Functional Outcome. *Am J Phys Med Rehabil* 1996;75:364–369.

121. Zuber M, et al. Botulinum antibodies in dystonic patients treated with type-A botulinum toxin—frequency and significance. *Neurology* 1993:1715–1718.

Chapter 10

Long-term Management of the Developmental Consequences of Child Physical Abuse

Cynthia Cupit Swenson, Ph.D., and
David J. Kolko, Ph.D.

Physically abused children appear to experience multiple behavioral, emotional, and cognitive impairments as a result of abuse. Long-term mental health management of the child and family is necessary. Unfortunately, we have little definitive data indicating which approaches work best, and management techniques must be determined on the basis of individual child and family needs. Because of the multiple causes of physical abuse, assessment and treatment should be comprehensive and should incorporate a variety of different methods. Cognitive behavioral therapy, effective with other populations, may play an important role. Long-term management must include work with the child, the parents, and the family, as well as coordination with other systems such as child protective services, law enforcement, and the schools. Work with the child should address trauma-related emotional symptoms, anger management, and social competence, and family sessions need to deal with attributions and clarification of the abuse.

GENERAL CONSIDERATIONS

Short-term management of child physical abuse focuses on reducing risk to the child, conducting a medical evaluation, completing the investigation, and resolving crises that may occur upon the disclosure or discovery of abuse. During this phase, services may be provided by law enforcement, child protection, medical, and mental health professionals. But the consequences of physical abuse of a child extend beyond these immediate concerns. This chapter addresses the long-term management of the developmental consequences of physical abuse, focusing primarily on interventions that target the impact of abuse on a child's development and adjustment.

Typically these interventions are provided through comprehensive mental health treatment of the child, parents, and family. Long-term mental health management also involves continued interaction with key systems that work to reduce child maltreatment, including child protection, law enforcement, and the schools. A collaborative working relationship with these systems is paramount for two reasons. First, some of the forensic and placement tasks begun in the initial phase of managing a physical abuse case continue for months and perhaps years and certainly can have an impact on children's development. Second, mental health services build on tasks completed in the early days of the case, with full disclosure and completion of a forensic and medical evaluation being the necessary prerequisites to abuse-focused treatment.

Based on a comprehensive treatment approach, this chapter reviews

- considerations for determining the appropriate course for long-term management;
- subsequent treatment of the child, parent, and family;
- the importance of collaborative work with all involved systems; and
- issues in empirical validation of treatment outcomes.

DETERMINING THE APPROPRIATE COURSE FOR LONG-TERM MANAGEMENT

Long-term management of child physical abuse begins with a determination of the most appropriate course of action for the child and family. The course of intervention is typically determined through assessment of a family's strengths and needs, characteristics of the abuse, and the traumatic impact of the abuse on the child and family. However, aspects of etiology and common developmental sequelae found in the research literature are also important for determining what types of intervention will be useful.

Child Physical Abuse Correlates

Physical abuse appears to be related to diverse child, parent, family, and social network factors. No single cause for child physical abuse has been identified. Existing correlational and longitudinal research indicates that child physical abuse is multidetermined.

Child Factors

Even though children are not responsible for an adult's violent behavior, several characteristics of child victims appear to place them at a higher risk for abuse. For example, younger and developmentally delayed children are more often victims of physical abuse than older or nondelayed children.[5,6,34] Behaviors such as child noncompliance[8] and prolonged crying[48] have been related to increased risk for parental abuse.

Parent Factors

At present, no psychiatric profile distinguishes physically abusive from nonabusive parents. However, parental social-emotional difficulties such as low self-esteem, poor impulse control, antisocial behavior, and substance abuse have been shown to be related to perpetration of physical abuse.[103,140]

Family Factors

The family factors related to perpetration of abuse mainly involve the marital or partner relationship. Single parents show a higher frequency of child abuse.[115] Among parents with partners, the quality of the relationship affects the occurrence of abuse. When partner domestic violence or frequent marital conflict exists, the child is at an increased risk for abuse.[135] On the other hand, a supportive relationship with a partner may reduce the risk for child maltreatment.[21]

Social Network Factors

Abusive families are commonly characterized as socially isolated.[114,122] They tend to have limited contact with friends, and express general dissatisfaction with social supports.[27,37] Abusive families derive little support from community resources because these families seldom use available resources[25] and display limited involvement in community activities.[50]

Recent ecological models suggest that the multiple factors related to child physical abuse are interactive and interrelated.[8,100] Given this relationship, considering all factors in treatment appears warranted. Treatment should focus on factors related to the child (noncompliance), parent (e.g., physical violence, depression, substance abuse), family (e.g., poor family communication, problem solving), and social network (e.g., extended family, community). In addressing child factors, it is important to consider not only child characteristics related to risk but also social and emotional consequences of abuse that may increase future risk.

Physical Abuse Developmental Sequelae

Although further research on abuse-related symptomatology is sorely needed, empirical support is growing for the negative developmental impact of physical abuse on children.[77] Physically abused children appear to experience multiple difficulties, including behavioral, emotional, and cognitive impairments.

Among existing studies assessing the symptoms exhibited by physically abused children, the most consistent finding is impairments in relationships and social or interpersonal behavior.[77] In part, relationships with adults and peers are impaired because of the tendency of physically abused children to exhibit higher levels of aggression than nonabused children.[60,64,111,114] However, positive relationships may also be minimal, because physically abused children have lower social competence and problem-solving skills than nonabused children.[49,62,65] For some individuals aggressive behaviors continue into adulthood and may be manifested in violent crimes.[96]

Many physically abused children may be ill equipped to manage the abuse-related emotional symptoms they experience. Studies assessing posttraumatic stress disorder (PTSD) among child physical abuse victims found rates of up to 50 percent. Greater numbers of children appear to experience some posttraumatic symptoms, without meeting criteria for the full disorder.[30,41,76,109] Many physically abused children also experience higher levels of depression and hopelessness and lower self-esteem than nonabused children.[69,74,75,109]

A third area of impairment for many physically abused children is cognitive or neuropsychological functioning. In early studies, physically abused children were thought to have lower intellectual functioning than their nonabused counterparts.[71,95] Later research on specific cognitive skills, rather than global functioning, indicates that physically abused children tend to have lower receptive language skills,[135] reading ability, and expressive language skills,[19] and poorer task initiation[1,4] comprehension, and abstraction.[130]

Overall, physically abused children are at risk for varied and serious mental health problems and developmental difficulties. Therefore long-term management and treatment should be individualized, yet multifaceted. Assessment of these children should then explore several potential areas of impairment.

TREATMENT OF THE CHILD, PARENT, AND FAMILY

There are no definitive answers to the question of how best to treat the impact of child physical abuse and how to stop subsequent abuse. Treatment of physically abused children and their families has received limited attention in the research literature, despite its widespread application in clinical settings. In the studies that have been done, information on efficacy of treatment is limited, because many of the studies were poorly controlled, few were based on experimental designs, and virtually none included follow-up data. Given that child physical abuse is multidetermined, focusing treatment solely on the parent or child may not be sufficient to effect meaningful changes in family functioning and reduce abuse risk. Treatment of the abuse victim, the offender, and the entire family are all considered equally important components of treatment.

The following sections focus on a comprehensive treatment model that includes the child victim, parents, and family. The importance of interactions with other key systems with which the family is involved will be briefly noted. Although a multifaceted assessment is certainly warranted to assist with developing treatment goals,[117] thorough discussion of a comprehensive assessment is beyond the scope of this chapter. Nonetheless, areas for assessment will be mentioned within each section.

Treatment of the Child

The symptoms of children who have been physically abused vary greatly from case to case. Thus, the focus of intervention is likely to vary from child to child and may target multiple symptoms. However, several common areas of impairment have been identified:

- trauma-related emotional symptoms,
- poor anger management, and
- limited social competence.

Few child treatment models that address the above noted symptoms have been empirically validated with physically abused children. Nevertheless, cognitive behavioral therapy (CBT) has been examined as a treatment for these same symptoms among sexually abused children[23,123] and children with social and behavioral difficulties.[72,73] CBT appears to have direct applicability to physically abused children and will be the basis for the following discussion of components for treating trauma-related emotional symptoms, poor anger management, and limited social competence.

Trauma-related Emotional Symptoms

Assessment. Trauma-related emotional symptoms include difficulties such as anxiety, depression, and posttraumatic stress that relate directly to the physical abuse. To determine the symptoms to be addressed, the child and parent or caregiver are interviewed, and they complete standardized measures. Information from the assessment is used to develop goals for a treatment plan.

Interview information is gathered on child and family history, general functioning, history of other traumatic events, and specific characteristics of the abuse. An assessment of facts and perceptions about the current case and history of other trauma can assist the therapist in understanding the child's attributions about the abuse and the effect on the family. The therapist will also want to explore the child's feelings about events he or she may be facing (e.g., court, removal from the home), and whether emotional symptoms are being exacerbated by current stressors.

In lieu of informally assessing potential trauma history, structured interviews may be used. For example, the Brief Assessment of Traumatic Events[86,87,88] assesses the occurrence of physical abuse, sexual abuse, and witnessing of family violence. Other structured interviews such as the child version of the Diagnostic Interview for Children and Adolescents[111] are used to diagnose PTSD. To date, these interviews have not been empirically tested but they may have clinical utility.[46]

Several standardized measures are commonly used for assessing children's anxiety, depression, and posttraumatic stress. The Revised Children's Manifest Anxiety Scale[112] and the State/Trait Anxiety Scale for Children[120] are widely used anxiety measures. The Children's Depression Inventory[83] is a common measure of childhood depression. Briere's Trauma Symptom Checklist for Children[16,38] assesses sequelae of childhood trauma, including subscales on posttraumatic stress, anxiety, depression, dissociation, anger, and sexual concerns. From the parent's perspective, measures such as the Child Behavior Checklist[3] or the Eyberg Child Behavior Inventory[39,40] provide ratings of how the child is externalizing and internalizing problems.

Trauma-focused treatment. Recent CBT studies with sexually abused children[23,31,123] have linked several treatment components to reductions in trauma-related emotional symptoms. Broadly, these include psychoeducation, anxiety management, and graduated exposure.

With physically abused children, psychoeducation could include the following activities:

- addressing the child's and family's views on violence and discipline,
- identifying attributions about the physical abuse, and
- safety planning and risk reduction.

These components were incorporated in a recent CBT protocol for children.[78] In addressing views on violence in that study, child physical abuse was defined and violent versus nonviolent ways to discipline were identified. Attribution-related activities involved having children identify their beliefs about why adults physically abuse children, whether children cause adult aggression, and, more specifically, whether they felt responsible for their parent's aggressive behavior. By addressing attributions, children may normalize feelings they are having about the abuse and correct thinking errors related to responsibility for an adult's behavior. In the final activity, coping styles are discussed[121] and children are given instructions on handling crises, such as those that would require first aid or some type of social support from a friend or adult. Children develop their own written safety and social support plan.

Physically abused children who have anxiety or other affective difficulties may benefit from anxiety management techniques, such as relaxation training, aimed at reducing the physiological manifestations of anxiety. For example, therapists may begin with an explanation of the physiological basis for controlled breathing[26] and progress to practice of diaphragmatic breathing. This skill may be difficult for children, but it can be simplified[82,127] by using aids, such as a paper cup. Specifically, the child lies on a mat, places a paper cup on his or her stomach, and is instructed to make sure the cup rises when inhaling and lowers when exhaling. Other relaxation techniques that may be added to the child's repertoire include deep muscle relaxation[107] and guided imagery.[11]

Graduated exposure is a technique used to break the link between anxiety and reminders of the abuse. This technique involves recapitulation of the abuse paired with anxiety management techniques. Graduated exposure has been validated with sexually abused children[31,123] and applied in individual[119] and group[127] treatment programs for physically abused children. Exposure is typically conducted after the child has learned anxiety management techniques. First, children are given a rationale for the use of exposure and instructed to use relaxation or controlled breathing during the process when they begin to feel anxious. A common exposure rationale compares talking about the abuse to turning a light on when children believe they see monsters in the dark.[29] Once the light is turned on, they see there are no monsters and they have, in effect, faced their fears with the result of no harm. A similar expectation is set up for discussing the abuse. For a more detailed discussion of this technique, see chapter 20.

Next, the child recapitulates the abusive incident(s), beginning with less anxiety-provoking details (e.g., where they were during the abuse) and eventually talking about more anxiety-provoking details (the actual assaultive behavior). During the recapitulation, the child is asked to talk about specific sights, sounds, or smells remembered from the abuse. As noted earlier, anxiety is countered with relaxation techniques. Telling about the abusive experience may be done by talking, drawing, using puppets, or any other method that works for the child. In a group setting, peers may assist with the telling of what happened and with the practice of anxiety reduction. A group activity used in exposure work involves making puppets that resemble the abuser. The puppet is instructed to tell about what he or she did that was physically abusive. Peers may then express their opinion about the abuse and give the child suggestions for safety and coping.

Anger Management

Assessment.   Since anger control difficulties and aggression are common problems among physically abused children, techniques that address this area may be a vital part of treatment. Standardized assessment tools measuring children's level of anger to given stimuli,[47,116] children's behavioral responses to anger,[63] and parents' observations of aggressive behavior[3,39,40] may be administered before and after treatment. But, assessment of anger-related cognitions, internal and external cues, and behavioral changes in the contexts where poor anger control usually occurs will be more informal and conducted on an ongoing basis.

Anger control training.   Outcome studies of existing models of anger control training have shown reductions in adolescents' disruptive and aggressive behaviors,[44,45,128] verbal aggression[28,44] and impulsiveness.[44] School-based group CBT for anger control has also produced increases in self-esteem and reductions in aggression among school-aged aggressive children.[90]

Techniques used in anger management programs include relaxation, assessment of physiological anger cues, development of coping statements, substitution of relaxation responses and coping statements for aggression, and self-evaluation.[44] Exploring the issue of violence as a route to power or self-esteem is a key component to encouraging children to use anger management. Violence is framed as a direct route to loss of power and control for the individual who commits violence and a means of gaining power for the provocateur.

Identification of "inside" and "outside" anger cues is one method for identifying warning signals.[78] To identify inside (i.e., physiological) cues, children may need examples of other children's discoveries, for example, increased heart rate, watering eyes, and the feeling of butterflies in the stomach. Outside cues may be context- or person-specific and will need ongoing assessment. For example, when the teacher corrects a behavior, the child may interpret correction as rejection and respond with escalating temper. Identification of the warning signals is vital, because these signals notify children when anger reducers should be implemented. Anger reducers include controlled breathing, relaxation, and specific cognitions. Cognitions that reduce anger arousal are developed by the child, and should be short and specific. For example, children may practice saying to themselves statements such as "let it go" or "take an ice break." Using the child's language and practice through role-playing is important to the child's actual implementation. Therapists must take care to advocate relaxation techniques that can be used in settings such as the classroom without disruption.

It should also be noted that some physically abused children may avoid overt expression of anger altogether. For these children, appropriate ways to express anger should be a focus. Some of the same techniques used for children with poor anger control (e.g., relaxation, cognitive substitution) may be useful to these children, but they will also need practice with verbal expression.

Social Competence

Assessment.   Social competence training models are based on the assumption that poor social competence results from skill deficits and that training will remediate these deficits.[98] As with anger control, a few standardized measures assess various social skills, such as children's ratings of their own assertiveness[14,98] and parents' observations of children's social skills.[54] However, direct observations and ratings by teachers and parents will be important for assessing specific changes in social competence during treatment.

Social competence training.   In addition to social skills models validated with young physically abused children,[42,43] a substantial body of literature exists on the effectiveness of social competence training (SCT) with children in general. A meta-analysis of social competence training studies conducted from 1981 to 1990[7] found that in the short term, social competence training is moderately effective with children. Individual studies evaluating the effectiveness of social skills training on children's social interaction abilities have reported increases in initiating positive peer interactions,[55] questioning peers, leadership skills,[84] knowledge of interpersonal problem solving and social overtures toward peers,[85] and social skills in role-playing.[9] Social skills training programs may include components focusing on positive peer and adult interactions and ways to handle problems or negative situations.[14,51,52,98]

Social problem solving is another common component of treatment for physically abused children and their parents[56,57] and also has been applied to nonabused children with behavior problems.[68,70,118,137] Initially this skill can be taught in a step-by-step didactic process. The social problem-solving steps may ask the following questions:

- Is there a problem?
- What is the problem?
- What do I want?
- What can I do?
- What are the consequences of each choice?
- What am I going to try?

Therapists can apply the steps to hypothetical and actual problems faced by the child and family. Follow-up is conducted with role-playing and actual practice in the family and school settings.

Other social competence skills are taught with brief didactics and extensive role-playing and practice in the home and school. These skills include ways to approach a group, making friends, giving compliments, making complaints, refusing others, assertiveness, and appropriate eye contact. To promote generalization, the parent should be a partner to the therapist in reinforcing appropriate social skills at home.

Treatment of Parent

Assessment

The focus of assessment and treatment of the parent will depend on whether or not the parent is the physical abuse offender. If the parent is not the offender, then an assessment of that parent should include considerations of the impact of the abuse on that parent, risk for child abuse by that parent, and parenting skills,[2,94,99,106] as well as any related psychiatric symptomatology.[20,32,97] This information is obtained through standardized measures, parent interview, and observation of parent and child interactions. Therapists will need specific knowledge of potential areas for intervention, such as the parent's expectation of the child, attributions about the child's behavior (e.g., personalizes child's behavior as hostility toward parent), strategies used to discipline (e.g., time-outs, praise, corporal punishment), and consistency in discipline.

The offending parent completes the same assessment as the nonoffending parent plus measures of other factors that may contribute to the risk for physical abuse, such as management of anger and relationship conflicts.[33,104,124–126] Edleson and Tolman's[36] ecological assessment of battering men offers an organization of assessment components that has direct applicability to male and female physical abuse offenders and augments information on risk and dangerousness. Although risk and dangerousness are important areas for assessment, the therapist should keep in mind that assessment in long-term management cases does not carry the forensic purpose of establishing guilt or innocence of an offender, but instead guides treatment.

Treatment Components

Self-management and child behavior management are two key targets for parent treatment. Self-management addresses anger control, social problem solving, and expectations and attributions about the child. Cognitive behavioral anger control training for parents[139] is similar to that for children and adolescents, and in fact may be conducted with the parent and child together. Topics specific to the physical abuse and to anger management include distinguishing firm from harsh discipline, identifying stress and violence precursors (inside and outside cues), identifying cognitive distortions the parent may make about the child's behavior, and determining when in the parenting context to use relaxation or coping statements. Identifying parents' source of blame for the abuse and determining whether they accept responsibility for their actions or minimize the importance or impact of the abuse may be important factors to lowering the risk for reabuse. Attributions and responsibility can be explored and changed through the clarification process described below. Some parents' self-management difficulties may be related to substance abuse or psychiatric disorders and may require specialized treatment or medication management. In such cases, a referral for additional services may be necessary.

Parent training has received primary attention in the child physical abuse literature, with the purpose of teaching nonphysical discipline and developmentally appropriate expectations.[136] A number of parenting books[22,102,108] and structured parenting group programs[35] are available to assist with skills training. Broadly, techniques are based on standard behavioral principles and include using praise and rewards, implementing time-outs and loss of privileges, use of contingencies and contracts, and encouraging the child socially and emotionally (i.e., developmental stimulation, play, talking, activities). Parent training has resulted in increased parental knowledge of normal child development and alternatives to physical punishment.[53] Moreover, abusive parents who have completed parent training, and their children, show reduced negative behaviors. A caveat to these results is that the improvements may not generalize from the therapist's office to the home setting. One study[142] addressed the generalization problem by teaching child management and self-control techniques to parents in the clinic with a follow-up rehearsal in the home. In this study, parents maintained improvements over a one-year follow-up period.

A more recent extension of this work emphasizes parent training in intrapersonal and interpersonal skills.[79] In addressing intrapersonal skills, training was directed toward understanding sources of stress, cognitive and affective contributors to the use of physical punishment (e.g., parental views on violence, expectations of children), and teaching self-control techniques (e.g., anger control, cognitive coping). The focus on interpersonal skills emphasized instruction in behavioral principles and contingency management procedures, such as withdrawing privileges and taking time-outs as alternatives to physical punishment.

A step beyond parent training, Parent-Child Interaction Training (PCIT) contains behavioral and systemic features and has proven beneficial to children with behavior problems. PCIT has not been evaluated with physically abusive parents and children, but its use may be relevant to this population in improving the commonly conflicted parent-child relationship.[133] Stages in PCIT include assessment, training of behavioral play skills, training of discipline skills, and booster sessions.

Family-based Treatment

Assessment

In addition to child and parent treatment, work with the family is important for changing the relationships and structure in the home that have supported family violence. With regard to assessment, much of the information about family relations and the impact of the abuse on the family and perception of it by the family will be obtained during the nonoffending and offending parent assessments. Standardized measures that assess family characteristics and relations,[61,101] as well as perceived social support,[24] can aid in determining family functioning and changes in that functioning.

Treatment

Although the development of family-based approaches with physically abusive families is in its infancy, current research is moving toward its inclusion in the treatment program. Important areas to target with the family include

- developing house rules,
- increasing general positive involvement with one another,
- minimizing use of blaming language,
- improving overall communication,
- setting up fair and predictable consequences, and
- problem solving and negotiation.

Problem solving may be taught didactically and then through practice involving the whole family. As problem solving is taught, the therapist can model appropriate verbal communication, such as clarifying a family member's perception of the problem and reframing the problem. Parents can then be coached to model the same behaviors.

Using the above noted techniques, Kolko[79,80] compared parallel cognitive behavioral individual treatment of the child and the parent to family therapy alone. Family therapy consisted of three therapeutic phases: engagement, skill building, and application/termination. In the engagement phase, the therapist assessed the family members' roles and interactions (e.g., genogram), sought to positively engage all family members using reframing to shift negative attributions of blame, reviewed the effects of physical force, and encouraged compliance with a no-violence agreement. In the skill-building phase, families developed a family problem list, participated in extensive training in problem solving and communication skills,[113] and identified individual responsibilities for problem-solving efforts at home. The application/termination phase was devoted to applying solutions and establishing family routines for problem solving in interactions likely to precipitate physical punishment,[113,129] some of which addressed problems in key systems (e.g., spousal/partner, school).

According to Kolko's findings, parents in the CBT condition reported less anger and use of physical discipline and force during treatment than parents in the family therapy condition. Children in the CBT condition reported less use of physical discipline and force by the parent during treatment and greater reduction in family problems over time than children in family therapy alone. Of particular importance, the average length of time reported until the first use of physical discipline or force was twice as long for parents in the CBT condition than for those in family therapy only.

A family and community focus has been examined through ecologically based intervention models that address multiple risk factors associated with physical abuse and neglect (e.g., child, parent, family, social network). Comprehensive family- and community-based interventions are important to treating physical abuse, because the child- or parent-focused programs delivered in traditional mental health settings may not generalize to the environments where the family and child must successfully adapt. Moreover, traditional interventions fail to address the multiple determinants of abuse. Two examples of ecologically based programs are multisystemic therapy (MST)[17,58] and Project 12-Ways.[91]

MST is an intensive family- and community-based treatment program with home-based service delivery focused on equipping parents and children with coping skills and supports. It has been evaluated with abusive families in one clinical trial[17] which randomly assigned families who had been investigated for abuse and neglect to home-based MST or office-based group parent training.[142] MST and parent training were effective in reducing parents' psychiatric symptoms and stress and improving family problems. Families who completed MST showed greater alleviation of family difficulties than did families who completed parent training only. No data exist on long-term follow-up of these families.

Project 12-Ways offers a range of services to families to teach parents and children how to cope with stresses without abuse or neglect. Several evaluations of Project 12-Ways have yielded promising results. In an early study, using a quasi-experimental design,[92] 50 abusive and neglectful families were randomly selected from 150 families who had participated in Project 12-Ways and were compared to 47 such families not served by the project. One Project 12-Ways family and five comparison families recidivated. A larger-scale evaluation[93] indicated positive short-term outcomes on recidivism but reduction in the effects over time. Recently Project SafeCare, an ecobehavioral program similar to Project 12-Ways was developed for families with children aged birth to 5 years who are at risk of abuse or neglect. Initial evaluations of Project SafeCare are comparing the efficacy of using videotaped training or in-home counselors to modify environmental and health risks[131] and promote improved parent-child interactions.[13] Results are forthcoming from these studies.

The Role of Clarification

In intrafamilial child maltreatment cases, discussing the offender's, victim's, and family's perception of the abuse and making a plan for reducing risk is considered an important part of treatment,[10,132] yet no standard method has been cited for accomplishing this task. Clarification is a process whereby offending parents acknowledge their responsibility for committing abusive behavior and for changing this behavior. In effect, the child victim and family have an opportunity to correct faulty attributions about their own role in the offender's abusive behavior. This process has not been evaluated empirically but has been presented in the abuse literature[89,132] and may provide families with a structured avenue for openly addressing the abuse. Considering the important role of parental attributions in subsequent risk for reabuse in physical abuse cases,[15,18] it would seem that clarification in physical abuse may also be important.

Prior to the clarification meeting, in which the offender apologizes and takes responsibility for abusive behavior, preparation work must be done with the offender, child victim, and other family members. Offenders must acknowledge all of their physically abusive behavior, view it as abusive, and not minimize the importance of the behavior or the impact on the child and family. They must understand and be able to state that the child is not responsible for the parent's violent behavior and to develop a plan for ways to parent without physical aggression. One means for preparing the offender and organizing the apology and declaration of responsibility is through a written letter. This letter is written by the offender, under the supervision of the therapist. Many drafts may be revised before the letter is in the final form that will be read to the child victim and family.

Preparation of the child for clarification can be done individually or with the nonoffending parent. Children will need assistance determining what they would like the offender to know about how the abuse affected them and what questions they would like the offender to answer. Nonoffending parents, if available, and other family members will need to discuss their own perceptions of the abuse, their feelings toward the offender and the child, and questions they would like answered by the offender. Preparation of all family members culminates in a clarification meeting in which the family hears the offender's letter, has a discussion based on the child's and family's questions, and develops a plan for decreasing the risk for further violence in the family.

School-aged children who have no cognitive delays should be able to participate in the clarification process. Ideally the meeting exemplifies new ways in which the family will communicate and solve problems. But, research incorporating this process into treatment is needed to determine its effectiveness.

INTERACTIONS WITH OTHER KEY SOCIETAL SYSTEMS

Certainly, the bulk of work during treatment with physically abusive families will take place with the family. However, with long-term management, therapists will likely interact with other key systems, such as family and criminal court, child protective services (CPS), and the child's school or day care provider.

Therapists can be an excellent resource to family court judges and guardians ad litem for assisting in recommendations about visitation and treatment. Although therapists may not be involved in the forensic process, they may be asked to give an opinion about the impact of the abuse on the child. Therapists' contacts with the criminal court system may involve criminal prosecution of the offending parent. The therapist may serve as an expert witness to educate the court on physical abuse research or may play a role more specific to the case. If the child victim has to testify in either family or criminal court, the therapist may assist with preparing the child.

In many cases CPS is involved with a family for an extended period. In some cases families view CPS as an adversary, so therapists may assist families and CPS in developing a positive working relationship. Therapists also may serve as resources for assisting CPS with treatment planning and visitation recommendations. Contact with the child's CPS caseworker can also provide the therapist with valuable information about the family, the status of the case, and resources in the community from which the family may benefit.

Many physically abused children have difficulties with aggression,[78] and their behavioral difficulties may impact their academic and social performance in school or day care. By working closely with the teacher, therapists may assist in developing classroom and behavior management plans. Therapists may also help the parent link up with school personnel; the parent can provide additional support in managing the child at school and the school may become a supportive resource for the parent.

EMPIRICAL VALIDATION

As noted throughout this chapter, no treatment model has been empirically validated with physically abused children and their families. Use of empirical designs that promote understanding of the effects of interventions and transportability of validated treatment models to real world settings is crucial. These goals may be realized through contributions from research, practice, and the combined efforts of the two.

Research Contributions

In the physical abuse area, studies on treatment with children, parents, and certainly families are in their infancy. However, the methodology for rigorous scientific evaluation of treatment outcome has been broadly developed and can readily be applied to physical abuse treatment studies. Experimental studies that use random assignment and assess internal and external validity are needed to increase confidence in the findings.[105] Important features for these studies to include are multiple measures completed by multiple informants, multivariate analyses, repeated measures, control or comparison groups, and follow-up evaluations.[78,81] Measures of treatment adherence, therapist competence, and client attrition and removal from treatment also should be evaluated. One problem inherent in conducting university-based research is that treatment conditions and clients are dissimilar to those in community- and clinic-based settings. To address this issue, researchers and practitioners should join to make research conditions more similar to practice conditions and to make practice methods more similar to research methods.

Practice Contributions

In clinical settings, high client caseloads and limited time and resources may preclude designing and conducting experimental studies.[12] However, data collection from individual cases with a pre- and posttreatment measure of outcome may be feasible, and may provide information regarding efficacy of a specific intervention with a specific client. Moreover, systematic assessment of individual clients may assist with operationalizing treatment goals and provide more objective measures for examining change and improving client care.[79,80,81] According to Kazdin,[67] ongoing assessment of individual cases may assist in development of more definitive observations on treatment course and outcome. Measures of clinical course may assist therapists in determining increased risk in abusive families that would require a change in intervention. For example, weekly child and parent ratings have been useful in determining individual differences among physically abusive families in response to intervention.[78]

Combining Research and Practice

As noted earlier and verified in meta-analyses,[138] children, interventions, and treatment conditions in university-based research are not representative of populations and conditions in community-based practice. According to Weisz et al.,[138] research-based clients often present with milder symptoms, are more homogeneous, and volunteer for treatment. Research therapists have smaller caseloads and conduct more structured, time-limited treatment. As a result of these differences, practitioners often view the resultant research as irrelevant to actual practice. Furthermore, these differences may reduce the external validity of research findings. In order to conduct clinically meaningful research, efforts must be made to conduct research in settings and with populations that are more similar to "real world" situations. To some extent, ecological models such as multisystemic therapy and Project 12-Ways have bridged the research-practice gap.[59,93] Further collaborative attention is needed to integrate important elements of research and practice and to develop and validate clinical services for physically abused children and their families.

CONCLUSION

Child physical abuse is a significant problem that may have a serious, detrimental impact on children and families. Children may be left with multiple psychiatric symptoms that accompany them into adulthood and place them at risk for abuse of their own children.[66] Because of the multidetermined nature of physical abuse, assessment and treatment should be comprehensive, incorporating multiple measures, methods, and participants.

Despite the seriousness of child physical abuse, from a research standpoint, little is known about case characteristics, social and emotional impact, and validity of treatment models.[105] No published accounts exist regarding components of a comprehensive assessment for physical abuse cases. At best, assessment techniques used in general child clinical and family interviews serve as a model for child physical abuse cases. But, these assessments do not address important abuse factors that may affect the child's and family's functioning.

Consistent with the assessment research, evaluation of treatment models for physically abusive families has been given limited attention. Based on existing research and clinical practice impressions, a comprehensive model of treatment is clearly indicated. Studies addressing child impact or parent behavior show some promise in the use of cognitive behavioral techniques with physically abused children and their parents. Extant comprehensive models that address multiple systems implicated in child physical abuse have been evaluated but lack follow-up data. Furthermore, comprehensive models have failed to evaluate child symptomatology other than parent-child relations. Research is needed to evaluate not only treatment techniques but also implementation of family reunification with physically abused children who are in out-of-home placements.

Professionals who evaluate, treat, and do research with physically abused children and their families have much work to do. This work must be based on the joint efforts of practitioners and researchers and assure professionals and families that services provided are clinically effective, cost effective, and promote child safety. Evaluation of treatment programs also should address external validity. That is, to increase the likelihood of implementation of validated treatment models in community-based practice, clients and conditions of research should resemble those of practice. To accomplish this, additional work is needed to integrate clinic and community procedures and approaches. Through the combined efforts of practitioners and researchers to provide assessment and treatment models that have passed the test of scientific rigor and are feasible in the "real world," significant progress in ameliorating the adverse consequences of child physical abuse can be made.

REFERENCES

1. Aber JL, Allen JP. Effects of maltreatment on young children's socioemotional development: An attachment theory perspective. *Dev Psychol* 1987;23:406–414.

2. Abidin RR. *Parenting stress index,* 3rd ed. Charlottesville, VA: Pediatric Psychology Press. 1990.

3. Achenbach TM. *Manual of the child behavior checklist and 1991 profile.* Burlington: University of Vermont, Department of Psychiatry. 1991.

4. Allen DM, Tarnowski KJ. Depressive characteristics of physically abused children. *J Abnorm Child Psychol* 1989;17:1–11.

5. Ammerman RT. Etiological models of child maltreatment. *Behav Modif* 1990;14(3):230–254.

6. Ammerman RT, Hersen M, Van Hasselt VB, McGonigle JJ, Lubetsky MJ. Abuse and neglect in psychiatrically hospitalized multihandicapped children. *Child Abuse Negl* 1989;13:335–343.

7. Beelmann A, Pfingsten U, Losel F. Effects of training social competence in children: A meta-analysis of recent evaluation studies. *J Clin Child Psychol* 1994;23(3):260–271.

8. Belsky J. Etiology of child maltreatment: A developmental-ecological analysis. *Psychol Bull* 1993;114(3):413–434.

9. Berler ES, Gross AM, Drabman RS. Social skills training with children: Proceed with caution. *J Appl Behav Anal* 1982;15:41–53.

10. Berliner L. Clinical work with sexually abused children. In Hollin CR, Howells K (eds.), *Clinical approaches to sex offenders and their victims.* New York: Wiley. 1991.

11. Berliner L, Wheeler JR. Treating the effects of sexual abuse on children. *J Interpers Viol* 1988;2:415–434.

12. Beutler LE, Williams RE, Wakefield PJ, Entwistle SR. Bridging scientist and practitioner perspectives in clinical psychology. *Am Psychol* 1995;50:984–994.

13. Bigelow KM, Kessler ML, Lutzker JR. Improving the parent-child relationship in abusive and neglectful families. In Kessler ML (Chair), *Treating Physical Abuse and Neglect: Four Approaches.* Symposium conducted at the 3rd Annual APSAC Colloquium, Tucson, Arizona, 1995.

14. Bornstein MR, Bellack AS, Hersen M. Social skills training for unassertive children: A multiple baseline analysis. *J Appl Behav Anal* 1980;10:183–195.

15. Bradley EJ, Peters RD. Physically abusive and nonabusive mothers' perceptions of parenting and child behavior. *Am J Orthopsychiatry* 1991;61:455–460.

16. Briere J. *Trauma Symptom Checklist for Children.* Odessa, FL: Psychological Assessment Resources. 1989.

17. Brunk M, Henggeler SW, Whelan JP. A comparison of multisystemic therapy and parent training in the brief treatment of child abuse and neglect. *J Consult Clin Psychol* 1987;55:311–318.

18. Bugental DB, Mantyla SM, Lewis J. Parental attributions as moderators of affective communication to children at risk for physical abuse. In Cicchetti D, Carlson V (eds.), *Child maltreatment: Theory and research on the causes and consequences of child abuse and neglect,* 254–279. New York: Cambridge University Press. 1989.

19. Burke AE, Crenshaw DA, Green J, Schlosser MA, Strocchia-Rivera L. Influence of verbal ability on the expression of aggression in physically abused children. *J Am Acad Child Adolesc Psychiatry* 1989;28:215–218.

20. Butcher JN, Dahlstrom WG, Graham JR, Tellegen A, Daemmer B. *Minnesota Multiphasic Personality Inventory-2 (MMPI-2): Manual for administration and scoring.* Minneapolis: University of Minnesota Press. 1989.

21. Caliso JA, Milner JS. Childhood history of abuse and child abuse screening. *Child Abuse Negl* 1992;16:647–659.

22. Clark L. *SOS! Help for parents.* Bowling Green, KY: Parents Press. 1985.

23. Cohen JA, Mannarino AP. A treatment outcome study for sexually abused preschool children: Initial findings. *J Am Acad Child Adolesc Psychiatry* 1996;35:42–50.

24. Cohen S, Mermelstein RJ, Kamarck T, Hoberman HM. Measuring the functional components of social support. In Sarason IG, Sarason B (eds.), *Social support: Theory, research, and applications.* The Hague, Holland: Martinus Nÿhoff. 1985.

25. Corse S, Schmid K, Trickett P. Social network characteristics of mothers in abusing and nonabusing families and their relationships to parenting beliefs. *J Community Psychol* 1990;18:44–59.

26. Craske MG, Barlow DH. *Therapist's guide for the mastery of your anxiety and panic (MAP) program.* Albany, NY: Graywind Publishing. 1990.

27. Crittenden PM. Social networks, quality of childrearing, and child development. *Child Dev* 1985;56:1299–1313.

28. Dangel RF, Deschner JP, Rasp RR. Anger control training for adolescents in residential treatment. Special issue: Empirical research in behavioral social work. *Behav Modif* 1989;13: 447–458.

29. Deblinger E. Child sexual abuse. In Freeman A, Dattilio FM (eds.), *Comprehensive casebook of cognitive therapy*, 159–167. New York: Plenum. 1992.

30. Deblinger E, McLeer SV, Atkins MS, Ralphe D, Foa E. Post-traumatic stress in sexually abused, physically abused, and nonabused children. *Child Abuse Negl* 1989;13:403–408.

31. Deblinger E, McLeer SV, Henry D. Cognitive behavioral treatment for sexually abused children suffering post-traumatic stress: Preliminary findings. *J Am Acad Child Adolesc Psychiatry* 1990;29(5):747–752.

32. Derogatis LR. *The SCL-90-R: Administration, scoring, and procedures manual-II.* Towson, MD: Clinical Psychometric Research. 1983.

33. DeRoma VM, Hansen DJ. *Development of the parental anger inventory.* Poster presented at the Association for the Advancement of Behavior Therapy Convention, San Diego, CA, 1994.

34. Diamond LJ, Jaudes PK. Child abuse in a cerebral-palsied population. *Child Abuse Negl* 1983;3:341–350.

35. Dinkmeyer D, McKay GD. *The parent's handbook: Systematic training for effective parenting.* Circle Pines, Minnesota: American Guidance Service. 1982.

36. Edleson J, Tolman R. *Intervention for men who batter: An ecological approach.* Newbury Park, CA: Sage Publications. 1992.

37. Egeland B, Breitenbucher M, Rosenberg D. Prospective study of the significance of life stress in the etiology of child abuse. *J Consult Clin Psychol* 1980;48:195–205.

38. Elliott D, Briere J. Forensic sexual abuse evaluations of older children: Disclosures and symptomatology. *Behav Sci Law* 1994;12(3):261–277.

39. Eyberg SM, Colvin A. *Restandardization of the Eyberg Child Behavior Inventory.* Poster presented at the annual meeting of the American Psychological Association, Los Angeles, CA, 1994.

40. Eyberg SM, Ross AW. Assessment of child behavior problems: The validation of a new inventory. *J Clin Child Psychol* 1978;7:113–116.

41. Famularo R, Fenton T, Kinscherff R. Child maltreatment and the development of posttraumatic stress disorder. *Am J Dis Child* 1993;147:755–760.

42. Fantuzzo JW, Jurecic L, Stovall A, Hightower AD, Goins C, Schachtel D. Effects of adult and peer social initiations on the social behavior of withdrawn, maltreated preschool children. *J Consult Clin Psychol* 1988;56:34–39.

43. Fantuzzo JW, Stovall A, Schachtel D, Goins C, Hall R. The effects of peer social initiations on the social behavior of withdrawn maltreated preschool children. *J Behav Ther Exp Psychiatry* 1987;18(4):357–363.

44. Feindler EL, Ecton RB, Kingsley D, Dubey, DR. Group anger-control training for institutionalized psychiatric male adolescents. *Behav Ther* 1986;17:109–123.

45. Feindler EL, Marriott SA, Iwata M. Group anger control training for junior high school delinquents. *Cogn Ther Res* 1984;8:299–311.

46. Finch AJ, Daugherty TK. Issues in the assessment of posttraumatic stress disorder in children. In Saylor CF (ed.), *Children and disasters*, 45–66. New York: Plenum. 1993.

47. Finch AJ, Saylor CF, Nelson WM. Assessment of anger in children. In Prinz RJ (ed.), *Advances in behavioral assessment of children and families*, 235–265. Greenwich, CT: JAI Press. 1987.

48. Frodi AM. Contribution of infant characteristics to child abuse. *Am J Ment Def* 1981;85:341–349.

49. George C, Main M. Social interactions of young abused children: Approach, avoidance, and aggression. *Child Dev* 1979;50:306–318.

50. Giovannoni JM, Billingsley A. Child neglect among the poor: A study of parental adequacy in families of three ethnic groups. *Child Welfare* 1970;84:196–214.

51. Goldstein AP. *The prepare curriculum.* Champaign, IL: Research Press. 1988.

52. Goldstein AP, Glick B. *Aggression replacement training: A comprehensive intervention for aggressive youth.* Champaign, IL: Research Press. 1987.

53. Golub J, Espinosa M, Damon L, Card J. A videotape parent education program for abusive parents. *Child Abuse Negl* 1987;11(2):255–265.

54. Gresham FM, Elliott SN. *Social Skills Rating System manual.* Circle Pines, MN: American Guidance Service. 1990.

55. Gresham FM, Nagle RJ. Social skills training with children: Responsiveness to modeling and coaching as a function of peer orientation. *J Consult Clin Psychol* 1980;48:718–729.

56. Haskett M. Social problem-solving skills of young physically abused children. *Child Psychiatry Hum Dev* 1990;21(2):109–119.

57. Haskett M, Kistner JA. Social interactions and peer perceptions of young physically abused children. *Child Dev* 1991;62:979–990.

58. Henggeler SW, Schoenwald SK, Borduin CM, Rowland MD, Cunningham PB. *Multisystemic treatment of antisocial behavior in children and adolescents.* New York: Guilford. 1998.

59. Henggeler SW, Schoenwald SK, Pickrel SG. Multisystemic therapy: Bridging the gap between university- and community-based treatment. *J Consult Clin Psychol* 1995;63:709–717.

60. Hoffman-Plotkin D, Twentyman CT. A multimodal assessment of behavioral and cognitive deficits in abused and neglected preschoolers. *Child Dev* 1984;55:794–802.

61. Hovestadt AJ, Anderson WT, Percy FP, Cochran SW, Fine M. A Family-of-Origin Scale. *J Mar Fam Ther* 1985;11(3):287–297.

62. Howes C, Espinosa MP. The consequences of child abuse for the formation of relationships with peers. *Child Abuse Negl* 1985;9:397–404.

63. Jacobs GA, Phelps M, Rohrs B. Assessment of anger expression in children: The Pediatric Anger Expression Scale. *Personality and Individual Differences* 1989;10(1):59–65.

64. Jaffe P, Wolfe D, Wilson S, Zak L. Similarities in behavioral and social maladjustment among child victims and witnesses to family violence. *Am J Orthopsychiatry* 1986;56:142–146.

65. Kaufman J, Cicchetti D. Effects of maltreatment on school-age children's socioemotional development: Assessments in day-camp setting. *Dev Psychol* 1989;25:516–524.

66. Kaufman J, Zigler E. Do abusive children become abusive parents? *Am J Orthopsychiatry* 1987;57:186–192.

67. Kazdin AE. Evaluation in clinical practice: Clinically sensitive and systematic methods of treatment delivery. *Behav Ther* 1993;24:11–45.

68. Kazdin AE, Esveldt-Dawson K, French NH, Unis AS. Problem-solving skills training and relationship therapy in the treatment of antisocial child behavior. *J Consult Clin Psychol* 1987; 55:76–85.

69. Kazdin AE, Moser J, Colubus D, Bell R. Depressive symptoms among physically abused and psychiatrically disturbed children. *J Abnorm Psychol* 1985;94(3):298–307.

70. Kazdin AE, Siegel T, Bass D. Cognitive problem-solving skills training and parent management training in the treatment of antisocial behavior in children. *J Consult Clin Psychol* 1992; 60:733–747.

71. Kempe CH, Silverman FN, Steele BF, Droegemueller W, Silver HK. The battered child syndrome. *JAMA* 1962;191:17–24.

72. Kendall PC. Treatment anxiety disorders in children: Results of a randomized clinical trial. *J Consult Clin Psychol* 1994;62:100–110.

73. Kendall PC, Braswell L. *Cognitive behavioral therapy for impulsive children.* New York: Guilford. 1993.

74. Kinard EM. Emotional development in physically abused children. *Am J Orthopsychiatry* 1980;50:686–695.

75. Kinard EM. Experiencing child abuse: Effects on emotional adjustment. *Am J Orthopsychiatry* 1982;52:82–91.

76. Kiser LJ, Heston J, Millsap PA, Pruitt DB. Physical and sexual abuse in childhood: Relationship with post-traumatic stress disorder. *J Am Acad Child Adolesc Psychiatry* 1991;776–783.

77. Kolko DJ. Characteristics of child victims of physical violence. *J Interpers Viol* 1992;7(2): 244–276.

78. Kolko DJ. Child physical abuse. In Briere J, Berliner L, Bulkley JA, Jenny C, Reid T (eds.), *The APSAC handbook on child maltreatment*, 21–50. Thousand Oaks, CA: Sage Publications. 1996.

79. Kolko DJ. Clinical monitoring of treatment course in child physical abuse: Psychometric characteristics and treatment comparisons. *Child Abuse Negl* 1996;20(1):23–43.

80. Kolko DJ. Individual cognitive behavioral treatment and family therapy for physically abused children and their offending parents: A comparison of clinical outcomes. *Child Maltreat* 1996;1(4):322–342.

81. Kolko DJ. Integration of research and treatment. In Lutzker JR (ed.), *Handbook on research and treatment in child abuse and neglect*, 159–181. New York: Plenum. 1998.

82. Kolko DJ, Swenson CC. *Psychosocial evaluation and treatment of physically abused children.* Workshop presented at the San Diego Conference on Response to Child Maltreatment, San Diego, CA, 1996.

83. Kovacs M. *The Children's Depression Inventory.* North Tonawanda, NY: Multihealth Systems. 1992.

84. Ladd GW. Effectiveness of a social learning method for embracing children's social interaction and peer acceptance. *Child Dev* 1981;52:171–178.

85. LaGreca A, Santogrossi D. Social skills training with elementary school students: A behavioral group approach. *J Consult Clin Psychol* 1980;48:220–228.

86. Lipovsky JA, Hanson RF. *Multiple traumas in the histories of child/adolescent psychiatric inpatients.* Paper presented at the annual meeting of the International Society for Traumatic Stress Studies, Los Angeles, CA, 1992.

87. Lipovsky JA, Hanson RF. *Traumatic event histories of child/adolescent psychiatric inpatients: What is being done to our children?* Paper presented at the annual meeting of the Association for the Advancement of Behavior Therapy, Boston, MA, 1992.

88. Lipovsky JA, Hanson RF, Hand L. *Sexual abuse, physical abuse, and witnessing violence in child/adolescent psychiatric inpatients: Relationship to psychopathology.* Paper presented at the San Diego Conference on Responding to Child Maltreatment, San Diego, CA, 1993.

89. Lipovsky JA, Swenson CC, Ralston ME, Saunders BE. The abuse clarification process in the treatment of intrafamilial child abuse. *Child Abuse Negl* 1998;22;7:729–741.

90. Lochman JE, Burch PR, Curry JF, Lampron LB. Treatment and generalization effects of cognitive-behavioral and goal-setting interventions with aggressive boys. *J Consult Clin Psychol* 1984;52:915–916.

91. Lutzker JR, Frame JR, Rice JM. Project 12-ways: An ecobehavioral approach to the treatment and prevention of child abuse and neglect. *Educ Treat Child* 1982;5:141–155.

92. Lutzker JR, Rice JM. Project 12-ways: Measuring outcome of a large in-home service for treatment and prevention of child abuse and neglect. *Child Abuse Negl* 1984;8:519–524.

93. Lutzker JR, Rice JM. Using recidivism data to evaluate Project 12-Ways: An ecobehavioral approach to the treatment and prevention of child abuse and neglect. *J Fam Viol* 1987;2:283–291.

94. Macmillan VW, Olson RL, Hansen DJ. Low- and high-deviance analogue assessment of parent-training with physically abusive parents. *J Fam Viol* 1991; 6:279–301.

95. Martin HP, Rodeheoffer MA. The psychological impact of abuse on children. *J Pediatr Psychol* 1976;1:12–15.

96. McCord J. A forty-year perspective on effects of child abuse and neglect. *Child Abuse Negl* 1983;7:265–270.

97. McLellan AT, Luborsky L, O'Brien CP, Woody GE. An improved evaluation instrument for substance abuse patients: The Addiction Severity Index. *J Nerv Ment Dis* 1980;168:26–33.

98. Michelson L, Sugai DP, Wood RP, Kazdin AE. *Social skills assessment and training with children: An empirically based handbook.* New York: Plenum. 1983.

99. Milner JS. *The Child Abuse Potential Inventory: Manual (2nd ed.).* Webster, NC.: Psytec. 1986.

100. Milner JS, Chilamkurti C. Physical child abuse perpetrator characteristics: A review of the literature. *J Interpers Viol* 1991;6:345–366.

101. Moos RH, Moos BH. *Family environment scale manual.* Palo Alto, CA: Consulting Psychologists Press. 1981.

102. Munger RL. *Changing children's behavior quickly.* Lanham, MD: Madison Books, 1993.

103. National Research Council. *Understanding child abuse and neglect.* Washington, DC: National Academy Press. 1993.

104. Novaco RW. *Anger control: The development and evaluation of an experimental treatment.* Lexington, MA: Lexington Books. 1975.

105. Oates RK, Bross DC. What have we learned about treating child physical abuse? A literature review of the last decade. *Child Abuse Negl* 1995;19:463–473.

106. O'Dell SL, Tarler-Benldo L, Flynn JM. An instrument to measure knowledge of behavioral principles as applied to children. *J Behav Ther Exp Psychiatry* 1979;10:29–34.

107. Ollendick TH, Cerny JA. *Clinical behavior therapy with children.* New York: Plenum. 1981.

108. Patterson GR. *Living with children: New methods for parents and teachers.* Champaign, IL: Research Press. 1976.

109. Pelcovitz D, Kaplan S, Goldenberg B, Mandel F, Lehane J, Guarrera J. Post-traumatic stress disorder in physically abused adolescents. *J Am Acad Child Adolesc Psychiatry* 1994;33:305–312.

110. Reich W. *Diagnostic Interview for Children and Adolescents—Child Version.* Unpublished manuscript. Washington University School of Medicine, St. Louis, MO. 1991.

111. Reid JB, Kavanagh K, Baldwin DV. Abusive parents' perceptions of child problem behaviors: An example of parental bias. *J Abnorm Child Psychol* 1987;15:457–466.

112. Reynolds CR, Richmond BO. "What I think and feel": A revised measure of children's manifest anxiety. *J Abnorm Child Psychol* 1978;51:674–682.

113. Robin AL, Foster SL. *Negotiating parent/adolescent conflict: A behavioral-family systems approach.* New York: Guilford. 1989.

114. Rosario M, Salzinger S, Feldman R, Hammer M. *Home environments of physically abused and control school-aged children.* Research presented at the Biennial Meeting of the Society for Research in Child Development, Baltimore, 1987.

115. Sack, WH, Mason R, Higgins JE. The single-parent family and abusive child punishment. *Am J Orthopsychiatry* 1985;55:252–259.

116. Saylor, CF, Benson B, Einhaus L. Evaluation of an anger management program for aggressive boys in inpatient treatment. *J Child Adolesc Psychother* 1985;2:5–15.

117. Schellenbach CJ, Trickett PK, Susman EJ. A multimethod approach to the assessment of physical abuse. *Violence Vict* 1991;6:57–73.

118. Shure MB. *I can problem solve: An interpersonal cognitive problem-solving program.* Champaign, IL: Research Press. 1992.

119. Smith DW, Swenson CC, Hanson R. Reducing trauma-related emotional symptoms through individual treatment for physically abused children. In Kessler ML (Chair), *Treating Physical Abuse and Neglect: Four Approaches.* Symposium conducted at the 3rd Annual APSAC Colloquium, Tucson, Arizona, 1995.

120. Spielberger CC. *Preliminary manual for the State-Trait Anxiety Inventory for Children ("How I Feel Questionnaire").* Palo Alto, CA: Consulting Psychologists Press. 1973.

121. Spirito A, Stark LJ, Williams C. Development of a brief checklist to assess coping in pediatric patients. *J Pediatr Psychol* 1988;13:555–574.

122. Starr RH Jr. A research-based approach to the prediction of child abuse. In Starr RH Jr. (Ed.), *Child abuse prediction: Policy implications,* 105–134. Cambridge, MA: Ballinger. 1982.

123. Stauffer LB, Deblinger E. Cognitive behavioral groups for nonoffending mothers and their young sexually abused children: A preliminary treatment outcome study. *Child Maltreat* 1996;1:65–76.

124. Straus MA. The Conflict Tactics Scale and its critics: Evaluation and new data on validity and reliability. In Straus MA, Gelles RJ (eds.), *Physical violence in American families. Risk factors and adaptations to violence in 8,145 families,* 49–73. New Brunswick, NJ: Transaction. 1990.

125. Straus MA. Measuring intrafamily conflict and violence: The Conflicts Tactics (CT) Scales. In Straus MA, Gelles RJ (eds.), *Physical violence in American families: Risk factors and adaptations to violence in 8,145 families,* 29–47. New Brunswick, NJ: Transaction. 1990.

126. Straus MB. Abused adolescents. In Straus MB (ed.), *Abuse and victimization across the life span,* 107–123. Baltimore: Johns Hopkins University Press. 1988.

127. Swenson, CC, Brown EJ. Cognitive-behavioral group treatment for physically abused children: A case study. *Cognitive and Behavioral Practice,* in press.

128. Swenson CC, Butler AC, Kennedy WA, Baum JG. *Group treatment for anger control with institutionalized adolescent offenders.* Paper presented at the annual conference of the Florida Association of School Psychologists, Tampa, Florida, 1988.

129. Szapocznik J, Kurtines W. *Breakthroughs in family treatment.* New York: Springer. 1989.

130. Tarter RE, Hegedus AM, Winsten NE, Alterman AI. Neuropsychological, personality, and familial characteristics of physically abused children. *J Am Acad Child Psychiatry* 1984;23:668–674.

131. Taub HB, Kessler ML, Lutzker JR. Teaching neglectful families to identify and address environmental and health-related risks. In Kessler ML (Chair), *Treating Physical Abuse and Neglect: Four Approaches.* Symposium conducted at the 3rd Annual APSAC Colloquium, Tucson, Arizona, 1995.

132. Trepper TS, Barrett MJ. *Systemic treatment of incest: A therapeutic handbook.* New York: Brunner/Mazel. 1989.

133. Urquizza AJ, McNeil CB. Parent-child interaction therapy: An intensive dyadic intervention for physically abusive families. *Child Maltreat* 1996;1:134–144.

134. Vondra JI. Sociological and ecological factors. In Ammerman RT, Hersen M (eds.). *Children at risk,* 149–170. New York: Plenum. 1990.

135. Vondra J, Barnett D, Cicchetti D. Self-concept, motivation, and competence among preschoolers from maltreating and comparison families. *Child Abuse Negl* 1990;14:525–540.

136. Walker CE, Bonner BL, Kaufman KL. *The physically and sexually abused child: Evaluation and treatment.* New York: Pergamon. 1988.

137. Weissberg RP, Gesten EL, Caplan M, Jackson AS. *Social problem-solving training for fourth graders: An abridged revision of the Rochester Social Problem-Solving Program.* Unpublished manual. New Haven, CT: Yale University. 1990.

138. Weisz JR, Weiss B, Han SS, Granger DA, Morton T. Effects of psychotherapy with children and adolescents revisited: A meta-analysis of treatment outcome studies. *Psychol Bull* 1995;117: 450–468.

139. Whiteman M, Fanshel D, Grundy JF. Cognitive-behavioral interventions aimed at anger of parents at risk of child abuse. *Social Work* 1987;November–December.

140. Widom CS. *Child abuse and alcohol use.* Prepared for the working group on alcohol-related violence, Fostering Interdisciplinary Perspectives, convened by the National Institute on Alcohol Abuse and Alcoholism, Washington, DC, 1992.

141. Wolfe DA, Mosk MD. Behavioral comparisons of children from abusive and distressed families. *J Consult Clin Psychol* 1983;51:702–708.

142. Wolfe DA, Sandler J, Kaufman K. A competency-based parent training program for child abusers. *J Consult Clin Psychol* 1981;49:633–640.

PART III

Neglect

Chapter 11

The Roots of Child Neglect

Maureen M. Black, Ph.D.

Child neglect is prevalent and has pervasive long-term effects, yet there is no generally accepted definition of it and in clinical manifestations it is often poorly distinguished from abuse. Neglect may be physical and/or emotional and different types of neglect require different types of interventions. Neglect interrupts normal development and the formation of secure attachment relationships. It is closely associated with poverty.

GENERAL CONSIDERATIONS

Neglect occurs when children's basic needs are not met. It is often defined as an act of omission rather than commission.[18,27,56] Although neglect lacks the sensationalism of abuse, it accounts for more than half of the substantiated reports of maltreatment,[52] almost half of maltreatment-related child deaths,[32] and often represents a chronic situation that leaves children feeling worthless.[32,33] Yet little is known about effective management of children who have been neglected, largely because there is no consensus regarding the definition of neglect.

DEFINING NEGLECT

Neglect is an interdisciplinary concept, of interest from multiple perspectives—medical, legal, and mental health professionals; social service agencies; the general public. Representatives from each perspective define neglect differently, depending on the conceptual basis and demands of their perspective. For example, legal definitions are relatively precise, because they are concerned with upholding specific laws regarding reports and consequences of child neglect.[26] On the other hand, health care providers often advocate for broader definitions of neglect, because they are concerned with the child's health and well-being, regardless of legal definitions.[17]

Many agencies and investigators rely on child protective services (CPS) to substantiate cases of child neglect.[27] However, referral biases suggest that families who are minority, low income, or already involved with social service agencies are disproportionately likely to be reported to CPS.[56] Moreover, once a report is made, decisions regarding investigation and substantiation often vary by local policies and interpretations. Because CPS-defined cases of neglect are a select subset of all neglect cases, management studies based on CPS-defined neglect are not necessarily representative.

Another definitional problem arises from the frequent co-occurrence of neglect and abuse,[38] making it difficult to differentiate the two problems. Because abuse is related to a clearly defined act, children who are both abused and neglected may be classified as abused rather than neglected. To the extent that management strategies for abuse and neglect differ, it may be difficult to extrapolate neglect issues from studies in which abuse and neglect are intertwined. Yet, from a clinical perspective, because most maltreated children have experienced multiple forms of maltreatment, it is important to consider management strategies that address children who have experienced both abuse and neglect.

Theoretically derived definitions of neglect are an attempt at standardization in order to make reliable and valid estimates of incidence and prevalence and to ensure that studies about the causes, consequences, and treatment of neglect are comparable. Although research definitions of neglect are often broad,[1] they also reflect the lack of consensus about this subject. For example, there is no agreement on how to operationalize a developmental perspective, despite the recognition that definitions of neglect should consider children's age or developmental skills.[1] In addition, investigators dispute the importance of harm, severity, and chronicity[10] and of caregiver intentionality and responsibility in definitions of neglect.[18] Finally, the definition of neglect is further complicated by the recognition that there are multiple subtypes of neglect. Several authors differentiate between physical and emotional neglect:[3,4,10] *Physical neglect* includes not meeting the child's need for food, clothing, shelter, and safety. *Emotional neglect* involves the interpersonal environment of the home and often includes negative aspects of the child's sense of security and psychological safety, acceptance, self-esteem, positive regard, and autonomy.[4] Zuravin has suggested 14 types of neglect:

- refusal to provide physical care
- delay in providing physical health care
- refusal to provide mental health care
- delay in providing mental health care
- supervisory neglect
- custody refusal
- custody-related neglect
- abandonment/desertion
- failure to provide a permanent home
- personal hygiene neglect
- inadequate housing standards
- inadequate housing sanitation
- nutritional neglect
- educational neglect[59]

Just as management strategies for abuse and neglect may differ, management strategies may differ depending on the type of neglect that the child has experienced.

THEORETICAL EXPLANATIONS OF NEGLECT

Child protection is a basic tenet of all theories of child development, particularly during children's early years, when they are dependent upon adult caregivers. Yet societies have struggled with their responsibilities for children. Examples throughout history and literature give evidence of children suffering long-term consequences as a result of abandon-ment and neglect by their parents.[48] Many societies have enacted legislation to guarantee children's protection and to terminate parental rights or to punish parents who do not protect their children.

Behavioral Theory

When management strategies for neglected children are based on theories of behavior or behavior change, clinicians and investigators are guided by general principles and are able to predict and interpret the outcome. Children's dependency needs vary, based on their age and developmental level. To develop long-term management strategies for indi-viduals who have experienced neglect during their childhood, regardless of the type, it is necessary to understand how neglect disrupts the expected developmental process.[54] For example, abandonment or inconsistent care of children ages 6 to 18 months may be partic-ularly difficult, for this is when children are forming attachment relationships.[46]

Attachment Theory

Attachment theory describes the emerging relationship between a child and attachment figure (usually a parent) from a developmental perspective. Children whose needs are met in a predictable, consistent, affectionate manner are likely to develop secure attachments. In contrast, children whose needs are not met consistently or whose caregivers are neither predictable nor reliable are likely to develop insecure, anxious attachments.[8,13,14] Bowlby describes inadequate parents as establishing a model in which they compensate for their inadequacies by demanding that their children view them as perfect and incapable of mak-ing a mistake.[8] Any transgressions in the relationship are regarded as the fault of the child. This process may undermine children's psychological development. For example, in an innovative study in which maltreated and nonmaltreated children responded to scenarios about parents and children, abused and neglected children justified parental unkind be-havior as punishment for their own inappropriate behavior.[16]

Early attachment relationships are linked to subsequent relationships, because children form internal working models of expectations regarding relationships and integrate these expectations into their personalities.[8] In other words, based on early attachment relation-ships, children develop expectations about relationships that are translated into roles for caregivers (or friends) and roles for themselves. It is not surprising that children who have been neglected early in life are more likely to display attachment disorders,[19,49] to have difficulty discriminating emotions in others,[22] to be avoidant in peer relationships,[30] and are at risk for long-term relationship problems.[20]

Cognitive-plus-Attachment Theory

One theory of neglect integrates attachment and cognitive therapy.[12] In this model, neglect is a deficit in information processing, and neglecting parents "experience reality differently, interpret its meaning differently, select different responses from different reper-toires of responses, and implement these responses under different conditions." Deficits can occur at any point in the information processing sequence. As parents and children develop an interactive communication system, children signal their need for caregiving (e.g., through cries) and parents respond. When parents do not respond to the signal it may be because

1. they do not perceive the signal,
2. they perceive the signal but do not interpret it as requiring a parental response,
3. they recognize that a response is needed but do not have a response available, or
4. they recognize that a response is needed and select one, but do not implement it.

An important component of this model is that each type of reaction calls for a specific intervention.[13] Parents who do not perceive their children's signals may be completely overwhelmed with their own affective needs. In addition to intervention into their own mental health needs, they may require specific intervention to recognize their children's signals as requests for caregiving. Parents who perceive their children's signals and interpret them correctly but are unable to select an appropriate response may need assistance in accessing appropriate sources of information. Finally, parents may perceive signals, interpret them correctly, and select a response but fail to implement it because their environment is not supportive. Parents may "know" what to do but be unable to implement appropriate caregiving due to insufficient resources, limited competence, or competing demands.

All four levels of the model can be conceptualized in parental reaction to the child who signals hunger by crying. A depressed parent or one who is engaged in other activities may not even "hear" the cries and thus not respond. At the next level, a parent may hear the cries, but misinterpret them as the child being irritable rather than hungry. At the third level, a parent may understand that the child is hungry and requesting food but may either not know what to do or do something that is inappropriate (e.g., offer a pacifier instead of food, offer food the child cannot eat). Finally, a parent may know that she should feed the child but fail to follow through because there is not enough food, she does not know how to prepare the food, she does not have the energy to prepare and offer the food, or she has other caregiving demands.

Development-Ecological Theory

An ecological model of development uses systems theory to emphasize that development occurs within an interactive social context.[9] When the social context does not provide adequate protection, neglect occurs and children may experience developmental problems.[23] For example, children who have experienced neglect may have problems in the acquisition of language skills,[2,21] cognitive development,[30,43,45,47] and academic performance.[55] Thus, both investigations and interventions into child neglect must consider children's social context, particularly their family and the influences on the family.

The integration of developmental-ecological models of child development highlights the interactive influences of children, caregivers, and the surrounding environment and culture on children's development.[5,6,9] Applied to child maltreatment, the developmental-ecological model suggests that neglect is the result of multiple interacting factors, including child, family, community, and cultural characteristics,[5,6,50] at differing levels of proximity to the child.[7]

A recent application of developmental-ecological theory and structural equation modeling among very low income, inner-city families of infants and toddlers found that the relationship between neglect and child and family function differed by the type of neglect.[29] Emotional neglect was associated with a path from family functioning through perceptions of child temperament. There were no direct links from family functioning, support, or life events to emotional neglect; but mothers who were involved in well-functioning families were less likely to regard their child as having a difficult temperament, and children who were perceived as being relatively easy were less likely to experience emotional neglect. These findings illustrate the importance of conceptualizing neglect from a developmental-ecological perspective that incorporates the family and the child's contribution through temperament. The link between mothers' perception of their children's temperament and child neglect suggests that maternal perceptions of children's temperament are an important component of neglect that should be incorporated into management strategies. In contrast, when physical neglect was considered, there were no associations with child temperament and family context. Thus, different factors may be associated with physical and emotional neglect.

CORRELATES OF NEGLECT

Child neglect is strongly associated with poverty[40,43] and with the correlates of poverty, including dependence on public assistance, low parental education, maternal depression, large numbers of children, crowding, and limited resources.[23,35,37,39,41,60] Poverty and child neglect are so closely linked that it is often difficult to differentiate the two.[40,57] Nevertheless, within their low-income communities, neglecting families are viewed as deviant,[42] and most children raised in low-income families do not experience neglect.[58]

Neglect has also been associated with a lack of social support and feelings of loneliness.[25,43,44] Although neglecting mothers often live in low-income communities with limited opportunities for social support,[53] they may have fewer social skills and be less likely to take advantage of available resources than non-neglecting mothers living in the same communities.[15,43] For example, although neglectful and non-neglectful mothers in one study were equally likely to live close to their own mothers, neglectful mothers reported fewer positive relationships and received less emotional support from their mothers.[11] Without social support, mothers may feel less satisfied and have less access to community norms of parenting.

Neglect has also been associated with maternal depression and mood disorders.[24,53,57] Neglecting mothers have been described with apathy-futility syndrome, a condition that resembles depression but does not meet criteria for clinical depression.[43] In addition, neglecting parents have been described as immature with a tendency toward role reversal and difficulties establishing boundaries with their children.[43]

Finally, children who are perceived by their mother as having a difficult temperament may be more likely to experience neglect.[29] Mothers who rate their children as having difficult temperaments spend less time playing with them and are less responsive to their cues.[28,31,36] In addition, mothers reporting that their children are easily upset also report more negative affect than mothers who report that their children are less easily upset.[34] It is unclear whether the potential link between temperament and neglect is related to the challenges of caring for a difficult child or to difficulties in information processing[12] or maternal functioning[42,51] whereby children are perceived as difficult. However, these findings suggest that children who are perceived as being difficult may be more likely to be neglected.

CONCLUSION

In order to develop strategies for the effective management of neglected children, a consensus regarding the definition of neglect is needed. However, child neglect, an interdisciplinary concept, is seen differently by the different disciplines that are involved with it; and at present there is no generally accepted definition, although a number of constructs have been suggested. Sometimes there is difficulty even in differentiating neglect, abuse, and poverty, as the three often occur concurrently, and treatment and management must consider these overlapping issues and needs. Once the emergency medical issues for the neglected child are addressed (see chapter 12), parent, family, and community issues must also be considered in context. There is a range of reasons why parents may not respond to a child's needs, and these reasons must be sorted out because each reason calls for a specific intervention. Interventions are discussed in detail in the next three chapters.

REFERENCES

1. Aber JL, Zigler E. Developmental considerations in the definition of child maltreatment. *New Dir Child Dev* 1981;11:1–29.
2. Allen RE, Oliver JM. The effects of child maltreatment on language development. *Child Abuse Negl* 1982;6:299–305.
3. Barnett D, Manly JT, Cicchetti D. Continuing toward an operational definition of psychological maltreatment. *Dev Psychopathol* 1991;3:19–29.
4. Barnett D, Manly JT, Cicchetti D. Defining child maltreatment: The interface between policy and research. In Cicchetti D, Toth SL (eds.), *Advances in applied developmental psychology*, vol. 8: *Child abuse, child development, and social policy.* Norwood, NJ: Ablex Publishing. 1993.
5. Belsky J. Child maltreatment: An ecological integration. *Am Psychol* 1980;35:320–335.
6. Belsky J. Etiology of child maltreatment: A developmental-ecological analysis. *Psychol Bull* 1993;114:413–434.
7. Belsky J, Vondra J. Lessons from child abuse: The determinants of parenting. In Cicchetti D, Carlson V (eds.), *Child maltreatment: Theory and research on the causes and consequences of child abuse and neglect*, 153–202. New York: Cambridge University Press. 1989.
8. Bowlby J. *Attachment and loss*, vol. 3: *Loss.* New York: Basic Books. 1980.
9. Bronfenbrenner U. *The ecology of human development: Experiments by nature and design.* Cambridge: Harvard University Press. 1979.
10. Cicchetti D, Barnett D. Toward the development of a scientific nosology of child maltreatment. In Grove W, Cicchetti D (eds.), *Thinking clearly about psychology: Essays in honor of Paul E. Meehl*, vol. 2: *Personality and psychopathology.* Minneapolis: University of Minnesota Press. 1991.
11. Coohey C. Neglectful mothers, their mothers, and partners: The significance of mutual aid. *Child Abuse Negl* 1995;19;885–895.
12. Crittenden PM. An information-processing perspective on the behavior of neglectful parents. *Crim Just Behav* 1993;20:27–48.
13. Crittenden PM. Internal representational models of attachment relationships. *Inf Mental Health J* 1990;11:259–277.
14. Crittenden PM. Quality of attachment in the preschool years. *Dev Psychopathol* 1992;4:209–241.
15. Crittenden PM. Social networks, quality of childrearing, and child development. *Child Dev* 1985;56:1299–1313.
16. Dean AL, Malik MM, Richards W, Stringer SA. Effects of parental maltreatment on children's conceptions of interpersonal relationships. *Dev Psychol* 1986;22:617–626.

17. Dubowitz H, Black MM. Medical neglect. In Briere J, Berliner L, Bulkley JA, Jenny C, Reid T (eds.), *The APSAC handbook on child maltreatment,* 227–242. Thousand Oaks, CA: Sage Publications. 1996.

18. Dubowitz H, Black M, Starr RH Jr, Zuravin S. A conceptual definition of child neglect. *Crim Just Behav* 1993:20;8–26.

19. Egeland B, Farber EA. Infant-mother attachment: Factors related to its development and changes over time. *Child Dev* 1984:55;753–771.

20. Erickson MF, Egeland B. Child neglect. In Briere J, Berliner L, Bulkley JA, Jenny C, Reid T (eds.), *The APSAC handbook on child maltreatment,* 4–20. Thousand Oaks, CA: Sage Publications. 1996.

21. Fox L, Long SH, Sanglois A. Patterns of language comprehension deficit in abused and neglected children. *J Speech Hear Dis* 1988;53:239–244.

22. Frodi A, Smetana J. Abused, neglected, and nonmaltreated preschoolers' ability to discriminate emotions in others: The effects of IQ. *Child Abuse Negl* 1984;8:459–465.

23. Garbarino J, Crouter A. Defining the community context for parent-child relations: The correlates of child maltreatment. *Child Dev* 1978:49;604–616.

24. Gaudin JM Jr. Effective intervention with neglectful families. *Crim Just Behav* 1993:20;66–89.

25. Gaudin JM Jr, Polansky NA, Kilpatrick AC, Shilton P. Loneliness, depression, stress, and social supports in neglectful families. *Am J Orthopsychiatry* 1993:1;597–605.

26. Giovannoni J. Definitional issues in child maltreatment. In Cicchetti D, Carlson V (eds.), *Child maltreatment: Theory and research on the causes and consequences of child abuse and neglect,* 3–37. New York: Cambridge University Press. 1989.

27. Giovannoni JM, Becerra RM. Defining child abuse. New York: Free Press. 1979.

28. Goodman-Campbell S. Mother-infant interactions as a function of maternal ratings of temperament. *Child Psychiatry Hum Dev* 1979:10;67–76.

29. Harrington D, Black MM, Starr RH, Dubowitz H. Child neglect: A model of temperament and family context. *Am J Orthopsychiatry* 1998;68:108–116.

30. Hoffman-Plotkin D, Twentyman CT. A multimodal assessment of behavioral and cognitive deficits in abused and neglected preschoolers. *Child Dev* 1984;55:794–802.

31. Houldin AD. Infant temperament and the quality of the childrearing environment. *Matern Child Nurs J* 1987:16:131–143.

32. Kadushin A. Neglect in families. In Wunnally EW, Chilean CS, Cox FM (eds.), *Mental illness, delinquency, addictions, and neglect,* 147–166. Newbury Park, CA: Sage Publications. 1988.

33. Lutzker JR. Behavioral treatment of child neglect. *Behav Modif* 1990;14:301–315.

34. Mangelsdorf S, Gunnar M, Kestenbaum R, Lang S, Andreas D. Infant proneness-to-distress temperament, maternal personality, and mother-infant attachment: Association and goodness of fit. *Child Dev* 1990;61:820–831.

35. Martin MJ, Walters J. Familial correlates of selected types of child abuse and neglect. *J Marr Fam* 1982;44:267–276.

36. Milliones J. Relationship between perceived child temperament and maternal behaviors. *Child Dev* 1978;49;1255–1257.

37. Nelson KE, Landsman MJ. Alternative models of family preservation: Family-based services in context. Springfield, IL: Charles C. Thomas. 1992.

38. Ney PG, Fung T, Wickett AR. The worst combination of child abuse and neglect. *Child Abuse Negl* 1994;18:705–714.

39. Pelton LH. The myth of classlessness. *Am J Orthopsychiatry* 1987;48:608–617.

40. Pelton LH. Poverty and child protection. *Protecting Children* 1991;7:3–5.

41. Pianta R, Egeland B, Erickson MF. The antecedents of maltreatment: Results from the Mother-Child Interaction Research Project. In Cicchetti D, Carlson V (eds.), *Child maltreatment: Theory and research on the causes and consequences of child abuse and neglect,* 203–253. New York: Cambridge University Press. 1989.

42. Polansky NA, Ammons PW, Gaudin JM. Loneliness and isolation in child neglect: Social casework. *J Contemp Soc Work* 1985;38–47.

43. Polansky NA, Chalmers MA, Williams DP, Buttenweiser EW. Damaged parents: An anatomy of neglect. Chicago: University of Chicago Press. 1981.

44. Polansky NA, Gaudin JM, Ammons PW, Davis KB. The psychology ecology of the neglectful mother. *Child Abuse Negl* 1985;9:265–275.

45. Reyome ND. A comparison of the school performance of sexually abused, neglected, and non-maltreated children. *Child Study J* 1993;23:17–38.

46. Rutter M[ichael], Rutter M[arjorie]. Developing minds: Challenge and continuity across the life span. New York: Basic Books. 1993.

47. Sandgrund A, Gaines RW, Green AH. Child abuse and mental retardation: A problem of cause and effect. *Am J Ment Def* 1974;79:327–330.

48. Scheuerle WH. Cries of the children in the novels of Charles Dickens. In Deats SM, Lenker LT (eds,), *The aching hearth: Family violence in life and literature,* 149–163. New York: Plenum Press. 1991.

49. Schneider-Rosen K, Braunwald KG, Carlson V, Cicchetti D. Current perspectives in attachment theory: Illustrations from the study of maltreated infants. In Bretherton I, Waters E (eds.), *Monographs of the Society for Research in Child Development* 50 (1–2, serial no. 209) 1985;194–210.

50. Starr RH Jr. The controlled study of the ecology of child abuse and drug abuse. *Child Abuse Negl* 1978;2:19–28.

51. Twentyman C, Plotkin R. Unrealistic expectations of parents who maltreat their children: An educational deficit that pertains to child development. *J Clin Psychol* 1982;38:497–503.

52. U.S. Department of Health and Human Services, National Center on Child Abuse and Neglect. *Child maltreatment 1994: Reports from the states to the National Center on Child Abuse and Neglect.* Washington, DC: U.S. Government Printing Office 1996.

53. Vondra JI. The community context of child abuse and neglect. *Marr Fam Rev* 1990;15:19–38.

54. Werner EE, Smith RS. Vulnerable, but invincible: A study of resilient children. New York: McGraw-Hill. 1982.

55. Wodarski JS, Kurtz PD, Gaudin JM, Howing PT. Maltreatment and the school-aged child: Major academic, socioemotional, and adaptive outcomes. *Soc Work* 1990;35:460–467.

56. Wolock I, Horowitz B. Child maltreatment as a social problem: The neglect of neglect. *Am J Orthopsychiatry* 1984;54:530–543.

57. Zuravin SJ. Child maltreatment and teenage first births: A relationship mediated by chronic sociodemographic stress? *Am J Orthopsychiatry* 1988;50:91–103.

58. Zuravin SJ. The ecology of child abuse and neglect: Review of the literature and presentation of data. *Violence Vict* 1989;4:101–120.

59. Zuravin SJ. Research definitions of child physical abuse and neglect: Current problems. In Starr RH Jr, Wolfe DA (eds.), *The effects of child abuse and neglect: Issues and research,* 100–128. New York: Guilford. 1991.

60. Zuravin SJ. Residential density and urban child maltreatment: An aggregate analysis. *J Fam Viol* 1986;1:307–322.

Chapter 12

Initial Treatment of Child Neglect: Medical, Psychosocial, and Legal Considerations

Cindy W. Christian, M.D.,
Toni Seidl, R.N., M.S.W., and
Frank P. Cervone, J.D.

Child neglect—most often manifested in the medical setting by illness, developmental delay, preventable injury, or malnutrition—can frequently be missed. Growth and developmental delays, lead poisoning, and failure to thrive are medical conditions that may be in part attributable to neglect. In addition to medical consequences, educational, emotional, and behavioral problems are often present in neglected children, and medical and psychosocial assessments will be related. Because of the complex issues involved with neglect, the best treatment is achieved with a team approach, and initial effort should focus on establishing a stable "medical home" for the child, while the initial health screening and assessment of the child's developmental, educational and emotional health are completed. Treatment for failure to thrive must emphasize both nutritional rehabilitation and social issues. Many parents of neglected children are needy and damaged themselves and must be approached nonjudgmentally; in-home involvement of a social service professional is essential for treatment to be successful. Legal involvement may come with civil efforts to remove a child from the home or with criminal prosecution. Crimes associated with neglect include reckless endangerment, endangering the welfare of a child, assault, aggravated assault, and manslaughter or homicide, although child neglect is rarely prosecuted.

GENERAL CONSIDERATIONS

Child neglect is not precisely defined (see chapter 11) and many neglected children are not identified by our present standards. Identification and treatment typically begins because neglect has resulted in an objective, definable consequence to the child, such as injury or illness. For example, the child may present to the physician with malnutrition, severe untreated dental caries, injuries, or untreated illnesses. In an educational setting, neglect may be recognized by inappropriate dress or by learning or behavioral problems. To the child welfare worker, neglect may be identified by an unsafe or dirty home without adequate food, heat, hot water, or beds.[25]

Regardless of the initially recognized problem, the treatment of neglect must begin with a comprehensive evaluation that addresses the medical, physical, educational, and psychosocial needs of the child.

MEDICAL EVALUATION OF THE NEGLECTED CHILD

Neglected children are at risk for a wide range of medical problems. In the medical setting, child neglect is most often manifested by illness, developmental delay, preventable injury, or malnutrition. While most families of neglected children can benefit from voluntary health and social services, severely neglectful families require intervention from the child welfare system. In practice, however, only a minority of neglected children are referred to that system.

Many of the health care risks seen in neglected children are also identified frequently in children living in poverty, underscoring the close association of these conditions.[48] Most information on the health of neglected children is derived from studies about children in foster care and therefore is biased towards children who have been removed from their biological homes—those most severely affected. However, many of the medical, developmental, and psychological problems identified in foster children are also likely to affect neglected children who remain with their biological families.

Evaluations of children entering foster care[16,26] or living in foster[16,24,32,37,40,43] or kinship care[14] identify significant health problems of neglected children, indicating a need for systematic evaluation in the acute postdiagnostic period. In one study, comprehensive medical evaluations of 5,181 abused and neglected children entering the foster care system found that 44 percent had health problems.[16] Anemia, infectious diseases, and asthma were the most common medical diagnoses. For neglected children, the most common diagnoses included lead poisoning, failure to thrive, and developmental delay—conditions at least in part attributable to neglect.

Studies of children who continue to live in foster care have repeatedly shown a high prevalence of chronic medical problems,[16,24,32,37,40,43] many of which were not diagnosed when the children entered the foster care system.[37] The problems related to a range of issues, including growth, developmental delay, learning, and behavior, as described below. The prevalence of emotional, behavioral, and relational problems was greater for children who entered foster care after 2 years of age.

Growth problems are more common in foster care children than in the general population. Approximately 10 to 15 percent of foster children are diagnosed with short stature or failure to thrive,[24,26,32,37,40] and in the first study of the health of children in kinship care, 18 percent of adolescents were obese.[14]

Developmental delays are also overrepresented in foster children.[24,26,32,37,40] One study reports developmental delay in 61 percent of 113 children under the age of 6 living in foster care.[40] Of the children with developmental delay, only 40 percent were involved in an educational or therapeutic program. Developmental problems may reflect the child's past emotional deprivation.

School-aged children with a history of neglect have high rates of educational problems. As many as 50 percent of school-aged children tested have cognitive problems or failing school performance.[24,32] These educational problems may also reflect the child's past emotional neglect.

Behavioral and psychological problems affect many foster children, with rates of at least 35 percent reported by most researchers.[24,26,32,37,40] Standardized developmental and emotional assessments of 213 foster care children evaluated in a comprehensive primary care center for vulnerable children identified developmental or emotional problems in 84 percent of the children evaluated.[24]

Routine health care is inadequate for many foster children. In early studies of the health care of foster children, the majority had not had vision or hearing testing.[43] When foster children are assessed, vision and hearing problems are frequently identified and often have been previously unaddressed.[14,26,37,43] Immunization delays are found in 45 to 70 percent of children in foster care,[14,32,37] and dental problems are common and often neglected.[14,21,26,37,43]

Between 40 and 90 percent of children in foster care have been shown to have at least one serious or chronic health problem, and many have more.[14,24,26,32,37,40] It is estimated that chronic health problems are three to seven times more prevalent among foster children than in the general population.[37] This high rate of chronic disease makes inadequate health care an even more significant deficiency for this population.

Compounding the multiple health problems that affect foster children is a medical and social service system unable to meet the child's needs. Few child welfare agencies have specific policies that address the medical and mental health needs of foster children. Medical care is often plagued by inadequate funding, planning, and coordination.[2] With the increasing numbers of children entering foster care during the past decade, the American Academy of Pediatrics has recently proposed guidelines for the health care of children in foster care.[2] These standards, if met, could improve the medical health of all neglected children, regardless of their living situation.

The first step is the establishment of a stable "medical home" for the child. The most important goal of health care is to establish continuity and ensure comprehensive and coordinated treatment.[2] Access to physician care is associated with improved health for children living in poverty,[48] yet many neglected children may not have a primary care physician at the time of diagnosis. During the first few months after diagnosis, initial and comprehensive health and psychosocial assessments are required.

The next step is a complete initial health screening to identify immediate medical needs and unrecognized health problems that will need attention in the future. Neglected children often have multiple health needs that cannot be addressed at a single visit. Addressing the most urgent needs initially and formulating a follow-up plan can make the child's medical care seem less overwhelming for the parent and physician. For children entering foster care, the initial visit will alert the foster parent and social worker to medical problems they may have been unaware of. Growth parameters should be measured and plotted on National Center for Health Statistics growth charts. Because neglected children also may be victims of physical or sexual abuse, a careful and complete examination should search for indications of inflicted trauma. In addition, communicable diseases should be recognized and treated.

Neglected children, whether living in a foster, kinship, or biological home, need frequent medical visits. Within a month after diagnosis of neglect, a comprehensive medical examination should be performed by a physician who will assume a continuing role as the primary care provider for the child. The child's past and present medical history should be recorded. The examination should include growth assessments, blood pressure, vision and hearing screening, and a complete physical examination. Screening tests for anemia, lead poisoning, and tuberculosis are essential. Additional screening for the human immunodeficiency virus (HIV), sexually transmitted diseases, and other medical problems may be done depending on the individual's case history and the results of physical examination. The child's immunization records should be reviewed if available (often they are not) and the appropriate immunizations administered. The child's eligibility for various federal programs, such as Medicaid, Supplemental Security Income (SSI), early intervention programs, food supplements through the Women, Infants, and Children program (WIC) and Head Start should be assessed and the appropriate referrals made.

In addition, the physician should attempt to assess the child's developmental, educational, and emotional health. Although the rates of reported problems vary, many neglected children require a comprehensive developmental and mental health assessment. Unfortunately, such assessments are not universally available or easily obtained, and the impact that welfare reform and managed health care will have on this disadvantaged population is not fully known. California researchers compared the utilization of health services by foster care children to that of the general Medicaid population by reviewing fee-for-service Medi-Cal (California's Medicaid program) claims for one year.[23] Utilization of both inpatient and outpatient services were similar in the two groups, except for mental health service utilization, which was much greater for foster children.

MEDICAL MANAGEMENT OF SEVERE NEGLECT

Chronic and severe physical neglect occasionally results in death and is probably underreported.[1,31,44] These infants and young children typically suffer from multiple complications of severe malnutrition, including infection and hypothermia, and have lived in catastrophic, severely dysfunctional homes. The prevalence of severe protein-calorie malnutrition in American children is not known, but it is surely underrecognized.[27] For example, a study found 16 children who had been hospitalized at an urban pediatric hospital in a four-and-one-half year period and who were eventually found to have primary severe malnutrition, based on weight-for-age criteria. The severity of their malnutrition was determined only retrospectively and was not recognized in any of the children during hospitalization.[27] Most of the children were living in poverty, were the most recent children born into large sibships, and had no ongoing source of medical care. Only three had been enrolled in the WIC program prior to hospitalization. The mean percentage of median weight for age was 55 percent, and during hospitalization, the average weight gain was 44 grams per day. Over half of the children were discharged to foster care.

The clinical patterns of severe malnutrition vary geographically.[45] Neglected American children seem to suffer more commonly from marasmus (protein-calorie deficiency) than kwashiorkor (primary protein deficiency).[27] In our experience, severely neglected infants rarely have been physically abused, in contrast to older children, whom we have found have often been both battered and starved.

Initial Medical Management of FTT

Failure to thrive (FTT) is the term given to malnourished infants and young children who fail to meet expected standards of growth. As most children with poor growth related to medical disease are identified early, the diagnosis is usually reserved for children whose malnutrition is related primarily to psychosocial and environmental problems. For many children with FTT, growth failure is but one manifestation of more significant family problems. Some researchers have suggested that the term be replaced with other generic terms, such as growth failure,[29] growth deficiency,[6] or with a specific etiologic diagnosis. Whatever the label, it is essential that the medical, nutritional, developmental, psychosocial, and environmental contributors be addressed during the initial management.

Because the possible causes of growth failure are so diverse, the management of FTT begins with a thorough search for its etiology. In a majority of cases, a comprehensive history and physical examination are sufficient to eliminate medical diseases as the cause for FTT. The appropriate laboratory evaluation is guided by the history and physical. An extensive, random laboratory search for medical diseases has no merit.[39] However, simple screening tests are recommended to screen for the common illnesses that may cause growth failure and to search for medical problems that result from malnutrition. The recommended laboratory tests include

- complete blood count (CBC) to screen for chronic blood loss, malignancy, infection, iron deficiency anemia, and lead toxicity
- urinalysis, urine culture, and serum electrolytes to assess renal infection or dysfunction
- PPD to screen for tuberculosis
- chemistry panel, which includes serum albumin, calcium, phosphorus, liver function tests, and a sedimentation rate (often but not invariably recommended)
- HIV testing (for selected children)
- stool for culture and ova and parasites (for children with diarrhea, abdominal pain, or malodorous stools)

For most children with FTT, treatment must emphasize both social issues and nutritional rehabilitation.[46] Initially, however, the therapy should focus on the nutritional and medical management of the patient and on engaging the family in the treatment plan. Parents of children with FTT may feel personally responsible and threatened by the diagnosis of malnutrition, or they may be so isolated, depressed, or dysfunctional that they cannot prioritize treatment of the child's growth failure.[12] Additionally, some parents misunderstand FTT as a physical or growth problem and do not identify family, psychosocial, or environmental factors as causative.[12] These differences in perception can greatly affect the long-term success of treatment.

A multidisciplinary approach to treatment is almost always warranted. Children with mild malnutrition and an identifiable cause may be successfully managed by the physician and family. However, even in seemingly straightforward cases, more significant causes may underlie the problem. For example, maternal illiteracy and impaired cognitive development are often associated with improper formula preparation, suggesting the need for additional family supports.[30] While the developmental and functional outcomes of different FTT treatment strategies have not been rigorously investigated, evidence exists that a team approach to treatment results in improved weight gain for children with FTT.[7] One study comparing the six-month weight gain of children with nonorganic FTT treated by a multidisciplinary team and by a primary care program found significantly better growth in children treated by the team. The children were classified as suffering from mild, moderate, or severe malnutrition. The multidisciplinary team consisted of a pediatrician or pediatric gastroenterologist, a nutritionist, developmental specialist, nurse practitioner, child psychiatrist, and social worker. Both the nurse practitioner and social worker made home visits. The hospital-based primary care program consisted of a pediatrician, pediatric resident, or a nurse practitioner. Children treated by the multidisciplinary team were more severely malnourished than those treated by the primary care program, yet for all classifications of malnutrition (mild, moderate, and severe), the children treated by the multidisciplinary team showed significantly better growth over the six-month period. Children treated by the multidisciplinary team also had significantly more contact with the treating team and had a better history of keeping referral appointments.

The majority of children with FTT can be managed in the outpatient setting, if the social issues can be adequately addressed. Hospitalization is indicated for children with severe malnutrition (less than 60% weight for age; less than 70% weight for height), those with serious intercurrent infections, when there is an immediate threat to the child's safety, if the child requires extensive multidisciplinary evaluation that is not available in the outpatient setting, or if intensive outpatient management has failed to result in catch-up growth.[17]

Initial goals of therapy for the malnourished child include

1. initiation of catch-up growth,
2. treatment of medical problems associated with FTT, and
3. initiation of parental education regarding nutrition and feeding.

Catch-up Growth

Because malnutrition is the biologic problem of all children with FTT, the cornerstone of treatment is nutritional management. Energy (caloric) requirements are greatest in early infancy and decline with advancing age. On average, infants in the first six months of life require approximately 90 to 110 kilocalories per kilogram of body weight per day (90–110kcal/kg/day) to meet their needs for activity and growth, and older infants and toddlers require slightly less. For any given child, however, additional factors may affect energy requirements, including body size, activity, illness, injury, and abnormal losses of nutrients. On occasion, a child's energy requirements are met, but dietary intake may be inadequate in specific nutrients, especially in deficiency states. Malnourished children may be ingesting enough calories to meet the requirements based on their weight and length but not for their age.[29]

In order to promote catch-up growth, children with FTT may require 1.5 times or more than the expected calorie and protein intake for their age.[9,47] In order to achieve these requirements, most children with FTT require calorically dense foods, as malnourished children may be anorexic and cannot be expected to double their food intake. For formula-fed infants, this is most easily accomplished by changing the concentration of formula, which increases the caloric density from 20 calories per ounce to 24 or 27 calories per ounce (see table 12.1). However, it is important to instruct parents not to independently adjust the formula composition, as concentrated formula can cause diarrhea or hypernatremia. For older children, dietary improvements should include increasing the caloric density of favored foods, with butter, margarine or oil, sour cream, peanut butter and other high caloric foods. High calorie oral supplementation formulas that provide 30kcal/oz are readily available, and are often well tolerated by the child.

Sometimes a less aggressive initial nutritional rehabilitation is necessary before more calorically dense regimens can be tolerated. Specific carbohydrates, fats, or proteins are also available as dietary additives. These preparations have the advantage of increasing the caloric density of foods without significantly increasing the volume consumed. Consultation with a clinical nutritionist is recommended to assist in choosing an appropriate and cost-effective additive.

As a general rule, the simplest and least costly effective approach to dietary change is

TABLE 12.1
Formula preparation for increasing caloric concentrations

Concentration	Amount of Powder/Liquid	Water (oz)
20kcal/oz	1 cup powdered formula	29
	4 scoops powdered formula	8
	13 oz liquid concentrate	13
24kcal/oz	1 cup powdered formula	24
	5 scoops powdered formula	8
	13 oz liquid concentrate	9
27kcal/oz	1 cup powdered formula	21
	5.5 scoops powdered formula	8
	13 oz liquid concentrate	6
30kcal/oz	1 cup powdered formula	18
	6 scoops powdered formula	8
	13 oz liquid concentrate	4

SOURCE: Adapted from Darby MH (ed.). *Department of Pharmacy Services pharmacy handbook and formulary,* 395. (Children's Hospital of Philadelphia) Hudson, OH: Lexi-Comp. 1995.

recommended. Depending on the severity of malnutrition, initiation of catch-up growth may take up to two weeks of refeeding.[9] Initially, weight gains of two to three times the normal growth rate for age may be observed. Care must be taken to ensure that initial rapid weight gain is not due to edema related to refeeding syndrome (see below). The normal growth rates for age documented by Guo et al. can serve as a guide for comparison.[22] During catch-up growth, weight gain will precede improvements in height. Months of refeeding are required to restore the patient's weight for height, stature, and head circumference.

In addition to providing adequate energy and protein, vitamin and mineral supplementation is essential. Many children with FTT are deficient in micronutrients, especially iron. In addition, all children with catch-up requirements need increased vitamins and minerals during the period of rapid growth. A multivitamin with iron and zinc is recommended for all malnourished children.

Associated Medical Problems

The interaction between malnutrition and infection is well known.[5,20] Malnutrition causes multiple defects in host defenses, involving abnormalities in epithelial barriers, complement, immunoglobulins, and cell-mediated immunity.[10] Additionally, infection increases the metabolic needs of the patient, and is often associated with anorexia. Therefore, children with FTT may suffer from a malnutrition-infection cycle, in which recurrent infections exacerbate the malnutrition, increasing the child's susceptibility to further infections.

During initial treatment, medical diseases that accompany FTT need to be identified and treated. Appropriate evaluations for otitis media, respiratory infections, and urinary and gastrointestinal infections should be based on the history and physical examination. It should be remembered that the signs of infection may be blunted in the malnourished child. The identified illnesses and the need for treatment should be carefully explained to the parent. It may be helpful to explain how the child's nutrition and infection relate to each other, to underscore the need to follow through with treatment. Again, the treatment regimen should be appropriate, but as simple as feasible in order to improve compliance.

Initiation of Parental Education

Successful long-term treatment of FTT requires a working relationship between the physician, the child, and the family. It has been recognized for decades that a punitive approach, in which the parent is blamed for the child's condition, can be damaging to both child and parent.[4] With some families, building a working relationship can be challenging for even the most skilled physician. Parents struggling with economic, social, and psychologic challenges may not be easily engaged, especially if alcohol or substance abuse is involved. Successful intervention is only possible, however, if the treating team approaches the family in a professional, nonjudgmental way. Expressions of anger, frustration, or hostility are neither necessary nor productive.

After the assessment, the diagnosis and causes of the malnutrition should be discussed with the parent in an open, supportive way. The physician should make very clear that malnutrition is not normal for a child nor due to an intrinsic disease. The risks of malnutrition for the child's future growth and development should be reviewed. Plans for initial nutritional management, medical therapy, and home support should be addressed. The importance of the parent's involvement in the child's management should be emphasized. The parent must understand that malnutrition may take months to correct and will require frequent contact with the medical community. Finally, it is important that the physician not separate himself from the personal relationship with the parents but work together with the social worker and other team members to engage the parent in the treatment plan.[4]

THE REFEEDING SYNDROME

During starvation, the body utilizes endogenous stores of glycogen, fats, and proteins to maintain metabolic requirements. Metabolic processes and growth are slowed to minimize the need for nutrients. Starvation is also characterized by decreases in total body potassium, magnesium, phosphorus, and other compounds. As the body attempts to maintain homeostasis during starvation, it is often capable of maintaining normal serum concentrations of electrolytes. This is partially related to the decreased blood volume commonly associated with malnutrition.

During rapid refeeding, fluid and electrolyte homeostasis may be lost and the body may be unable to maintain normal serum concentrations of vital electrolytes. Rapid expansion of the contracted blood volume may overwhelm the heart, inducing congestive heart failure and fluid retention, further altering serum electrolyte concentrations. This may further depress myocardial function. These changes and the associated complications resulting from the shifts that occur in malnourished patients undergoing overly rapid and aggressive refeeding are collectively termed the refeeding syndrome. The changes affect phosphorus, potassium, calcium, and magnesium and can result in life-threatening cardiac, pulmonary, or neurologic problems. Infants and children at risk for refeeding syndrome are those with marasmus, kwashiorkor, anorexia nervosa, and those who have experienced prolonged fasting.[41]

Ideally, the refeeding syndrome should be prevented, but more commonly it remains simply unrecognized. A significant disturbance that contributes to refeeding syndrome is hypophosphatemia. Refeeding hypophosphatemia is thought to result from total body depletion during starvation, coupled with increased cellular influx of phosphorus during anabolic refeeding. In turn, marked hypophosphatemia may result in cardiac (arrhythmia, congestive heart failure), hematologic (hemolytic anemia, thrombocytopenia, and hemorrhage), neurologic (coma and seizures), and pulmonary abnormalities.[41] Cardiac, neurologic, and pulmonary complications are the most clinically important.

The refeeding syndrome in severely neglected infants recovering from starvation has not been reported but likely has occurred. Avoidance of the refeeding syndrome should be the standard of care and is best accomplished by slow refeeding of severely malnourished children, with meticulous attention to fluid and electrolyte status.

Nutritional therapy should begin slowly. Although in general, enteral feeds are preferred, infants with life-threatening malnutrition suffer from villous atrophy, decreased secretion of pancreatic enzymes, and intestinal malabsorption,[42] and the use of parenteral nutrition may be required. We generally begin feeds at approximately 50 to 75 percent of the child's estimated needs and increase by 10 to 20 percent each day as tolerated. A balanced regimen of carbohydrate, protein, and fats is provided, and electrolyte and mineral requirements, based on daily requirements for age, are supplied. Serum glucose, sodium, potassium, phosphorus, calcium, and magnesium are monitored every eight hours, and adjustments in fluids and electrolytes are made as needed. Extra phosphorus, potassium, and magnesium are commonly required. It must be remembered that these oral supplements are generally hyperosmolar, irritating to the gastrointestinal tract, and therefore may not be well absorbed. All infants are given multivitamins and are assessed for vitamin deficiencies as indicated. As feedings are increased and catch-up growth initiated, it may be useful to provide twice the recommended daily allowance of vitamins and minerals. Daily weights are recorded, and weekly measurements of serum prealbumin are used to assess protein and calorie intake during the past week. During parenteral feeding, enteral feeds are slowly begun. As the patient improves, enteral feeds are advanced and parenteral feeds are decreased accordingly. Significant electrolyte abnormalities and significant edema are indications to either decrease the caloric delivery or slow the increase in caloric delivery, until further vitamin or mineral supplements correct the deficiency or the edema begins to resolve.

CHILD PROTECTIVE SERVICES INVOLVEMENT

Ongoing involvement of a social service professional to work with the child and family in the home is essential to the success of treatment. In some communities, hospital-based multidisciplinary programs include social workers and public health nurses who are available to work intensively with families at home.[7] In other communities, private social service agencies can be enlisted by the medical community to provide home services and ongoing feedback to the medical team. However, in some locales, social services to families in need can only be obtained through referrals to the local child welfare agency, who in turn may contract services out to a private agency. For some communities, therefore, child protective services (CPS) involvement is common and not necessarily indicative of severe neglect.

In communities that do not require a referral to CPS to obtain home services, CPS involvement is still occasionally required. Referrals to CPS should be made immediately for any child with evidence of inflicted injury or whose safety with the family is in doubt. Children often need to be placed in an alternative home if parents are actively drug addicted, psychotic, or have intentionally withheld food from them. Finally, families may be referred to child welfare after attempts at engaging the family and providing for improved functioning have failed and the child's well-being is judged to be at continued jeopardy.

The decision to refer a family to CPS should be made carefully and should be discussed with the family prior to doing so. As always, the discussion with the parent should not be punitive but should focus on the concern for and well-being of the child.

PSYCHOSOCIAL CONSIDERATIONS

Whatever the presentation or severity of a child's neglect, his or her illness represents the failure of society's safety net. The medical manifestations of neglect are many and distinct. The common elements in each case are parents or caretakers who are emotionally fragile and isolated.[35] With the identification of neglect, and the ensuing medical, psychosocial, and legal crises this represents, parents may become further stressed and alienated from their support network.

Although the medical sequelae of neglect require specific medical interventions, the initial assessment and treatment of the family is, in fact, usually more generic. The expectations we make of parents are similar regardless of the severity of the neglect. What is likely to differ, however, is the pace and order of the interventions. The number of external systems called on to respond may differ, depending on the clinical situation. For example, mild malnutrition may be sufficiently handled by the physician and the medical social worker, but neglect that has become more serious or protracted often requires child protective services intervention. When the threshold for criminality is reached, as it is in the severest forms of neglect, referrals to the criminal justice system will be necessary.

Regardless of the severity or chronicity of the neglect, the health care team's identification of a problem and its subsequent response create a crisis for the family. Time-honored thinking about crisis intervention informs us that although painful and profoundly challenging, personal crises have the potential to promote growth and create an enhanced level of functioning in those affected. From this positive perspective, a crisis can be perceived as a catalyst that disrupts previously dysfunctional modes and patterns of functioning and evokes new and more constructive responses from an individual or a family.[19] The goal of intervention, therefore, is to create an atmosphere that does more than merely acknowledge past problems, but allows for hopefulness and constructive problem solving. This can be a daunting task for all involved. The eventual plan crafted for change must be comprehensive and focus on immediate and long-term changes. Needs may range from parental education and access to entitlement services to mental health, drug, and alcohol treatment. In order for a plan to be useful and relevant, it must be created mutually by parents and practitioners. The formation of a plan takes place only after thorough assessment of the patient and family.

The evaluation begins by establishing a therapeutic alliance with the family, in the context of the discussion of the child's medical management. We approach the conversation as if we have two patients, the ill child and the family. Caring for the parents requires understanding their emotional state and present circumstances.[36,38] Deference, a show of empathy, and respect are the key attitudes required in assessing those who are in an emotional state of crisis. Parents often have tremendous difficulty appreciating that the child they see as normal and appropriate is, in fact, in danger. This misperception is influenced by many psychological and environmental factors, including mental illness (most commonly maternal depression), drug and/or alcohol abuse, and distraction and lack of energy resulting from domestic violence, poverty, illiteracy, under- or unemployment, substandard housing, and overwhelming child care responsibilities. When we raise issues regarding the quality of parenting, regardless of the contributing factors, we expose the parent's vulnerability. In response, some parents withdraw from involvement with the team and others become defensive. If done carefully, however, the initial assessment can begin to build a positive, rather than adversarial, relationship between the parent and the providers.

The initial assessment centers on the condition of the child and on clarifying discrepancies between the parent's perception and the objective assessment of the child's condition. Parents are asked to relate their perception of the child's presenting problem and how the problem evolved. They are asked to describe the child and the circumstances around which care was sought, if it was sought. To accomplish this task, the treatment team needs to join with the family by reaching out to them as individuals who, along with the child, are the center of the team effort. Since our approach to history taking tends to be excruciatingly detailed, we allow ourselves a good deal of time and are prepared with a good deal of patience. History taking can be a nonlinear and emotional event for the family.

Through a process of empathic questioning we begin with general questions about the child and move toward more specific details of his or her care and illness. The pace of this interview will be determined by the parent's openness or reticence to discussion of these details. Even parents of critically neglected children are often open initially to discussing their child's condition. Precise information regarding feeding schedules, nutritional intake, persons responsible for feeding and caretaking, child behaviors, and patterns of daily living can all be gleaned at this point.

If unchallenged, parents are likely to allow the practitioner to inquire further about the following areas of family life:

- support systems (friends and relatives)
- housing
- social networks (including child welfare)
- means of financial support
- source of health care
- characteristics of the relationship with an intimate partner
- personal goals including education and career

Depending on the response, more direct questions can be posed, such as the parent's schooling and grade-level attainment, experience with drugs and alcohol (past, present, and by family members). A complete psychosocial history should also include inquiry into experience with personal loss as well as general stressors, such as overwhelming responsibility for other persons and the illness of family members.

The histories offered by neglectful families are often disturbing. They are likely to reveal misunderstandings about the child's development, dietary intake, and behavior. They often embrace myriad unrealistic expectations about the child's needs and perceptions about interactive cues. What may be missing from the history is the presence of any empathy for the child's condition.[15] In our experience, lack of empathy is a very poor prognostic sign, indicative of parents' inability to appreciate the seriousness of the child's condition. It also suggests that they will not be able to conscientiously follow through on recommendations. Unfortunately, many of the parents we see are so needy and damaged themselves that they have little internal reserve to offer in parenting their own children. In many cases, parents of neglected children present as neglected themselves. The old maxim applies: one cannot give what one does not have. The level of parental attachment is usually apparent during the first hours and days of treatment. Our concern escalates when we observe parents who deny or minimize the child's condition, are not empathic and appear detached from the child's hospitalization and accompanying procedures, or are more concerned with themselves than with the child's well-being.

Through this evaluative process, the professionals will begin to assess the parent's cognitive resources, emotional state, and whether the risk to the child is reversible. We cannot stress how important this is in formulating a plan that will eventually lead to timely and well-suited recommendations. The recognition of active mental illness, drug or alcohol addiction, domestic violence, or mental retardation at the earliest stage of an assessment will prevent misplaced efforts and frustration for both the team and the family.

After hearing the history from the family, the practitioner is obligated to share with parents any findings that differ from the parent's narrative. By stating our concerns about the child up-front in a clear, precise, and thoughtful way, we can give comfort and direction at the time when the parent is most undefensive, and consequently most open to engagement. Parental response to this direct and potentially threatening information serves to be diagnostic on several fronts. It reveals whether or not the family has the potential to move forward in an unreserved manner, with assistance from the community agencies. It also tells us how well the parent appreciates the seriousness of the child's plight.

We would be remiss not to mention how counterintuitive this approach is to us as pediatric practitioners when confronted with a devastatingly neglected child. It is certainly easier and less emotionally conflicting to banish parents, report them to the child protective services system, and focus undistractedly on the medical needs of the acutely ill child. However severe the neglect, conversation with parents should be gentle and nonaccusatory, without the assignment of blame. At the same time, however, we do firmly establish the concept that the parents are responsible for their children. This is, in fact, our first psychosocial intervention, and one that gives us a framework for exploring the family's history, values, culture, coping mechanisms, level of function, ecology, resources, and social supports. These data form the basis of our clinical impression regarding the etiology of the illness, the affective quality of the parent-child relationship, and the parent's potential to form a collaborative trusting alliance with providers.

In our practice, the medical and psychosocial assessments are interrelated and are obtained in an integrated fashion as much as possible. Assessing and treating neglect from an interdisciplinary perspective has long been accepted as the sine qua non of the experienced practitioner.[8,28] This approach helps the family know that their family is cared for by practitioners with specific but overlapping roles and responsibilities. It also prevents family members from dividing the practitioners and lessens the likelihood of their undermining the treatment plan. It is rare that we consider a solo meeting with a parent. When we do, it is purposeful and determined by the team.

Acceptance by parents and caretakers of their past difficulties in parenting and the associated implications for the child is a requisite ingredient for change. Parents who are not able to confront their vulnerabilities tend to be unavailable for participation in the change process. On the other hand, when parents acknowledge and assume responsibility for the omissions in care that have caused risk to their child, we consider that a positive prognostic sign. This very ownership of the problem is a characteristic that suggests a level of self-awareness and openness that is predictive of a successful outcome. Over the years, we have encountered families who can be engaged in lifestyle changes for themselves and their children. These families tend to be future oriented and not stymied by the predictable hard work of exposing their lives to outsiders at an almost microscopic level. They are able to form partnerships with the providers who offer them concrete referrals and direct services as well as emotional support. (For more on long-term management, see chapter 14.)

There are times when our team completes a biopsychosocial and environmental family history and is amazed that the situation before us is not far worse than it is. Whatever the case, our approach always needs to be flexible enough to address the individual needs of each family. No assessment focused exclusively on vulnerabilities gives us the true picture of a parent's potential to change. Assessments must focus on strengths as well as vulnerabilities,[11] so that we can begin interventions at a point where parents can meet with an initial success rather than an initial failure.

LEGAL CONSIDERATIONS

Legal definitions of neglect depend on the context and usage of the term.[18] Many states include neglect in the statutory definition of child abuse. For example, the Pennsylvania Child Protective Services law defines the term *child abuse* as including "serious physical neglect by a perpetrator constituting prolonged or repeated lack of supervision or the failure to provide essentials of life, including adequate medical care, which endangers a child's life or development or impairs the child's functioning."[33] Few jurisdictions designate "child neglect" as a crime; instead they focus on offenses such as child endangerment, assault, or even manslaughter or homicide.

CIVIL NEGLECT AND CHILD WELFARE

In most neglect cases, both the courts and social service systems work within a construct of incremental intrusion into the life of a child and family. Sometimes the child remains with the neglectful parent, with supportive services and oversight offered by a public or private child welfare agency. A child will be removed from the home only after less drastic interventions have been tried and have failed. Since removal of a child from his or her parent is a severe intrusion into the civil rights of the parent, a higher legal standard must be met: Is the child at risk of harm? Does the child need to be placed in foster or kinship care, or would court-ordered cooperation of the parent be sufficient to provide the child with needed care?

Likewise, there are different points of intervention, and not every part of the legal system is involved in every case. The case of an unsupervised child might begin with a phone call to the police from a neighbor who believes the child is home without supervision. Law enforcement could prosecute criminally for endangerment of the child but more typically will go no further than to take the child to the local child welfare agency for intervention in the situation. If the abandonment resulted in some severe injury or deprivation, the case might go from the police to the hospital and to the arrest of a parent.

Neglect cases require civil court action when a coercive authority is needed to gain control of a child's care. Cases that meet the threshold for civil proceedings are known in various jurisdictions as dependency, supervision, abuse, or care-and-protection cases. The parties include representatives for the parent, the child, and the state or county child welfare agency. The court will be asked to find that the parent has not met or cannot meet the child's needs, and the court may determine that state intervention is required. Depending on local law, the court will find that the child is a "person in need of supervision" or a "dependent child." However, the immediate intervention in a neglect case rarely results in termination of parental rights. Rather, the legal steps are incremental, justifying state intrusion into the life of this child and family. Parents remain involved and even in control of many decisions.

In order to substantiate a neglect case as child abuse, one must have substantial evidence that the abuse occurred. Yet, even in the eyes of the law, neglect cases are ambiguous. Consider the child with so little nurturance in his life that he fails to show any signs of attachment or affect. When does the emotionally needy child become the emotionally neglected child? When does neglect become criminal?

CRIMINAL NEGLECT

In contrast to the civil child welfare case, a criminal prosecution for neglect is rare. Crimes associated with neglect include reckless endangerment, endangering the welfare of a child, assault, aggravated assault, and manslaughter or homicide.

From a practical viewpoint, the law and its functionaries—child protective services workers, prosecutors, judges—will find important distinctions in the severity of neglect. Severely ill children who present acutely occasionally necessitate a police report and an arrest. Chronic, less severe deprivation seldom results in criminal proceedings, even though the damage may be profound and lasting. Neglect rises to the level of criminal behavior when a public official with the authority to arrest or charge believes that the person responsible should be punished and there is sufficient evidence to prosecute successfully.

The elements of a crime include an act, an intention, and, typically, a harm. The act requirement focuses on the conduct of the accused. Since the criminal law is about punishment for violations of societal rules, it rarely mandates affirmative actions. Parents and other caregivers hold a special duty to provide care and supervision, especially for young children who cannot sustain themselves. In this way neglect is different from most crimes, as it focuses on the inaction of a caregiver.

Under most crimes, the actor must have known or should have known the effects of his actions. For example, the crime is not simply that the child lost weight precipitously but that the child was in the parent's care and the parent had reason to know the effects of failing to feed the child. Compare the situation of a medical illness which results in malnutrition; such "organic" causes are not attributed to the intention of the caregiver, even when the caregiver is aware of the medical problem. Some crimes also have a "recklessness" standard: the perpetrator acts with such reckless disregard for life as to make the specific state of mind irrelevant.

Much of neglect practice involves inferences of causation. One concept of inferential proof is "exclusive control" and the doctrine of *res ipsa loquitur* (the thing speaks for itself). The classic res ipsa case involves a sack of flour falling from a second story window and hitting a passerby on the head. If there was only one person in the room with the window, we can reasonably infer that he somehow caused the sack to reach the window sill and—on purpose or by accident or negligence—fall to the ground. How can we make the child neglect case inferentially? Here is an example: A young child fell from the window of a homeless shelter. The window was well above the height of the child's crib, and with the window pane opened into the room, the child would have had to pull him- or herself up and over the window frame. Witnesses placed the mother in the room around the time of the fall. The child's fall was broken by a shrub at ground level and she sustained two broken legs. Mother eventually pled guilty to a charge of reckless endangerment of the child.

The criminal standard of "proof beyond a reasonable doubt" presents a much higher burden than the civil benchmarks of "preponderance of the evidence" or "clear and convincing evidence." In neglect cases, the possibility of confounding medical and environmental factors and the difficulty in proving specific parental intention usually make it difficult to meet the criminal standard of proof.

DOCUMENTATION

The challenge of preparing medical and psychosocial information for use in the courtroom requires a high level of ongoing collaboration among professionals from all disciplines involved. Immediately following the identification of neglect, the treating physician should identify and document a course of evaluation and treatment that will both respond to the child's needs and provide a written record for possible later use in the court system. The medical social worker should create a record of the team's interactions with the family, including the recommendations and referrals made. The chief legal consideration for the non-lawyer in the immediate postdiagnostic period is to make a record that a court might later be able to rely upon and a lawyer could use. When hospital staff create a record, they must be mindful that the record has uses other than immediate communication of medical treatment information. Like most recordkeeping, medical records have the dual purpose of informing the present caregivers and making the record of one's present care available for future accountability.

The record should speak for itself, in time, content and accuracy. The notes should document who was present, what questions were asked, and, if possible, when the recording was made. Because a neglect case may involve proof of some degree of parental resistance or inability to provide needed care, that information should be documented objectively. The participation and awareness of the parent may be relevant, as team members and the court may be considering what the person knew and when he or she knew it. What was the form and content of the plan developed with the family? Who participated in the formation of the plan? What parent-child interactions were observed? Did the parent express an understanding of the problem and the proposed interventions?

If and when medical records are used in a legal proceeding, the lawyer using them will have to contend with several rules that are designed to ensure the integrity and reliability of the records. Someone must demonstrate who was responsible for and in control of the record. The record must be authenticated as the actual document produced by the hospital. Lastly, because the records are hearsay evidence, that is, out-of-court statements brought in second-hand, they will be admissible only if they qualify under the recognized exceptions of records maintained in regular course of business. These rules help to define the terms of creating and managing information. (Hearsay rules and other legal concepts are discussed more fully in chapter 23.)

THE CHILD ADVOCATE

Both civil and criminal interventions can be frustrated by a simple structural impediment: there is often no medical, child welfare, or legal continuity of care for the neglected child. The systems involved have no long-term memory with which to act, thwarting adequate preparation for court proceedings. For civil proceedings, the lawyer will need time to identify, collect, and study the relevant evidence, interview the treating professionals and consult with experts, and schedule and subpoena witnesses. While a child sexual or physical abuse case may consume 2 to 5 hours of preparation time in order to bring the case to a civil trial, a neglect case might require 10 to 50 hours' effort. In the criminal context, there are laws that govern the amount of time allowed before trial, so preparation time is pressured.

Some jurisdictions provide a lawyer or other person to represent the child's needs and interests in the legal arena, and this advocacy is helpful. Lawyers for children (the child advocate) may attend both the civil dependency hearing and criminal hearings and trials. Working with social workers, they can assess the child's safety by conducting home visits, reviewing relevant documents such as police reports, child welfare files, hospital records, school records, and psychological reports, and by contacting service providers to investigate or press for the provision of needed services.

The child advocate should maintain contact with the child and the child's caregivers. According to the American Bar Association, "establishing and maintaining a relationship with a child is the foundation of representation."[3] Child clients who are old enough need to be taught what to expect when they go to court or to an interview, and they should be accompanied and supported throughout court testimony. Some jurisdictions offer court school programs to make the legal proceeding more familiar to a child witness.

Pro bono attorneys and lay volunteers, known in many areas as court-appointed special advocates, or CASAs, offer resources to child welfare systems. Compared to lawyers for the county agency and for the parents, the child advocate can often focus more time and attention on the case. While there is some risk of micromanagement, the attention to the details of a neglect case can make a positive difference in service delivery and parental accountability.

CONCLUSION

The health issues of the neglected child may encompass a range of medical problems, including malnutrition, failure to thrive, preventable injury, and developmental delay. The complexity of neglect cases usually necessitates a team approach, and medical practitioners may also find themselves concerned with psychological, social, and legal issues. Indeed, these issues often play into the medical treatment of neglect. The emotional fragility and isolation of parents or caretakers of neglected children is a common thread and must be addressed. This is doubly important when the child is to remain in the biological home. Medical practitioners also have an important role to play in the documentation of the neglect, which is likely to be an important part of any ensuing legal actions, either civil or criminal.

REFERENCES

1. Adelson L. Homicide by starvation. *JAMA* 1965;186:458–460.
2. American Academy of Pediatrics. Health care of children in foster care. *Pediatrics* 1994; 93:335–338.
3. American Bar Association. Standards of practice for lawyers who represent children in abuse and neglect cases, 1996, § C-1.
4. Barbero GJ, Shaheen E. Environmental failure to thrive: A clinical view. *J Pediatr* 1967; 71:639–644.
5. Berkowitz FE. Infections in children with severe protein-energy malnutrition. *Pediatr Infect Dis J* 1992;11:750–759.

6. Bithoney WG, Dubowitz H, Egan H. Failure to thrive/growth deficiency. *Pediatr Rev* 1992;13:453–460.

7. Bithoney WG, McJunkin J, Michalek J, et al. The effect of a multidisciplinary team approach on weight gain in nonorganic failure-to-thrive children. *J Dev Behav Pediatr* 1991;12:254–258.

8. Bross D, Krugman R, Lenhrr N, et al. *The New Child Protection Team Handbook.* New York: Garland. 1988.

9. Casey PH. Compensatory growth in severe FTT. *South Med J* 1985;78:1057–1060.

10. Chandra RK. Nutrition, immunity, and infection: Present knowledge and future directions. *Lancet* 1983;1:688–691.

11. DeJong P, Miller S. How to interview for client strengths. *Soc Work* 1995;40:729–736.

12. Drotar D, Sturm L. The role of parent-practitioner communication in the management of non-organic failure to thrive. *Fam Sys Med* 1988;6:304–316.

13. Dubowitz H, Black M. Child neglect. In Reece RM (ed.), *Child abuse medical diagnosis and management,* 279–297. Malvern, PA: Lea and Febiger. 1994.

14. Dubowitz H, Davidson N, Feigelman S, et al. The physical health of children in kinship care. *Am J Dis Child* 1992;146:603–610.

15. Feshbach N. The construct of empathy and the phenomenon of physical maltreatment of children. In Cicchetti D, Carlson V (eds.), *Child maltreatment: Theory and research in the causes and consequences of child abuse and neglect.* Cambridge: Cambridge University Press. 1989.

16. Flaherty EG, Weiss H. Medical evaluation of abused and neglected children. *Am J Dis Child* 1990;144:330–334.

17. Frank D, Silva M, Needlman R. Failure to thrive: Mystery, myth, and method. *Contemp Pediatr* 1993;114–133.

18. Gaudin J. Defining and differentiating child neglect. *APSAC Advisor* 1995;8:16–19.

19. Golan N. *Treatment in crisis situations.* New York: Free Press. 1978.

20. Gordon JE, Scrimshaw NS. Infectious disease in the malnourished. *Med Clin North Am* 1970;54:1495–1508.

21. Greene P, Chisick M, Aaron G. A comparison of oral health status and need for dental care between abused/neglected children and nonabused/non-neglected children. *Pediatr Dent* 1994; 16:41–45.

22. Guo S, Roche AF, Fomon SJ, et al.. Reference data on gains in weight and length during the first two years of life. *J Pediatr* 1991;119:355–362.

23. Halfon N, Berkowitz G, Klee L. Children in foster care in California: An examination of medicaid reimbursed health services utilization. *Pediatrics* 1992;89:1230–1237.

24. Halfon N, Mendonca A, Berkowitz G. Health status of children in foster care. *Arch Pediatr Adolesc Med* 1995;149:386–392.

25. Helfer RE. The neglect of our children. *Pediatr Clin North Am* 1990;37:923–942.

26. Hochstadt NJ, Jaudes PK, Zimo DA, Schacter J. The medical and psychosocial needs of children entering foster care. *Child Abuse Negl* 1987;11:53–62.

27. Listernick R, Christoffel K, Pace J, Chiaramonte J. Severe primary malnutrition in U.S. children. *Am J Dis Child* 1985;139:1157–1160.

28. Ludwig S. A multidisciplinary approach to child abuse. *Nurs Clin North Am* 1981;16:161–165.

29. Maggioni A, Lifshitz F. Nutritional management of failure to thrive. *Pediatr Clin North Am* 1995;42:791–810.

30. McJunkin JE, Bithoney WG, McCormick MC. Errors in formula concentration in an outpatient population. *J Pediatr* 1987;111:848–850.

31. Meade JL, Brissie RM. Infanticide by starvation: Calculation of caloric deficit to determine degree of deprivation. *J Forensic Sci* 1985;30:1263–1268.

32. Moffatt MEK, Peddie M, Stulginskas J, et al. Health care delivery to foster children: A study. *Health Soc Work* 1985;129–137.

33. Pennsylvania Child Protective Services Law. *Pennsylvania consolidated statutes annotated.* Title 23, § 6303 (b).

34. Polansky N, Chalmers MA, Buttenweiser E, et al. Isolation of the neglectful family. *Am J Orthopsychiatry* 1979;49:149–152.

35. Polansky N, Gaudin JN, Ammons P, et al. The psychological ecology of the neglectful mother. *Child Abuse Negl* 1985;9:265–275.

36. Rank O. Fate and self-determination. In Moustakas CE (ed), *The self.* New York: Harper and Row. 1956.

37. Schor EL. The foster care system and health status of foster children. *Pediatrics* 1982; 69:521–528.

38. Shulman L. *The skills of helping: The preliminary phase of the work,* 3rd ed., 53–78. Itasca, IL: F. E. Peacock. 1992.

39. Sills RH. Failure to thrive: The role of clinical and laboratory evaluation. *Am J Dis Child* 1978;132:967–969.

40. Simms MD. The foster care clinic: A community program to identify treatment needs of children in foster care. *J Dev Behav Pediatr* 1989;10:121–127.

41. Solomon SM, Kirby DF. The refeeding syndrome: A review. *J Parenter Enter Nutrit* 1990; 14:90–97.

42. Suskind RM. Gastrointestinal changes in the malnourished child. *Pediatr Clin North Am* 1975;22:873–883.

43. Swire MR, Kavaler F. Health supervision of children in foster care. *Child Welfare* 1978; 57:563–569.

44. Trube-Becker E. The death of children following negligence: Social aspects. *J Forensic Sci* 1977;9:111–115.

45. Waterlow JC. Classification and definition of protein-calorie malnutrition. *Br Med J* 1972; 3:566–569.

46. Waterlow JC. Some aspects of childhood malnutrition as a public health problem. *Br Med J* 1974;4:88–90.

47. Whitehead RG. Protein and energy requirements of young children living in the developing countries to allow for catch-up growth after infections. *Am J Clin Nutr* 1977;30:1545–1547.

48. Wise PH, Meyers A. Poverty and child health. *Pediatr Clin North Am* 1988;35:1169–1186.

Chapter 13

Prevention and Ongoing Medical Management of Child Neglect

Howard Dubowitz, M.D.

There are key principles physicians should follow to prevent and treat child neglect. Prevention of neglect involves principles of management, including early identification of risk factors and warning signs. Long-term treatment requires knowledge of the family dynamics, consideration of parental and family issues as well as those issues directly focused on the child, and, often, utilization of community resources. It is necessary that physicians articulate goals of treatment, back these up with a written treatment plan that the family agrees to, assume the role of advocate for the child, and accept that treatment is likely to be protracted, with no quick fixes available.

GENERAL CONSIDERATIONS

For many physicians, involvement in the area of child maltreatment has focused on recognizing and reporting suspected child abuse and neglect. The subsequent responsibilities for these children are often seen as the domain of community agencies and social workers as they investigate the reports and develop plans for protecting the children and serving their families. But physicians need to be involved in the ongoing, long-term health care and psychosocial needs of children who have been neglected as well as those at risk for neglect.

Neglect is a heterogeneous phenomenon that can manifest in very different ways: failure to obtain child health supervision and preventive care, noncompliance with an asthmatic child's regimen, nonorganic failure to thrive—each example illustrates a different manifestation of possible neglect. Underlying contributory factors may vary enormously. Even medical neglect encompasses several different circumstances and problems.[7] Inevitably, management must be tailored to the needs of an individual child and family, and specific approaches will vary greatly. This makes it difficult to delineate the specific measures a physician should employ in all or most of such varied situations, but there are at least 14 key principles involved in the ongoing treatment of child neglect. Many of these principles may appear mundane at first, but too often they are not implemented, for sometimes it seems that our problem is not what we don't know but that we ignore what we do know.

The treatment of child neglect should include the following principles:

1. Identify early warning signs of neglect.
2. Develop a family portrait.
3. Clearly define neglect.
4. Declare an interest in helping the family.
5. Begin with the least intrusive approach.
6. Consider informal supports and resources.
7. Consider the needs of child, parent, and family.
8. Offer extra support and monitoring.
9. Consider the need for long-term services.
10. Know the community's resources.
11. Articulate treatment and prevention goals.
12. Specify clear interventions, in writing.
13. Build on strengths.
14. Individualize the treatment plan.
15. Be an advocate.

IDENTIFY EARLY WARNING SIGNS

Neglect is often difficult to stop or treat, particularly in families with multiple and chronic problems. Recidivism rates of 50 to 70 percent have been found in demonstration projects.[4,24] Primary or secondary prevention can only be accomplished by being able to predict which families are at risk for neglect before it has occurred.[24] Although sensitive and specific predictors have proved elusive, we do know several risk factors that are associated with neglect. These include maternal depression, cognitive limitations, and substance abuse; families who are stressed and have few supports; and children with chronic disabilities.[1] In keeping with our pediatric mandate concerned with the "new morbidity,"[13] an expanded review of systems should probe for potential risk and protective factors.

The following are examples of questions that probe for such factors:

- How have you been feeling lately?
- You seem a little down today. How are you doing?
- I've been seeing lots of folks with drug problems. Is this a problem in your family?
- Has anyone criticized you for drinking too much?
- Do you have any big problems these days?
- Whom do you talk to when things are tough?
- What kind of time do you get to yourself, without the kids?

When red flags appear in such a review of the psychosocial system, physicians should inquire further and intervene early to help address the problem.

Discussions with parents in the course of supervising a child's health care give the physician another opportunity to think ahead and offer guidance on potential problems. For example, when physicians explain the natural curiosity and advancing mobility of toddlers and recommend safety precautions, this is a way of preventing injuries that might occur as a result of inadequate supervision, a form of neglect. Another is explaining the needs of older children for certain limits. For children with identified health problems (e.g., asthma), we can be careful to educate families about the condition, what to expect, when to seek help, and what they can do at home. These small steps can make a big difference in children's receiving the health care they need and in preventing a form of neglect.

As suggested earlier, many of the families at risk for neglect require social and mental health services. Physicians may reasonably be expected to do the following:

Schedule more frequent visits to provide counseling and monitoring. This is often done when, for example, growth appears to be faltering or a behavioral problem like enuresis is uncovered.

Give a little more time to ensure that instructions are clear, and in writing. One contributor to noncompliance is when the treatment plan is poorly conveyed or understood.

Consider the needs of the parent(s). The value of nurturing the parents—both for themselves as individuals and to bolster their parenting abilities—is too often overlooked.

Consider the needs of the family. A family focus is helpful for understanding the child's immediate environment and for encouraging the use of informal resources. Inviting fathers in and reinforcing their participation in childrearing is one example.

DEVELOP A FAMILY PORTRAIT

In order to provide optimal pediatric care generally, not only for evaluating possible child maltreatment, it is helpful to have a good understanding of what it is like for a child in his or her family. This includes information about

- who lives at home,
- what the caregiving arrangements are,
- what the major stresses and supports are,
- what the family's strengths and weaknesses are, and
- significant cultural issues.

It is especially helpful to include in this picture those who are considered family, defining the term liberally. In developing such a portrait we are able to better understand the underpinnings of possible neglect, and to intervene appropriately.

This effort requires time; the portrait can be built over the course of several visits. Circumstances frequently change, however, and there is a need to periodically update the portrait. If we are really going to make pediatrics more family focused,[12] there should be a "Family Portrait" section in a child's medical chart.

CLEARLY DEFINE NEGLECT

Definitions of neglect vary and are often hazy.[8] The child welfare system and many physicians focus on omissions in parental or caregiver care, but neglect is broader than that, a situation in which a child's basic needs are not being met. In order to determine medical neglect, a few key questions should be answered.

Is there actual or probable harm due to a lack of medical care? If yes, a basic need has been neglected. If not, it is questionable whether a fuss should be made. For example, missing a follow-up appointment after an ear infection when the child appears well probably does not qualify as neglect. Even several such missed appointments are unlikely to be consequential. In contrast, a serious delay in receiving care for bacterial meningitis in an obviously ill child, contributing to severe sequelae or death, is medical neglect.

Does the recommended medical care offer a significant net benefit? This requires weighing the anticipated benefits (e.g., shortened duration of illness) with the possible costs (e.g., the risk of side effects from the treatment). Again, if the answer is not clearly yes, it is difficult to justify considering this neglect. The courts are understandably reluctant to force treatment that does not offer a major net benefit.[2]

Does the parental or professional behavior not meet reasonable expectations? It is critical that efforts to identify neglect be driven by our interest in ensuring children's adequate care, not in placing blame. We need to apply the reasonableness test, to assess whether it is reasonable to expect the desired behavior. A child with a very high blood lead level may appear healthy and one would not expect a parent to recognize the problem. Similarly, professionals should not be deemed negligent when unforeseen complications arise. In contrast, parents and professionals may act in ways that contribute to a child's neglect, as when parents refuse a strongly recommended treatment or when a hurried physician fails to carefully explain the regimen for an asthmatic child.

These criteria are key for defining medical neglect. There are multiple possible explanations which are important for understanding *why* the neglect occurred and for intervening. The determination of neglect, however, is based on the child's experience, whatever the underlying reasons. Interventions must be guided by an understanding of the *why*.

DECLARE INTEREST IN HELPING

Families in which neglect is a problem may be very difficult and frustrating to work with and change very hard to achieve. Not surprisingly, many physicians do not enjoy this challenge and may feel quite negative about such families. If a practitioner's negative feelings are extremely strong, it may be preferable to recommend another provider. If one is going to work with the family, by choice or otherwise, it is useful to explicitly declare one's interest in helping the family. This helps establish the rapport and trust on which successful interventions depend.

BEGIN WITH THE LEAST INTRUSIVE APPROACH

The approach needs to fit the underlying problems and risks, but, in general, it is advisable to respect the importance our culture places on a family's privacy and to start with the least intrusive intervention. For example, when faced with a child failing to thrive, initial strategies might be to provide counseling on feeding and a suitable diet. Additional measures might include building parenting capabilities and social supports. If the problem persists, a home visitor or parent aide may be necessary; and if this still proves inadequate, a referral to child protective services (CPS) may be appropriate.

Taking the least intrusive approach is also important when dealing with a family with different cultural practices. There are profound ethical and practical implications in judging a different cultural practice as "bad" or neglectful. This is not to suggest that all behavior should be accepted because someone sincerely believes it to be right; clearly, there are actions that are harmful or dangerous to children. But, it is important to establish that the family's approach is indeed harmful and that the criteria for neglect have been met.

It is always advantageous to maintain a respectful and constructive approach to seek an adequate compromise. For example, children raised on a vegan diet can be adequately nourished provided there is appropriate attention to all nutrients. A heavy-handed approach should also be avoided when confronting families with different religious beliefs, such as Jehovah's Witnesses. Here too, compromise can be sought—"bloodless surgery" when the potential need for blood transfusions is at issue. Child protective services and legal remedies should be used as last resorts in such cases. However, in some instances the harm or risks to the child are so great as to warrant immediate CPS involvement, such as when death might ensue without urgent treatment. In these rare instances, the court may transfer custody of the child to the state (i.e., CPS) and mandate treatment, over the family's objections. Most states, however, have religious exemptions to their child maltreatment statutes, whereby failure to provide medical care due to religious reasons is *not* considered abuse or neglect.[7]

CONSIDER INFORMAL SUPPORTS AND RESOURCES

Social isolation has been identified as a frequent problem in families where neglect is a problem.[5] Professionals are inclined to think of other professionals when considering resources for providing support services to families, overlooking informal help available from family, friends, and religious institutions with which the family may be connected. Families who are resistant to interventions from a public agency or a mental health professional might be far more accepting of support from an institution or individual they trust and already have a relationship with.

Fathers are naturally important for the emotional and material support they can offer to mothers, as well as for their contributions to children's development and well-being.[12] Physicians can encourage a father's involvement in childrearing by inviting him to accompany mother and child to office visits. Similarly, other key kin or support persons should be included in a family-focused approach.

CONSIDER CHILD, PARENT, AND FAMILY

Pediatrics has long focused on children while often ignoring parental and family issues. It is important to appreciate that healthy parents and a well-functioning family are important per se, as well as being critical determinants of children's health, development, and well-being.[10,12] The family is the critical environment in which children are raised. It follows that a concern for a child cannot ignore this family context. For example, it is very difficult for a mentally retarded parent to take good care of a child. It follows that evaluations and treatment plans need to include this broader perspective. It may often prove to be an effective strategy to address family and parental issues first so that the child can be better nurtured.

OFFER EXTRA SUPPORT AND MONITORING

Recent changes in the reimbursement for health care make it increasingly difficult for physicians to provide the more frequent or lengthier appointments that neglect situations often require. Physicians can face a major ethical dilemma as they balance patient needs with corporate dictates for "productivity."

What do increased support and monitoring entail? This could mean extra time spent explaining to a parent how to manage a child's atopic dermatitis. It could involve helping a parent cope with a toddler's tantrums. It might mean time with other family members, the father or a grandmother, to ensure a shared understanding of and approach to a problem. It might focus on prevention, as when parents with borderline intelligence prepare for their children's puberty and adolescence. Monitoring could be to ensure that a child's growth keeps on track or that obesity is diminishing. All of this requires time, at least, and this suggests another principle.

CONSIDER THE NEED FOR LONG-TERM SERVICES

It seems natural for clinicians to wish to see cures or improvement, and quickly. Conversely, it is frustrating when problems appear recalcitrant, with little progress toward resolution. Physicians need to come to terms with the reality that many families where neglect has been identified will need long-term support, akin to that required for a chronic medical disease. We recognize that individuals with cystic fibrosis require lifelong additional services; some psychosocial disabilities are similar. The lure of "quick fixes" is felt not only by physicians. The enthusiasm for brief and intensive interventions in many family preservation initiatives attests to this phenomenon in the child welfare system.

KNOW THE COMMUNITY'S RESOURCES

There are many times and situations when physicians need to recognize what they cannot do. Physicians play an important role by facilitating an appropriate referral to another professional or agency. For primary care providers there remains an important role as liaison between the family and others involved in their care, and managed care usually demands this. A stronger relationship between families and their primary health care providers may be a valuable benefit of managed care. The trust in such relationships may encourage families that are ambivalent, as so often is the case in neglectful situations, to accept (or at least to try) other services. At the same time, physicians should convey that referral is not abandonment. Rather, rooted in the physician's concern and caring, referral may be the optimal way to provide the help the family needs.

ARTICULATE GOALS

It is useful to set clear goals for preventing or remedying a problem, and the goals should be realistic and attainable. For example, one might aim to decrease episodes of diaper rash with better hygiene. Visits to the emergency department may be reduced with improved compliance with the anti-asthma regimen. It is important to avoid setting goals that are unlikely to be met. It is also important that the goal resonate with the family. Giving numbers for spirometry might mean little; preventing hospitalization or enabling participation in sport should be much more appealing. Finally, it is crucial for the goals to be understood and agreed upon.

SPECIFY CLEAR INTERVENTIONS, IN WRITING

Much talk and loose arrangements are destined for misunderstanding and frustration. The treatment plan needs to be clearly conveyed and in writing. This "contract" helps ensure joint acknowledgment by the physician and the client of what needs to happen. There is also a need to probe possible disagreement or concerns about the plan. For example, a parent's hesitation about using a medication could jeopardize the treatment plan.

As an example, a plan to improve care for an asthmatic child might be:

1. No one will smoke in the home.
2. John will receive nebulized X every morning (around 8), afternoon (around 4), and night (before going to bed).
3. If he has a cold or starts wheezing, he will also receive nebulized Y at around the same times, and will continue to do so for a week after the cold or wheezing stops.
4. Prescriptions will be renewed before they run out.
5. If John continues to have difficulty breathing even after taking his medications, he will be brought in to see Dr. Z.

BUILD ON STRENGTHS

Too often we focus on problems without seeking out and building on strengths.[10] This deficit model, based on the medical model centered on pathology, can inhibit use of more constructive approaches to working with families. For example, parents' expressions of concern for their child's well-being provide an opportunity for urging them to comply with a treatment recommendation. A new orientation seeking what is positive is a much needed, major change.

INDIVIDUALIZE TREATMENT PLANS

Because no two families are alike, treatment plans should be based on a clear understanding of the family and tailored to their individual needs. Simplistic formulae are unlikely to yield optimal outcomes.

It is also helpful to simplify treatment plans, recognizing the need to establish priorities. One contributor to noncompliance is a complex demand, such as to medicate a child four times a day; if possible, less frequent dosages should be prescribed. Compliance with recommendations for children with complex medical conditions will also be enhanced by prioritizing the most important aspects of their care and deferring less critical issues until a more opportune time.

BE AN ADVOCATE

Returning to the context in which child neglect occurs, advocacy is needed at various levels: the individual child, parent, family, community, and the society.[6] Helping a diabetic teenager come to terms with her disease is a form of advocacy. When we educate parents about the need to monitor toddlers around a swimming pool, we are advocating on the toddlers' behalf, explaining what they cannot. Acknowledging the stress a parent may feel and facilitating help is also advocacy. Efforts to strengthen a family and recognizing the importance of its healthy functioning are also forms of advocacy. Physicians advocate on behalf of the community when they are active in developing new programs and resources, and, in the broadest sense, we advocate for our society when we help shape health and social policies that benefit children and families. Each of these levels of advocacy is valuable in addressing the problems underpinning child neglect.

CONCLUSION

Helping address the problems of child neglect is very challenging, but, motivated by the ramifications for children and their families, there are many things physicians can do that will make a difference. Together with colleagues in other disciplines, physicians can enhance the care of children, ensure that their basic needs are met, and reduce the neglect of children.

REFERENCES

1. Benedict MI, White R, Wulff LM, Hall BJ. Reported maltreatment in children with multiple disabilities. *Child Abuse Negl* 1990;14:207–217.
2. Bross DC. Medical care neglect. *Child Abuse Negl* 1982;6:375–381.
3. Crouch JL, Milner JS. Effects of child neglect on children. *Crim Just Behav* 1993;20:49–65.
4. Daro D. *Confronting child abuse.* New York: Free Press. 1988.
5. DePanfilis D. Social isolation of neglectful families: A review of social support assessment and intervention models. *Child Maltreat* 1996;1:37–52.
6. Dubowitz H. The pediatrician's role in preventing child maltreatment. *Pediatr Clin North Am* 1990;37:989–1001.
7. Dubowitz H, Black M. Medical neglect. In Briere J, Berliner L, Bulkley J, Jenny C, Reid T (eds.), *The APSAC handbook on child maltreatment.* Thousand Oaks, CA: Sage Publications. 1996.
8. Dubowitz H, Black M, Starr R, Zuravin S. A conceptual definition of child neglect. *Crim Just Behav* 1993;20(1):8–26.
9. Erickson MF, Egeland B, Pianta R. The effects of maltreatment on the development of young children. In Cicchetti D, Carlson V (eds.), *Child maltreatment: Theory and research on the causes and consequences of child abuse and neglect,* 674–684. New York: Cambridge University Press. 1989.
10. Gaudin J. Child neglect: A guide for intervention. Washington, DC: U.S. Department of Health and Human Services, National Center on Child Abuse and Neglect. 1993.
11. Giovannoni JM, Billingsley A. Child neglect among the poor: A study of parental adequacy in families of three ethnic groups. *Child Welfare* 1970;49:196–204.
12. Green M. Bright futures: Guidelines for health supervision of infants, children, and adolescents. Arlington, VA: National Center for Education in Maternal and Child Health. 1994.

13. Haggerty RJ, Roghmann KJ, Pless IB. *Child health in the community,* 94–116. New York: John Wiley and Sons. 1975.

14. Hanson DJ, Pallotta GM, Tishelman AC, Conaway LP, McMillan VM. Parental problem-solving skills and child behavior problems: A comparison of physically abusive, neglectful, clinic, and community families. *J Fam Viol* 1989;4:353–368.

15. Kendall-Tackett KA, Eckenrode J. The effects of neglect on academic achievement and disciplinary problems: A developmental perspective. *Child Abuse Negl* 1996;20(3):161–170.

16. Polansky NA, Gaudin J, Ammons PW, Davis KB. The psychological ecology of the neglectful mother. *Child Abuse Negl* 1985;9:265–275.

17. Regan DO, Ehrlich SN, Finnegan LP. Infants of drug addicts: At risk for child abuse, neglect, and placement in foster care. *Neurotoxicol Teratol* 1987;9:315–319.

18. Reisinger KS, Bires JA. Anticipatory guidance in pediatric practice. *Pediatrics* 1980;66:889.

19. Rivera B, Widom CS. Childhood victimization and violent offending. *Violence Vict* 1992;5:19–35.

20. Seagull EA. Social support and child maltreatment: A review of the evidence. *Child Abuse Negl* 1987;11:41–52.

21. U.S. Department of Health and Human Services, National Center on Child Abuse and Neglect. *Child maltreatment 1994: Reports from the states to the National Center on Child Abuse and Neglect.* Washington, DC: U.S. Government Printing Office. 1996.

22. U.S. Department of Health and Human Services, National Center on Child Abuse and Neglect. *Executive summary of the Third National Incidence Study of Child Abuse and Neglect.* Washington, DC: National Clearing House on Child Abuse and Neglect Information. 1996.

23. Wiese D, Daro D. *Current trends in child abuse reporting of fatalities: The results of the annual 50-states survey.* Chicago: National Committee to Prevent Child Abuse. 1995.

24. Wolfe DA. Prevention of child neglect. *Crim Just Behav* 1993;20:90–11.

Chapter 14

Long-term Psychological Management of Neglect

Maureen M. Black, Ph.D.

While we still lack much in the way of systematic evaluation of programs to treat the long-term psychological consequences of child neglect, it is evident that the application of a number of principles will be of value. Intervention should be early—optimally, before neglect has occurred. It should be directed toward the child's specific needs but also address parenting deficits with accessible and innovative teaching techniques and tie into community programs and agencies that can provide additional support. Intervention efforts should appreciate cultural diversity and look to the long term by encouraging community activism and advocating social policy to reduce poverty. Evaluation must be built into all interventions, so that successful programs can be applied on a larger scale.

GENERAL CONSIDERATIONS

An understanding of the consequences of neglect is the bedrock upon which successful management strategies rest. The effects of child neglect on children's development can be pervasive. Not only are neglected children more likely to demonstrate lower scores on measures of intellectual, emotional, social, academic, and psychological functioning,[1,14,21,32–34,46] but they are learning inappropriate patterns of parenting. Social learning theory predicts that children learn the behavior they see modeled by their parents. Thus, it is not surprising that neglected children have been described as passive and socially withdrawn.[18,40]

CONSEQUENCES OF NEGLECT

Much of what is known about the long-term consequences of neglect has come from the Minnesota Mother-Child Project, a prospective, longitudinal study of 267 children born into low-income families with multiple sociological risk factors.[13] When the children were 2 years of age, they were classified by type of maltreatment, including both physical and emotional neglect. Using systematic data collection procedures, they have been evaluated into their early adolescent years with a comprehensive assessment battery, including measures of cognitive and emotional functioning, academic performance, peer interactions, and behavior.

Not only were neglected children more likely to be anxiously attached, but during their preschool years, they were characterized as showing little enthusiasm during interactive play and were often avoidant of early school opportunities.

The consequences for children who were emotionally neglected (those raised with a psychologically unavailable mother) were particularly devastating.[13] In comparison with their nonmaltreated peers (who had been recruited from the same cohort), the emotionally neglected children demonstrated lower academic performance, more emotional problems, and lower peer acceptance. They were also more withdrawn and inattentive than the children who had been physically abused. Emotional neglect may be harder to recognize than physical neglect, because the children may be receiving material care but not have their emotional needs met. Yet, the consequences of early emotional neglect interfered with children's adjustment in every aspect of their life, including family, peers, and school.[13]

Another method for examining the long-term consequences of neglect is adult recall of childhood experiences. A recent study of 512 college students illustrated that in comparison with a history of abuse, a history of neglect was more strongly associated with current psychological and relationship difficulties (anxiety, depression, somatization, paranoia, and hostility).[17] Although these findings are theoretically defensible and consistent with other research, caution is warranted in relying on retrospective accounts, particularly given Williams' findings regarding the variability of recall validity among women who had been sexually abused as children.[44]

A third method of examining the long-term consequences of child neglect is through matching child protective services records with juvenile and adult crime reports. In a recent investigation, approximately one-fifth of the adults who had been victimized as children by abuse (21%) or neglect (20%) were arrested for a violent offense during their adolescent or adult years, as opposed to arrest rates of 14 percent among a control group matched by age, race, sex, and family social class.[28] Thus, the long-term consequences of neglect include an increased likelihood to engage in violent crimes.

Despite the general acceptance of the negative effects of neglect on children's development, some neglected children develop well, with few apparent residual consequences. One of the most extensive investigations of vulnerability and resilience among children raised in poverty and at risk for neglect found that families with strong support systems were more able to provide the nurturance and guidance necessary to promote optimal development.[43] In addition, children with well developed cognitive and social skills who were encouraged to participate in educational opportunities and who achieved success and satisfaction from academic achievements have been able to escape many of the negative consequences associated with neglect.[2,25,27] These factors increase the likelihood of resilience and can be built into long-term management programs.

INTERVENTIONS AMONG NEGLECTED CHILDREN

Intervention and long-term management of child neglect should follow the assessment of neglect within the family and should consider the type of neglect, the potential causes of neglect, the theories surrounding neglect, and the possible disruptions to children's development. For example, the intervention for children who have experienced physical neglect following a sudden loss of resources would differ from the intervention for children who have been emotionally neglected throughout their life. The former might benefit from crisis intervention, vocational counseling, stress management, or temporary public assistance. In contrast, the latter might require a long-term, comprehensive intervention—an example is Project 12-Ways, which provides direct assistance in specific areas of need, such as child care or skills training.[26]

Intervention programs for neglected children have been found to be successful only half the time.[16] For example, a review of 19 demonstration projects involving neglecting families funded by the National Center on Child Abuse and Neglect from 1978 to 1982 noted minimal success.[12] Two-thirds of the families had additional reports of neglect during the intervention, and 70 percent were assessed as likely to recidivate. Improvement in overall functioning was evident in only half the families (52%), often because the families were experiencing multiple problems that required intensive and comprehensive intervention strategies.

However, there are some bright spots. Evidence is emerging about encouraging programs such as the Nurturing Program and Project 12-Ways. The Nurturing Program provides group training for parents in effective strategies for caring for their children.[4] Project 12-Ways is designed to help neglecting families make major changes in their parenting strategies by assisting them with basic skills such as menu planning, grocery shopping, and home safety. Evaluations, primarily single subject, suggest that families have been able to acquire and maintain basic home maintenance and parenting skills.[26,35]

Home intervention has attracted national attention as an effective strategy in promoting the health and development of young children.[8,29,41,42] Although home visiting programs are often directed toward children, rather than toward parents and families, a recent evaluation involving low-income children who were born healthy but experienced growth deficiency in their first two years of life found that early home intervention was effective in promoting a nurturant home environment and reducing the developmental delays often experienced by low-income, urban children.[5]

RECOMMENDATIONS FOR LONG-TERM MANAGEMENT

Although many clinicians and investigators have used main effect models to develop intervention strategies, Bronfenbrenner has argued that the relationship between contextual factors, such as neglect, and development often varies as a function of personal characteristics (e.g., age), processes (e.g., family structure), or both.[7] For example, early home intervention among children with failure-to-thrive led to better cognitive development and interactional skills at age 4, but only in those children whose mothers reported few depressive symptoms.[22] Thus, Bronfenbrenner argues against a "one-size-fits-all" intervention and recommends that, in developing management strategies, clinicians and investigators focus on the child but also consider the child's family, community, and culture, as well as intervening variables that may alter the impact of the management strategy on the child and family.[7]

The following recommendations are based on the theories explaining neglect and the interventions that have been successful.

Direct intervention services toward child's specific needs. Most interventions for neglect have focused on the family and have not offered services directly to the child.[9] Although family focused intervention programs are consistent with the theories explaining neglect, because they attempt to make changes in children's proximal environment, children who have been neglected may need intervention services directed toward their specific needs. Children who have clear developmental delays or emotional problems may require special education or therapeutic intervention. For example, children who have cognitive or language delays or academic difficulties may benefit from tutoring or special education. Children of parents who have modeled a lack of motivation and a disregard for learning may lack basic learning skills. They may require additional assistance to help them with the learning process, instruction in being inquisitive, asking questions, using feedback from others, and using unstructured time for learning or homework. As children get older, they may benefit from vocationally oriented intervention to help them set short- and long-term attainable goals and plan for their future.

Therapeutic intervention may be available through individual, group, or family counseling, depending on the needs of the child and family. A child with emotional problems who has never experienced secure and stable caregiving may need individual therapy. Group therapy has been effective in helping neglected children develop socially appropriate interaction skills.[12] Group therapy may be particularly helpful for school-age children, so they develop better interactive skills before they are confronted with the demands of adolescence. Family therapy may be useful to families that are not confronted with multiple problems and are committed to remedying their relationship with their child.

Address parental concerns regarding the child's behavior.   Mothers may describe their neglected children as being temperamentally difficult. Clinicians should ask parents to describe their children's behavior and should listen to what they say. Although parents' descriptions of their children's behavior may not be consistent with reports from teachers or other observers,[39] the descriptions from parents may provide insight into their parenting behavior. Thus, when parents describe behavior problems in their children, they may be asking for assistance for themselves, particularly with parenting and family functioning. Dealing with parental concerns regarding children's behavior through parent support and education may reduce maternal anxiety, enrich parent-child relationships, and prevent emotional neglect.

Provide maternal education about the needs of the child.   Neglect has also been associated with maternal depression, apathy-futility syndrome, and psychological immaturity.[32] Mental health treatment may enable mothers to feel more empowered, have more energy, and be more nurturant of their children. However, mothers often require ongoing and direct assistance to learn how to parent their children, particularly if they have never been adequately parented themselves. Mothers who have difficulty recognizing, interpreting, and responding to their children's signals may benefit from the information-processing interventions described by Crittenden.[10] These strategies enable mothers to increase their awareness of their surroundings, the needs their children are communicating, and their ability to fulfill those needs.

The home visiting programs are very encouraging, because they provide direct modeling and enable mothers to practice their caregiving skills within their home environment. Olds and Kitzman recommend that home intervention require an ongoing supportive therapeutic alliance between the primary caregiver and the home visitor, with direct opportunities to model and practice developmentally appropriate, culturally sensitive parenting behavior.[31] Although short-term intervention can be effective, most high-risk families probably require frequent and long-term involvement to develop and implement the changes necessary to promote and maintain healthy development in their children over time.

Intervene before neglect occurs.   Intervention programs directed toward families and children should be introduced during early childhood *before* the negative effects of neglect on the child have become pervasive.[19] Evidence from early home and center-based intervention programs among children at risk for developmental delays illustrates that the developmental delays often seen among low-income children during their preschool years can be averted.[5,23,47] Children who begin school with readiness skills are more able to benefit from academic programs and less likely to require special education. The link between early Head Start intervention programs for low-income children and the prevention of problems during adolescence[47] is very encouraging and provides additional evidence for early intervention.

Make a comprehensive evaluation of intervention success.   Rigorous evaluation procedures that examine the impact of the intervention on youth behavior should be incorporated into the intervention design.[20] Evaluations should include outcomes using multiple strategies and from multiple sources (e.g., parents, schools, observations, etc.) rather than relying exclusively on self-reports. In this way, effective interventions can be replicated and implemented on a large scale and ineffective interventions can be modified or abandoned.

Appreciate cultural diversity.   Interventions should be responsive to the cultural and developmental needs of the children and families. It is important for families to identify with ethnic models and to learn developmentally and culturally appropriate behaviors.[3] Ethnic pride should be incorporated into interventions with an emphasis on mutual respect for ethnic and cultural diversity.

Teach parents how to parent.   Families often want to provide nurturance and care for their children, even if they are not successful. Intervention programs should provide parents with realistic and relevant strategies by which to learn about their children's developmental needs and be involved with their children. Parenting programs and parent aides may provide the support and guidance to help parents adopt more nurturant, effective parenting practices.[30]

Volunteering in schools, churches, or neighborhoods alerts parents to the issues prevalent in the community, provides positive role modeling, provides a positive example to their children, and enables parents to monitor their children's activities and friends. To the extent possible, families should be integrated into the planning, implementation, and evaluation of interventions to ensure that the programs meet the needs of their children and are well integrated into the community, so that if they are successful, they can be sustained.

Support programs promoting stable families.   Youth in stable families are less likely to exhibit the negative effects associated with neglect.[15] Thus, social programs and policies that promote family stability should also benefit children. For example, programs and policies that encourage fathers to stay involved with their children and that help fathers build parenting skills should reduce the likelihood of neglect.

Use accessible and innovative teaching modalities.   Innovative techniques, such as videotapes, can be used to involve families and to extend interventions beyond clinical or educational sites into homes. Videotapes have been used effectively with adolescent mothers to alter parenting skills[6] and to enhance attitudes and knowledge regarding AIDS risk-behaviors.[24,37,45] Using the principles of social learning theory,[3] videotapes can be culturally sensitive and include realistic portrayals of alternatives to situations that could result in neglect.

Enlist child protective services as an ally in intervention. When neglect is suspected, it is necessary to report that suspicion to child protective services for an investigation. Intervention programs are often coordinated by protective services workers, who attempt to ensure children's protection and preserve the unity of the family. Family preservation programs can be very intensive (multiple home visits per week) and provide direct services to teach parents to protect and nurture their children.

If children are endangered, they can be removed from the family for placement in kinship or foster care. Children's plasticity and adaptability, together with the power a nurturing home can have on their development, produce optimistic outcomes from such placements. For example, Skuse reported that children who had been severely neglected during their early years and had cognitive skills below chronological expectations were able to achieve age-appropriate cognitive skills after they were placed in more nurturing environments.[36] Although developmental recovery from neglect is not universal, these findings provide convincing evidence for the need to develop a management system that includes multiple levels of intervention that depend on the need of the child and family, including the possibility of foster care. Although many programs are guided by principles of family preservation, when families are unable to provide the level of protection and nurturance required by the child, it may be necessary to provide an alternative environment through foster care. Even children who have been severely neglected can benefit from a nurturing environment.

Advocate for social policy to reduce poverty. Because neglect is often associated with poverty, programs that reduce poverty should reduce the likelihood of neglect. Job training, vocational counseling, and increased job opportunities should increase household income. In addition, programs to improve housing and neighborhood standards and safety may prevent injuries associated with neglect; emergency food aid and affordable food stores may prevent nutrition related neglect; child care may prevent supervision-related neglect; and medical and mental health care services that are affordable and accessible may prevent medical neglect.

Encourage activism to improve community services. Community institutions often recognize that neglect can undermine the integrity of the entire community.[15,32] For long-term success, intervention strategies should move beyond individual level strategies. Attainability is dependent upon the commitment of community organizations.

Many communities offer programs for youth such as Boy Scouts and Girl Scouts, church programs, sports, and recreational centers. These programs expose youth to normative activities within their community, provide positive role models, and help youth develop positive social skills. However, there are at least three barriers to community services. First, low-income communities, where neglected children are most likely to live, are least likely to have community services for youth. Advocacy with community leaders may be an effective strategy to help them recognize the importance of community programs so youth are helped to become productive members of the community. The second barrier is that neglecting parents may have difficulty encouraging and supporting their children's involvement in community activities. Although parental involvement often enhances community programs—which are usually not well funded and rely on volunteers—children should not be penalized by their parents' inability or unwillingness to participate. Thus, advocacy and support may be necessary to help community programs recognize the critical role they play for children, regardless of parental involvement. Finally, children who have been neglected may not have learned to use community resources. Because neglecting parents are often isolated and not well integrated into their communities, their children may not know about or recognize the value of community resources. In addition, neglected children who are withdrawn and lack interaction skills and motivation may require additional support and encouragement to become involved in community programs. Volunteer programs such as Big Brothers and Sisters may be helpful in enabling children to take advantage of community programs. These programs can provide children with an advocate and provide personalized support.

METHODOLOGICAL CONSIDERATIONS IN NEGLECT

In addition to the lack of consensus regarding the definition of neglect, there are no agreed-upon or commonly accepted measurement strategies. Clinicians, teachers, and others rely on observable signs that children are not being adequately protected, such as failure to grow, poor hygiene, injuries, and failure to attend school or to comply with necessary health or medical recommendations. However, there are no standards, and investigators often develop their own operational definitions and measurements of neglect. Straus and colleagues have recently developed a 20-item self-report measure of four types of neglect (physical, emotional, cognitive, and supervisory) that can be administered to adolescents.[38] The authors have begun to collect data on the internal consistency and construct validity of the scale.

There is little empirical evidence available for developing effective programs. Most programs have not been systematically evaluated. Thus, there is a need not only for a stronger consensus regarding the definition of neglect and better measurement strategies but also for more systematic evaluations of the programs that are in place.[11]

CONCLUSION

Child neglect is a complex and long-term problem, but it is not clearly defined, and this adds to the difficulties of long-term psychosocial management. Early and preventive intervention should be emphasized. Short-term intervention can be effective, but most high-risk families require frequent and long-term involvement to develop and implement the changes necessary over time to promote and maintain healthy development in children who have been neglected. While initial and continuing efforts must be devoted to the specific needs of the child, to be effective, treatment efforts must eventually encompass the parent and the community.

REFERENCES

1. Allen RE, Oliver JM. The effects of child maltreatment on language development. *Child Abuse Negl* 1982;6:299–305.

2. Augoustinos M. Developmental effects of child abuse: Recent findings. *Child Abuse Negl* 1987;11:15–27.

3. Bandura A. Social foundations of thought and action: A social cognitive theory. Englewood Cliffs, NJ: Prentice-Hall. 1986.

4. Bavolek S, Comstock CM, The nurturing program for parents and children. Eau Claire, WI: Family Development Associates. 1983.

5. Black MM, Dubowitz H, Hutcheson J, Berenson-Howard J, Starr RH. A randomized clinical trial of home intervention for children with failure to thrive. *Pediatrics* 1994;94:1404–1408.

6. Black MM, Teti LO. Videotape: A culturally sensitive strategy to promote communication and healthy nutrition between adolescent mothers and infants. *Pediatrics* 1997;99:432–437.

7. Bronfenbrenner U. Ecological systems theory. In Wozniak R, Fisher K (eds.), *Specific environments: Thinking in contexts,* 3–44. Hillsdale, NJ: Erlbaum. 1993.

8. Carnegie Corporation. *Starting points: Meeting the needs of our youngest children.* New York: Carnegie Corporation. 1994.

9. Cohn AH, Daro D. Is treatment too late: What ten years of evaluation research tell us. *Child Abuse Negl* 1987;11:433–442.

10. Crittenden PM. An information-processing perspective on the behavior of neglectful parents. *Crim Just Behav* 1993;20:27–48.

11. Crouch JL, Milner JS. Effects of child neglect on children. *Crim Just Behav* 1993:20;49–65.

12. Daro D. Confronting child abuse, New York: Free Press, 1988.

13. Erickson MF, Egeland B. Child neglect. In Briere J, Berliner L, Bulkley JA, Jenny C, Reid T (eds.). *The APSAC handbook on child maltreatment,* 4–20. Thousand Oaks, CA: Sage Publications. 1996.

14. Fox L, Long SH, Sanglois A. Patterns of language comprehension deficit in abused and neglected children. *J Speech Hear Dis* 1988;53:239–244.

15. Garbarino J. Raising children in a socially toxic environment. San Francisco, CA: Jossey-Bass. 1995.

16. Gaudin JM Jr. Effective intervention with neglectful families. *Crim Just Behav* 1993;20: 66–89.

17. Gauthier L, Stollak G, Messe L, Aronoff J. Recall of childhood neglect and physical abuse as differential predictors of current psychological functioning. *Child Abuse Negl* 1996;20:549–559.

18. Giovannoni J. Definitional issues in child maltreatment. In Cicchetti D, Carlson V (eds.), *Child maltreatment: Theory and research on the causes and consequences of child abuse and neglect,* 3–37. New York: Cambridge University Press. 1989.

19. Helfer RE. The neglect of our children. *Pediatr Clin North Am* 1990;37:923–942.

20. Hennggler SW, Smith LA, Schoenwald SK. Key theoretical and methodological issues in conducting treatment research in the juvenile justice system. *J Clin Child Psychol* 1994;23:143–150.

21. Hoffman-Plotkin D, Twentyman CT. A multimodal assessment of behavioral and cognitive deficits in abused and neglected preschoolers. *Child Dev* 1984;55:794–802.

22. Hutcheson J, Black MM, Winslow M, Dubowitz H, Berenson-Howard J, Starr RH, Thompson BS. *Risk status and home intervention among children with failure to thrive: Follow-up at 4 years of age.* Baltimore: Department of Pediatrics, University of Maryland. 1996.

23. Infant Health and Development Program. Enhancing the outcomes of low-birth-weight, premature infants. *JAMA* 1990;263:3035–3042.

24. Kalichman SC, Kelly JA, Hunter TL, Murphy DA, Tyler R. Culturally tailored HIV-AIDS risk reduction messages targeted to African-American urban women: Impact on risk sensitization and risk reduction. *J Consult Clin Psychol* 1993;61:291–295.

25. Luthar SS, Zigler E. Vulnerability and competence: A review of research on resilience in childhood. *Am J Orthopsychiatry* 1991;61:6–21.

26. Lutzker JR. Behavioral treatment of child neglect. *Behav Modif* 1990;14:301–315.

27. Masten AS, Garmezy N, Tellegen A, Pellegrini DS, Larkin K, Larsen A. Competence and stress in school children: The moderating effects of individual and family qualities. *J Child Psychol Psychiatry* 1988;29:745–764.

28. Maxfield MG, Widom CS. The cycle of violence revisited 6 years later. *Arch Pediatr Adolesc Med* 1996:150:390–395.

29. National Commission on Children. *Opening doors for America's children: Interim report.* Washington, DC. 1990.

30. Nelson KE, Landsman MJ. Alternative models of family preservation: Family-based services in context. Springfield, IL: Charles C. Thomas. 1992.

31. Olds DL, Kitzman H. Review of research on home visiting programs for pregnant women and parents of young children. *Future Child* 1993;3:53–92.

32. Polansky NA, Chalmers MA, Williams DP, Buttenweiser EW. *Damaged parents: An anatomy of neglect.* Chicago: University of Chicago Press. 1981.

33. Reyome ND. A comparison of the school performance of sexually abused, neglected, and non-maltreated children. *Child Study J* 1993;23:17–38.

34. Sandgrund A, Gaines RW, Green AH. Child abuse and mental retardation: A problem of cause and effect. *Am J Ment Def* 1974;79:327–330.

35. Sarber RE, Halasz MM, Messmer MC, Bickett AD, Lutzker JR. Teaching menu planning and grocery shopping to a mentally retarded mother. *Ment Retard* 1983;21:101–106.

36. Skuse D. Extreme deprivation in early childhood. II. Theoretical issues and a comparative review. *J Child Psychol Psychiatry* 1984;25:543–572.

37. Stevenson HC, Davis G. Impact of culturally sensitive AIDS video education on the AIDS risk knowledge of African-American adolescents. *AIDS Educ Prev* 1994;6:40–52.

38. Straus MA, Kinard EM, Williams LM. *The neglect scale.* Durham, NH: Family Research Laboratory, University of New Hampshire. 1996.

39. Tein J, Roosa MW, Michaels M. Agreement between parent and child reports on parental behavior. *J Marr Fam* 1994;56:1–15.

40. Twentyman C, Plotkin R. Unrealistic expectations of parents who maltreat their children: An educational deficit that pertains to child development. *J Clin Psychol* 1982;38:497–503.

41. U.S. Advisory Board on Child Abuse and Neglect. *Creating caring communities: Blueprint for an effective federal policy on child abuse and neglect.* Washington, DC: U.S. Government Printing Office. 1991.

42. U.S. General Accounting Office. *Home visiting: A promising early intervention strategy for at-risk families* (report no. GAO/HRD-90-83). Washington, DC: U.S. Government Printing Office. 1990.

43. Werner EE, Smith RS. *Vulnerable, but invincible: A study of resilient children.* New York: McGraw-Hill. 1982.

44. Williams LM. Recall of childhood trauma: A prospective study of women's memories of child sexual abuse. *J Consult Clin Psychol* 1994;62:1167–1176.

45. Winett RA, Anderson ES, Moore JF, et al. Efficacy of a home-based human immunodeficiency virus prevention video program for teens and parents. *Health Educ Q* 1993;20:555–567.

46. Wodarski JS, Kurtz PD, Gaudin JM, Howing PT. Maltreatment and the school-aged child: Major academic, socioemotional and adaptive outcomes. *Soc Work* 1990;35:460–467.

47. Zigler E, Muenchow S. *Head Start: The inside story of America's most successful educational experiment.* New York: Basic Books. 1992.

Chapter 15

Emotional Abuse and Neglect

Stephanie Hamerman, M.D., and
Stephen Ludwig, M.D.

Emotional or psychological abuse of children accompanies all physical forms of abuse and also can occur independently. It can cause longer-lasting injury than physical abuse. However, this type of abuse is not precisely defined and is greatly underreported. The key is parental behavior that injures a child's emotional or psychological health, and it may take several forms. Types of emotional abuse include confinement, verbal assault, and exploitive or punitive behavior. While several parental assessment tools exist that might be helpful in measuring psychological or emotional abuse, the scarcity of specific work in this area makes it difficult to point to specific or specialized treatment strategies. However, considerable study has been done on the emotional effects of divorce on children, and the divorce model may provide insights for further understanding and treatment of emotional abuse and neglect.

GENERAL CONSIDERATIONS

Coupled with every instance of physical trauma inflicted on a child and every episode of sexual abuse is an emotional or psychological injury.[8] Although much medical attention is paid to the resultant bruises, broken bones, head injuries, and sexually transmitted diseases, the lasting impact of abuse results from the psychological injury.[5] Even when children sustain only psychological injury, such injury can have a life-threatening potential. Instances of isolated or pure psychological/emotional abuse are not often reported but probably account for the greatest burden of abuse morbidity. This chapter explores psychological/emotional abuse in its various forms and considers treatment strategies.

DEFINING PSYCHOLOGICAL ABUSE

Perhaps the greatest barrier to understanding and treating psychological abuse has been our inability to clearly define it. The concept at its core is that a parental behavior (or behaviors) has the impact of injury to the child victim's psychological health. However, we have difficulty operationally defining psychological abuse beyond this core concept.[15] Issues that cloud the definition have to do with parental intent, child resiliency,[4] defense mechanisms,[13] other cofactors, and a general lack of certainty about psychodynamic mechanisms. As a result, the definition of psychological abuse remains unclear and the use of psychological abuse provisions of most state laws continues to be minimal.

National Incidence Study Definitions

The Third National Incidence Study of Child Abuse and Neglect (NIS-1993)[11] defined emotional abuse in terms of a harm standard and an endangerment standard. The harm standard states that a child must have suffered "demonstrable" harm as a result of maltreatment. This includes "moderate" harm by abuse, versus "serious" harm by neglect. The study classified three types of emotional abuse:

- close confinement
- verbal or emotional assaults
- nonspecific abuse

Close confinement includes tying, binding, and other inappropriate confinement or physical restriction. For more extreme forms of tying and binding, the harm standard guidelines permit the assumption that serious emotional injury occurred, so explicit symptoms are not required for the child to qualify as emotionally abused under the harm standard.

Verbal or emotional assault has two categories. The first is systematic patterns of belittling, denigrating, scapegoating, or other forms of overtly rejecting treatment. The second is threats of other forms of maltreatment, for example, abandonment, beatings, or sexual assault.

Nonspecific abuse encompasses all varieties of abusive, exploitative, or overtly punitive behaviors where actual physical contact has not occurred. This includes:

- intentional withholding of food, shelter, sleep, and other necessities
- assigning excessive responsibilities
- making excessive demands for income-producing work

The central feature of the endangerment standard is that it includes children who have not yet been harmed by maltreatment but who have experienced abuse that put them in danger of being harmed, according to views of community professionals or child protective service agencies. Thus, the endangerment standard estimates include all harm-standard children but add others as well, by relaxing the definitional requirements in several respects.

Federal Statutory Definitions

Under the Federal Child Abuse Prevention and Treatment Act 42,[16] *psychological maltreatment* means a repeated pattern of caregiver behavior or an extreme incident or incidents of behavior that conveys to children that they are worthless, flawed, unloved, unwanted, endangered, or only of value in meeting another's needs. Psychological maltreatment includes acts of commission (e.g., verbal attacks by a caregiver) as well as acts of omission (e.g., emotional unavailability of a caregiver). The term *psychological,* instead of *emotional,* is used because it better incorporates the cognitive, affective, and interpersonal conditions that are the primary concomitants of this form of child maltreatment.

Professionals should be aware of legal definitions of psychological maltreatment that are applicable in their community. Definitions specific to a particular state will generally be found in one or more of its civil or criminal statutes.

APSAC Definitions

A third set of definitions comes from the American Professional Society on the Abuse of Children.[1] Six forms of psychological maltreatment are described:

- spurning
- exploiting/corrupting
- terrorizing
- denying emotional responsiveness
- isolating
- unwarranted denial of mental health care, medical care or education

A repeated pattern or extreme incident(s) of these conditions constitutes psychological maltreatment. Such conditions convey the message that the child is worthless, flawed, unloved, endangered, or only valuable in meeting someone else's needs.

SPURNING (hostile rejecting/degrading).   Verbal and nonverbal caregiver acts that reject and degrade a child; includes

- belittling, degrading and other nonphysical forms of overtly hostile or rejecting treatment
- shaming and/or ridiculing the child for showing normal emotions such as affection, grief, or sorrow
- consistently singling out one child to criticize and punish, to perform most of the household chores, or to receive fewer rewards
- public humiliation

EXPLOITING / CORRUPTING.   Caregiver acts that encourage the child to develop inappropriate behaviors (self-destructive, antisocial, criminal, deviant, or other maladaptive behaviors); includes

- modeling, permitting, or encouraging antisocial behavior (e.g., prostitution, performance in pornographic media, initiation of criminal activities, substance abuse, violence to or corruption of others)
- modeling, permitting, or encouraging developmentally inappropriate behavior (e.g., parentification, infantilization, living the parent's unfulfilled dreams)
- encouraging or coercing abandonment of developmentally appropriate autonomy through extreme overinvolvement, intrusiveness, and/or dominance (e.g., allowing little or no opportunity or support for child's views, feelings, and wishes; micromanaging child's life)
- restricting or interfering with cognitive development

TERRORIZING.   Caregiver behavior that threatens or is likely to physically hurt, kill, abandon or place the child or child's loved ones/objects in recognizably dangerous situations; includes

- placing a child in unpredictable or chaotic circumstances
- placing a child in recognizably dangerous situations
- setting rigid or unrealistic expectations with threat of loss, harm, or danger if they are not met

DENYING EMOTIONAL RESPONSIVENESS (ignoring). Caregiver acts that ignore the child's attempts and needs to interact; fail to express affection, caring, and love for the child; and show no emotion in interactions with the child; includes

- being detached and uninvolved through either incapacity or lack of motivation
- interacting only when absolutely necessary
- threatening or perpetrating violence against the child
- threatening or perpetrating violence against a child's loved ones or loved objects
- failing to express affection, caring, and love for the child

ISOLATING. Caregiver acts that consistently deny the child opportunities to meet needs for interacting/communicating with peers or adults inside or outside the home; includes

- confining the child or placing unreasonable limitations on the child's freedom of movement within his or her environment
- placing unreasonable limitations or restrictions on social interactions with peers or adults in the community

MENTAL HEALTH, MEDICAL, AND EDUCATIONAL NEGLECT. Unwarranted caregiver acts that ignore, refuse to allow, or fail to provide the necessary treatment for the mental health, medical, and educational problems or needs of the child; includes

- ignoring the need for or failing or refusing to allow or provide treatment for serious emotional/behavioral problems or needs of the child
- ignoring the need for or failing or refusing to allow or provide treatment for serious physical health problems or needs of the child
- ignoring the need for or failing or refusing to allow or provide treatment or services for serious educational problems or needs of the child

Family Function Definitions

Ludwig and Rostain[9] have taken a more functional approach, defining the areas of family function as provision for (1) physical needs; (2) developmental, behavioral, and emotional needs; and (3) social relationships. Families may injure children in either the oversupply or the undersupply of these tasks. Psychological abuse may fall into several of the subcategories, as shown in table 15.1.

The terms *emotional abuse* and *psychological abuse* are often used interchangeably. However, O'Hagan[12] has written about the problem of defining the terms and makes an important distinction between them. O'Hagan proposes the following definitions:

Emotional abuse is the sustained, repetitive, inappropriate emotional response to the child's experience of emotion and its accompanying expressive behavior. Emotional abuse repeatedly inflicts emotional pain upon the child (e.g., fear, humiliation, distress, despair, etc.). It inhibits the child from spontaneous, appropriate, positive,

TABLE 15.1
Family dysfunction

Task	Dysfunctional Inadequacy	Dysfunctional Excess
Supplying Physical Needs		
Protection	Failure to protect Child abuse	Overprotection and overanxiety
Food	Underfeeding Failure-to-thrive	Overfeeding, obesity
Housing	Homelessness	Multiple residences "Yo Yo"/vagabond children
Health care	Medical neglect	Excessive medical care Munchausen syndrome by proxy
Providing Developmental, Behavioral, *Emotional Needs*		
Stimulation: developmental and cognitive	Understimulation Neglect	Overstimulation ("hothousing") Parental perfectionism
Guidance: approval and discipline	Inadequate approval Overcriticism Psychological abuse	Overindulgence ("spoiled child")
Affection: acceptance and intimacy	Inadequate affection Emotional neglect Rejection Hostility	Sexual abuse Incest
Socialization		
Intrafamilial relationships	Attenuated family relationships Distanced parents	Parenting enmeshment Overinvolved relationships
Extrafamilial, community relationships	Boundaryless families Deficiency in training in extrafamilial relationships	Excessive restriction from extrafamilial relationships

SOURCE: Ludwig and Rostain. Used with permission.

NOTE: Dysfunction in families may occur through either excessive or inadequate attention to normal family tasks.

emotional feeling and emotional expression. It impairs emotional development, that is, the child's continuing ability to experience an increasing range of emotions, to regulate and modulate emotional experiences, and to express them appropriately. Emotional abuse will minimize the child's learning about, and experience of, the increasing subtleties of emotional life. The child's perception and understanding of emotion become distorted, whether it be the child's own emotional experiences or the emotional expressivity of others. Emotional abuse will have serious adverse effect on the child's social development and social life.

Psychological abuse is the sustained, repetitive, inappropriate behavior which damages or substantially reduces the creative and developmental potential or crucially important mental faculties and mental processes of a child; these faculties and processes include intelligence, memory, recognition, perception, attention, imagination, and moral development. Examples of such sustained, repetitive, and pervasive behavior may be domestic violence, desertion, unpredictability, lies, deception, exploitation, and various other forms of abuse (particularly sexual abuse, violence, and neglect). Psychological abuse impedes and impairs the child's developing capacity to understand and manage her environment to the degree that age and development should normally enable her to understand and manage it. Psychological abuse greatly confuses and/or frightens the child, renders her more vulnerable, less confident, and will adversely affect her education, general welfare, and social life.

These examples illustrate the varied definitions of this form of abuse. That a condition is defined in so many different ways implies a lack of full understanding and, more importantly, a lack of operational facility with the terms. Unclear definitions leads to decreased reporting, which in turn leads to decreased understanding about effective therapy. Wissow[21] has written about the "reluctance to recognize emotional maltreatment." Reluctance is evident when we explore incidence data concerning emotional abuse.

INCIDENCE

The true incidence of emotional abuse is impossible to determine. Regional and national incidence surveys reflect the child abuse reporting process, not the true incidence. For example, in the state of Pennsylvania reporting system, in 1990, there were more than 12,000 substantiated reports of abuse of all forms, and less than 1 percent of the cases reported were filed under the emotional abuse statute.

The Third National Incidence Study of Child Abuse and Neglect (NIS-3) indicated 1,553,800 cases of all forms of maltreatment, a rate of 23.1 per 1,000 children, including 204,500 cases of emotional abuse (3.0 per 1,000 children) and 212,800 cases of emotional neglect (3.2 per 1,000 children). These rates are significantly higher than the two previous national incidence surveys. Because the NIS-3 considered endangerment, rather than true harm, the incidence rates increased.

MANAGEMENT CONSIDERATIONS

Quantification and Assessment

There have been several attempts to assess parental functioning and to quantify parents' ability to meet their child's needs. Mrazek, Mrazek, and Kinnert[10] have reported on their Parenting Risk Scale (PRS), an interviewing tool that assesses parents in five key dimensions:

- emotional availability
- control
- psychological disturbances
- knowledge base
- commitment

The authors used the scale in a substantial cohort of children and found it to be a reliable and valid assessment of parenting.

Another attempt at quantifying psychological maltreatment was executed by Brassard, Hart, and Hardy.[3] These authors developed a more specific scale to measure psychological maltreatment in order to overcome some of the aforementioned definitional problems. The Psychological Maltreatment Rating Scale (PMRS) evaluates mother-child dyads and is moderately reliable and valid in discriminating between maltreating parents and comparison parents. Three factors emerged from the authors' analysis. Two are prosocial—the quality of emotional support and the facilitation of social cognitive development. The third factor relates to hostility directed toward the child. Thus, psychological abuse was noted to be not only the presence of hostility directed toward the child but also the lack of the two positive parenting factors.

Sanders and Becker-Lausen[14] have described the Child Abuse and Trauma Scale (CAT), another quantitative index of the frequency and extent of various types of negative experiences. This is a self-reporting scale that was used on college students. The CAT has three subscales that examine sexual abuse, punishment, and neglectful/negative home atmosphere.

All three of these assessment tools are focused at operationalizing psychological abuse in ways that it can be measured reliably. They add to our understanding of the subelements of emotional abuse and are steps in the direction of gaining tools that are as helpful as the radiograph for skeletal injury or the standard growth curve for failure to thrive.

Treatment

As case definitions of psychological abuse are not precise and the number of case reports is small, it is difficult to point to specific or specialized treatment strategies. There are few treatment programs that "specialize" in psychological/emotional abuse. All types of therapies have been used in individual abuse cases, including individual psychotherapy, family therapy, group therapy, and therapeutic schools and preschools. Some courses of therapy have been brief, others extended over years. No one therapy stands out as the best; indeed, few have undergone any scientific examinations of their effectiveness.

Junewicz[6] examined five categories of children who sustained psychological abuse. These included those whose parents

- were preoccupied with interpersonal conflicts
- had mental illness
- had borderline or inadequate personalities
- had drug or alcohol problems
- had stressful conflicts within the family

Children in the last category probably represent the most common setting for psychological abuse. Children witness the intense conflict between their parents and are often brought in to take sides. In considering treatment strategies for psychological abuse, it may be worthwhile to look at children who fall into the Junewicz categories and use the categories as models of varieties of abuse.

DIVORCE AS A MODEL

One model available is the study of the impact of divorce on children. Divorce is a definable event that has emotional impact on parents and children. The effect of divorce on children has been reported often and studied in depth. Klosinski[7] has reported on the mechanism of psychological maltreatment in the context of separation and divorce. Wallerstein writes that "the psychological effect of divorce and the disturbances in parent-child attachment are similar to those where the child is the direct target of abuse."[18] Using divorce as a model for emotional abuse may give some insights into treatment that might be applied more broadly.

Divorce has traumatic emotional effects on children. Children may experience the loss of an intact family, the absence of a noncustodial parent, or the loss of familiar friends, neighborhood, and school. Three areas of emotional trauma involve

- the divorce itself
- the effects of divorce on the parent's ability to parent the children
- the effect of litigation on the children

Children may feel powerless.[22] They may suffer cognitive dissonance about loyalty and betrayal. They may be unable to trust. They may feel disillusioned because their concept of family is shattered. The family structure that gives nurturance and protection has collapsed. In middle-class families, divorce may be the central issue of childhood. According to Wallerstein and Kelly,[20] preschoolers fear abandonment. Children aged 5 to 8 openly grieve for the departed parent. Children aged 8 to 12 are likely to feel anger. Children may have fantasies of catastrophe. They may worry for themselves and for their parents. Benedek[2] lists experiences of fear, sadness, anger, "guilt over causing the divorce," loneliness, rejection, and wishing for parental reconciliation.

Wallerstein and Kelly[20] showed a gender difference in children's psychological adjustment to divorce. Although boys and girls did not differ in their overall psychological adjustment at the time of the marital breakup, 18 months later the psychological adjustment of the boys had deteriorated whereas the psychological adjustment of the girls had improved. In adolescence, both girls and boys have an increased need for their father. There is evidence that adolescent girls in divorced and remarried families are especially affected.[19]

Adults who are regressing themselves secondary to divorce have difficulties parenting.[2] They may involve children inappropriately in marital issues, for example, as a confidant. They may "parentify the children" by reversing roles with them. They may overburden children with responsibility, or, in response to their own feelings of guilt, prevent children from assuming adequate responsibility. In attempting to fill every minute of their children's time with activities, parents can deprive them of emotional availability, so that the children cannot express their feelings.

Witnessing parents verbally abusing each other in the adversarial process of divorce litigation can cause deleterious effects that may not surface immediately. This is especially true for adolescent girls, who may have significant problems with romantic relationships later in life. If, in a custody battle, a parent succeeds in punishing a spouse by precluding the child from a relationship with that spouse, then the child "loses" a parent. In addition, the narcissistic injury of the divorce can bind parents in an unhealthy dynamic of proving their correctness and innocence, with the child caught in the middle, forced to take sides. Being constantly beseeched to "take a side" or being used as a pawn for revenge places the child in a double bind, causing tremendous emotional conflict over loyalty and betrayal in children.

Treatment for the emotional trauma of divorce involves successful completion of Wallerstein's six psychological tasks:[17]

1. acknowledging the marital rupture
2. disengaging from parental conflict and stress to resume customary pursuits
3. resolution of losses
4. resolving anger and self-blame
5. accepting the permanence of the divorce
6. achieving realistic hope regarding relationships

To avoid children's emotional abuse from divorce, Benedek[2] has suggestions for parents. First, parents should spend time with their children and encourage expression of their feelings, not overload them with activities as a substitute. Second, parents should not fight in front of the children and should try to minimize spousal conflict by cooperating. Third, parents should not punish children for regressive behavior; children will abandon regressive behavior if consistent parenting is provided. Parents should focus on building a child's self-esteem by listening attentively to the child and helping the child deal with loneliness by accepting responsibility, for example, the responsibility of caring for a pet.

Applying the lessons of the divorce model to other categories of abuse by parents is not easy. The first step of any therapy must always be an attempt to stop the abuse. The second effort aims at normalizing the child's life so that normal growth and development may occur. The third task is an effort to remediate injury that has already occurred and, finally, as children grow towards maturity to have them understand their parents' failings from an adult perspective. The ways that these therapy goals can be accomplished remain ill defined. Before more specific treatment can be recommended there is a need for much more precision in defining psychological abuse, reporting it, and understanding its dynamics. Only once these steps have been accomplished, can there be a meaningful inquiry into therapy.

REFERENCES

1. *APSAC practice guidelines: Psychosocial evaluation of suspected psychological maltreatment in children and adolescents.* Chicago: American Professional Society on the Abuse of Children. 1995.

2. Benedek EP, Brown CF. *How to help your child overcome your divorce.* Washington, DC: American Psychiatric Press. 1995.

3. Brassard MR, Hart SN, Hardy DB. The psychological maltreatment rating scales. *Child Abuse Negl* 1993;17:715–729.

4. Cicchetti D, Rogosch FA, Lynch M, Holt KD. Resilience in maltreated children: Processes leading to adaptive outcome. *Dev Psychopathol* 1993;5:629–647.

5. Clausen AH, Crittenden PM. Physical and psychological maltreatment: Relations among types of maltreatment. *Child Abuse Negl* 1991;15:5–18.

6. Junewicz WI. A protective posture toward emotional neglect and abuse. *Child Welfare* 1983;62:243–252.

7. Klosinski G. Psychological maltreatment in the context of separation and divorce. *Child Abuse Negl* 1993;17:557–563.

8. Ludwig S. Child abuse and neglect. In Fleisher G, Ludwig S (eds.), *Textbook of pediatric emergency medicine,* 3rd ed. Baltimore: Williams and Wilkins. 1993.

9. Ludwig S, Rostain A. Family function and dysfunction. In Levine MD, Carey WB, Crocker AC (eds.), *Developmental-behavioral pediatrics,* 2nd ed. Philadelphia: W. B. Saunders. 1992.

10. Mrazek DA, Mrazek DM, Kinnert M. Clinical assessment of parenting. *J Am Acad Child Adolesc Psychiatry* 1995;34(3):272–282.

11. National Clearinghouse on Child Abuse and Neglect Information. *Reports from the states to the National Child Abuse and Neglect Data System* (NCANDS). http://child.cornell.edu. 1994.

12. O'Hagan KP. Emotional and psychological abuse: Problems of definition. *Child Abuse Negl* 1995;19(4):449–461.

13. Rostain AL, Shumway WE. Acute psychiatric manifestations. In Ludwig S, Kornberg AE (eds.), *Child abuse: A medical reference,* 2nd ed. New York: Churchill Livingstone. 1992.

14. Sanders B, Becker-Lausen E. The measurement of psychological maltreatment: Early data on the Child Abuse Trauma Scale. *Child Abuse Negl* 1995;19(3):315–323.

15. Thompson AE, Kaplan CA. Childhood emotional abuse. *Br J Psychol* 1996;168:143–148.

16. *United States Code 5106g(4): Federal Child Abuse Prevention and Treatment Act 42.* Washington, DC: U.S. Government Printing Office. 1974.

17. Wallerstein JS. Children of divorce: The psychological tasks of the child. *Am J Orthopsychiatry* 1983;53:230–243.

18. Wallerstein JS. Changes in parent-child relationships during and after divorce. In Anthony EJ, Pollock GH (eds.), *Parental influences in health and disease.* Boston: Little, Brown. 1985.

19. Wallerstein JS, Blaksee S. *Second chances: Men, women, and children a decade after divorce.* New York: Ticknor and Fields. 1989.

20. Wallerstein JS, Kelly JB. *Surviving the breakup: How children and their parents cope with divorce.* New York: Basic Books. 1980.

21. Wissow LS. *Child advocacy for the clinician: An approach to child abuse and neglect.* Baltimore: Williams and Wilkins. 1990.

22. Wolmar R, Taylor K. Psychological effects of custody disputes on children. *Behav Sci Law* 1991;9:399–417.

PART IV

Munchausen by Proxy

Chapter 16

Munchausen by Proxy: Definitions, Identification, and Evaluation

Catherine C. Ayoub, R.N., M.N., Ed.D., Robin M. Deutsch, Ph.D., and Robert Kinscherff, J.D., Ph.D.

Munchausen by proxy (MBP) is both a pediatric and a psychiatric entity. It is a form of child abuse in which a parent or caregiver (usually a mother) exaggerates, fabricates, or induces illness in a child. The primary motivation of the parent—who is often diagnosed with factitious disorder by proxy—is to present herself as an exceptional mother. Assessment can be difficult because of the elaborate deception involved. Such deception underscores the necessity for an assessment that considers the complex physical and mental health aspects of this interactional disorder, which also draws the health care provider into the web of deceit. MBP affects the whole family; often the father is an enabler, siblings are involved, and the extended family play active roles. Child victims experience significant psychological problems during childhood and frequently into adulthood. Ongoing, coordinated individual therapy is imperative for the child's emotional health. Prognosis for effective intervention with the perpetrator is often poor and significant risks to the child frequently endure after the detection of MBP.

GENERAL CONSIDERATIONS

Munchausen syndrome and its diagnostic counterpart, *factitious disorder,* are terms used to describe psychiatrically disturbed adults who intentionally produce or feign illness or psychological signs or symptoms in themselves. In such cases, the primary motivation is to assume the role of patient.[2] The name Munchausen is a reference to the antics of Baron Karl Frederich Hieronymus von Münchhausen, an eighteenth-century German mercenary cavalry officer who was famous for lies and elaborate fabrications of war exploits.

Munchausen by proxy (MBP) was originally seen as an extension of Munchausen syndrome or factitious disorder. However, more recent work suggests that the two disorders are distinct[2] and should be described as separate entities. The phrase "Munchausen by proxy" has been used in the recent literature to describe the falsification of illness—physical, psychiatric, and/or psychoeducational—in a child resulting from deliberate exaggeration, fabrication, or inducement of symptoms by a parent or significant adult. Between 93 percent to 98 percent of parents or caregivers with factitious disorder by proxy are mothers or mother surrogates, making the psychiatric disorder primarily a disease of women.[16]

It is critical to acknowledge that MBP is both a pediatric and psychiatric entity.[4] It is an interactional disorder, requiring a focus that extends beyond each individual to the consequences of the interaction between them. The term *MBP* has been used to describe the symptoms of the child victim; the parent's psychiatric disorder; the interactional triad of parent, health care provider, and child; and the family's dysfunction. All are valid facets of the disorder. However, neither medical nor mental health diagnostic systems are fully equipped to describe the full picture of the disorder. Each approach draws upon the other in order to more accurately characterize the medical and psychiatric dimensions of MBP. Definitions published by a working group of the American Professional Society on the Abuse of Children[4] described the two components of MBP. The component that describes the child victims reads: "Pediatric Condition (illness, impairment, or symptom) Falsification (PCF) is a form of child maltreatment in which an adult falsifies physical and/or psychological signs and/or symptoms in a victim, causing the victim to be regarded as ill or impaired by others."[4] The document says this about the perpetrating parent: "Persons who intentionally falsify history, signs, or symptoms in a child to meet their own self-serving psychological needs have been diagnosed with Factitious Disorder by Proxy (FDP) and should be coded as such (Factitious Disorder Not Otherwise Specified—300.19, see DSM-IV, [2] p. 475)."[4]

Although there are no scientifically robust studies on the incidence of MBP, interest in the disorder has increased tremendously in the last ten years. Applied to the United States, the findings of a conservative British study of several of the most common pediatric presentations of MBP would suggest that there are more than 600 new cases per year in the United States.[9] A number of experts now believe that the condition is more common than suspected but difficult to detect because of the elaborate deception at the core of the malady. Estimates of mortality rates in MBP vary from 9 percent[5] to 22 percent[6] in identified children. Morbidity to the child is close to 100 percent, both physical and psychological. In Rosenberg's study[13] sibling death was estimated to be 4.8 percent.

Children with falsified symptoms of illness tend to make dramatic physical recoveries upon separation from their parents. However, child victims appear to fare far less well in the psychiatric realm. In the only long-term follow-up study to date, survivors reported serious emotional difficulties in childhood, including insecurity, faulty reality testing, avoidance problems, and posttraumatic stress symptoms that for most endured into adulthood.[8] One of the most striking findings of this study was that the abuse did not stop until the child left home, and in a number of cases it continued well into the victim's adult life, suggesting that the life cycle of MBP is much longer than previously suspected. This finding raises doubt about the widely held belief that older children are able to better protect themselves from this form of abuse.

ASSESSMENT

An accurate assessment of MBP requires an integrated approach. One of the most common reasons for failure to diagnose and for misdiagnosis is the reliance upon assessments that are compartmentalized and conducted without information about the child's past history and pattern of victimization and the parent's history of emotional and social functioning. Mental health evaluations based primarily on individual interviews and/or psychological testing with one or both parents can be not only misleading but also dangerous. A second reason for diagnostic errors is assessment by persons who are unfamiliar with MBP or who consider it to be so rare that they fail to include it as a differential diagnosis. Although interviews and psychological testing may raise the suspicion of MBP, they are typically not adequate to confidently rule it in or out. Interviews and psychological testing must be conducted with an appreciation of the medical records and observations that give rise to the pediatric or psychiatric suspicion of MBP. MBP parents do not demonstrate a consistent psychological profile that can be detected by current psychological tests and they are adept liars and imposters—capable of fooling mental health professionals. Most medical and mental health professionals are not trained to obtain the amount of objective medical, historical, and/or psychological data necessary to confidently comment on the presence or absence of MBP. Furthermore, medical, social, and child protection systems are not structured to make such assessments easy. Consequently, we strongly argue for knowledgeable, integrated, multidisciplinary input into investigation and assessment of the alleged child victim and the parent perpetrator[7] whenever MBP is suspected. This is the best method for confidently identifying actual cases of MBP while avoiding false diagnoses.

An adequate assessment requires clear documentation of each of the components that contribute to a comprehensive overview of the parent, child, family, and provider networks. Mental health professionals assigned to either a preliminary or more detailed court ordered assessment must have active, ongoing contact with the pediatric assessors and care providers. They should have detailed information about what gave rise to the suspicions of child abuse in each case and about the ways in which the child has allegedly been maltreated. "Blind" or fragmented assessments are strongly contraindicated. However, failure to psychiatrically assess the parents should not preclude primary practitioners from identifying and reporting child abuse after examining the alleged child victim.

When MBP is suspected, the initial focus should be on the child victim. Victimization through the exaggeration, fabrication, and/or inducement of a physical or psychological illness is child abuse, which has been identified as "pediatric condition falsification."[4] Child abuse may be present regardless of the motivation of the parent. It does not require a DSM-IV[1] diagnosis of factitious disorder by proxy in the parent in order to be called abuse. Indeed, not all cases in which a parent presents with a child with falsified pediatric condition or illness will constitute MBP. However, the consequences to the child may be equally dangerous. The child's falsified symptoms require careful assessment and documentation (see chapter 18). If child abuse by illness or condition falsification is suspected, then health care providers are obligated to follow their state guidelines for mandatory reporting to state child protection authorities with or without confirmation of a psychiatric diagnosis in the parent.

There are some situations in which falsification of illness may be present but factitious disorder by proxy is not the diagnosis of the perpetrator. Mothers with factitious disorder by proxy should be differentiated from mothers who directly injure their children out of anger or frustration. Overwhelmed parents who exaggerate their child's symptoms to get help for the child or frightened parents who do the same are not diagnosed with FDP. Mothers who are delusional or psychotic, where the psychosis encompasses the illness issues, are not exhibiting FDP. However, there have been several MBP mothers described in the literature who had psychotic features that were unrelated to the MBP. These mothers were given diagnoses of FDP.[3]

Pediatric condition falsification may take a number of forms. Common presentations include recurrent apnea, poisoning, intestinal disorders, seizures, infections, vomiting, and diarrhea. However, only the imagination and sophistication of the perpetrator limit the nature of the presenting symptoms. (Additional information on the pediatric component of MBP can be found in chapter 18.)

PSYCHOLOGICAL AND DEVELOPMENTAL PRESENTATION OF THE CHILD

Child abuse by pediatric condition or illness falsification is not a diagnosis of exclusion, but evidence is often circumstantial. The most striking evidence in these cases includes either direct observation or laboratory evidence of inducement of illness, such as observation by video surveillance of deliberate contamination of central lines by the mother or the presence of nonprescribed medication in the child's bloodstream. Less-direct evidence also can be compelling but often requires careful documentation of changes in the child's health status when the parent is present or of the child's presentation over time with symptoms involving vague, contradictory, or improbable medical or psychiatric histories. Although falsification of physical symptoms is the most common form of MBP, falsification of psychological or developmental symptoms is not unheard of.[14] In some cases, the child's symptoms may have some genuine physical basis, but children with concurrent real illness should not be excluded from consideration for MBP if a number of their medical or psychiatric symptoms could be the result of falsification.[15] For example, a child who genuinely has diabetes mellitus may be subjected to intentional misuse of insulin in order to induce a more brittle presentation of the disease. Additionally subjecting children to repeated sexual abuse evaluations where the motivation of the parent is to attract attention for "good mothering" has been identified as a form of MBP.[12]

Abuse may involve one child in the family or several children serially or simultaneously.[1] Not infrequently there is a history of another child in the family being ill or dying of a mysterious illness. In a number of cases where only one child is the target, that child is more often the second or youngest child rather than the oldest. In these families, older siblings are frequently groomed to serve as caregivers and helpers. Parentified siblings are common and tend to take on a pseudo-mature stance which mimics that of their mothers. Their ambivalence can be transparent, however, as they struggle to compete for attention with the "sick" child. In cases of psychological or educational MBP, it is more likely that several children are victims simultaneously.

Although psychological assessment of and support for the child during evaluation is important, the mental health provider should be careful to assess the current emotional responsiveness of the child in light of the physical and developmental findings. Parent-child interaction may appear superficially appropriate. Parents with factitious disorder by proxy tend to do well on pencil-and-paper parenting assessments. Observation of the child's behavior with each parent and family can be helpful but it is not diagnostic. Many of these children are quiescent in the face of their mother's commitment to their illnesses and seldom expose the deception directly.

In spite of the close relationship often witnessed between mother and child prior to their separation, powerful findings show that the child often experiences dramatic improvements in health status once the parent and child are separated. If children have some legitimate component to their physical or emotional difficulties, or if they have been co-opted into internalizing the sick role, they may show some lingering physical symptoms that should not be taken as an indication of an improper diagnosis of child abuse. Children who present as dependent and ill spontaneously embrace physical wellness upon separation from their mothers. Their psychological and social functioning, particularly in terms of normalization—peer, school, recreational activities—improves as well.

Psychological responses of the children are surprising. Many school-age child victims of MBP do not appear to be distressed at prolonged separation from their mothers. If they are in a familiar place, like the hospital, they do not appear acutely anxious or preoccupied with their mother's absence. Many do not ask for their parents and simultaneously begin to explore their surroundings in proactive and health-directed ways.

Although these children do not often ask for their mothers after separation, they do remain loyal to their parents. They are also careful to conceal new attachments with others from their parents for fear that they will be challenged. The threat of rejection and reprisal from parents is considerable. In addition, it is often difficult for these children across the age span to acknowledge that their primary caregiver has repeatedly injured them in the name of caring and concern. As a consequence, a number of MBP child victims insist that their mothers are "always right" despite considerable evidence to the contrary.

Continued risk of physical harm to the target child is considerable even under closely supervised circumstances.[13] Professionals working with the child should be aware that the risk of serious harm to the child from the inducing parent *increases* as access is restricted or when confrontation occurs. Many mothers persist almost obsessively to make contact with and influence the child in some way. From the beginning of suspicions by hospital staff or other guardian, the child's safety should be considered in light of the serious and possibly lethal consequences. For example, an increased risk of abduction when mothers are separated from their children has been documented, as has increased potential for violence by a mother or her designee toward the child or the providers. A shift of parental focus to a sibling after the target child is placed elsewhere is also not uncommon. It is imperative that the medical, mental health, and child protective professionals who are involved with either parent or child be clearly aware of these risks and able to consider children's safety as first priority.

The child identified as a victim of MBP who has lived with the inducing parent frequently presents with underlying psychiatric symptomatology.[14] Libow and Schreier[16] point out that violation of trust by a parent is a more powerful predictor of psychological consequences for the child than the form of abuse or the distinction between active induction and symptom fabrication. The extent and longevity of psychological symptoms among MBP child victims are variable, as are their timing and presentation. Significant problems during childhood include: eating disorders, behavioral growth problems, nightmares, self-destructive fantasies, oppositional-defiant disorder, identity and attachment difficulties, school concentration problems.

Across the developmental spectrum, children victimized by MBP exhibit considerable need for extensive control over their environments, which can supersede their desire to form attachments. They often continue to be hypervigilant long after they are in a safe alternative placement. The child's sense of safety is often directly related to contact with his mother and should be evaluated in this light; the role of extended family members as messengers for the mother should also be painstakingly evaluated before contact with them is allowed.

Notable is the "chameleon" quality of many of MBP children's responses to those around them. They often react differently in different contexts and seem to be attempting to anticipate and conform to the expectations of the adult or child with whom they are speaking. Lying is not an uncommon finding nor is sadistic behavior toward other children and animals by some of the more chronically abused MBP children. Sexualized behavior in these child victims has been observed in a number of cases, but the origin of such behavior is unclear. Some additional behavioral observations include issues with physical space, lack of respect for the possessions of others, social immaturity and lack of social skills, and lack of awareness of basic social interactions. Children in MBP frequently develop a view of the world as negative and adults as untrustworthy. In some cases, the child's behavior improves significantly when contact is completely severed between mother and child. In other cases, symptomatic behaviors persist, even with minimal or no contact with mother.

School-age children removed from their parents initially appear remarkably nonreactive and unaffected. They frequently go on to do well physically and have few behavioral difficulties in alternative placement if protected from unsupervised contact with the perpetrating parent. However, further evaluation often reveals deep identity issues and a striking compartmentalization of events that keeps them from being integrated across time. Often, if asked how they went from being sick to being well, these school-age victims say they do not know and they resist inquiry that directs their attention to this issue. If they are in a safe environment, as they approach adolescence, this "black hole" in their cognitive awareness may begin to crumble. As they begin to use abstract reasoning they become more anxious and behavioral symptoms may develop around identity issues and the dilemma that their health creates given their past illness.

The child victim of MBP who has lived with the inducing parent for an extended period of time and whose illness has been chronic is at the highest risk for behavioral difficulties. This child has a tendency to be at increased risk for serious reality distortions, poor self-esteem, and a view of self as special and above compliance with social rules. Such children have considerable difficulty in alternative placements, because of aggressive and sexual behaviors and serious issues with trust. Many of these children can be seen as attachment disordered.[3] In children where prolonged victimization is suspected, special foster care or alternative special placement with additional psychological supports should be considered.

Careful psychological evaluation is important for understanding the impact of the victimization and for treatment planning for children of all ages. Although the number of therapists trained to treat MBP children is limited, ongoing individual therapy is imperative for the child's emotional health.

PSYCHOLOGICAL AND SOCIAL PRESENTATIONS OF WOMEN WITH FACTITIOUS DISORDER BY PROXY

The second component to the identification of MBP is the focus on the suspected perpetrator. There is no particular psychological profile or list of symptoms that indicates a diagnosis of factitious disorder by proxy. However FDP is a perversion of mothering, and the core motivation of the FDP mother is to present herself not only as a good mother but as an exceptionally attentive, self-sacrificing, and committed mother, in order to meet her own psychological needs.[4] In order to maintain and heighten this role, the mother, by inflicting injury either directly or indirectly on her child, perpetuates situations in which she can act as this "special" mother.

This "imposturing"[16] involves using the child as an object through which to obtain the attention and interest of one or more individuals seen by the mother as powerful. The mother's focus may be directed at the physician or physicians involved with her child's care, as well as toward nursing staff and ancillary personnel who care for the child. In some cases mothers tend to "doctor shop," especially if they are confronted with questioning of the nature or severity of the child's illness. However, when a physician is particularly responsive to the mother and uses her input to plan and order care, MBP mothers may form a strong and longlasting alliance with the health care provider.

Mothers not only gain the trust of professionals but often step over the usual boundaries established between health care provider and patient. As a consequence, they are given additional responsibilities for performing technical tasks usually reserved for health care personnel. For example, one mother with a child with a gastrostomy tube, which repeatedly became obstructed, bragged about how when the button came out she was able to surgically reimplant it at home with step-by-step instruction from the child's doctor. Other boundary violations include an extension of professional relationships into the personal lives of providers.

According to Schreier and Libow,[16] lying (in the service of imposturing) plays a number of roles for the FDP perpetrator. First, it transforms difficult realities into ones that not only are bearable but also provide support, identify the perpetrator as a victim, and evoke positive attention. Second, this lying allows the mother to borrow some of the attitudes and beliefs and even imitate the actions of those she sees as powerful. This emulation is a way for mothers to gain for themselves the power and control they so seriously lack internally. Third, the creation of a "fantasy life" provides external structure and internal meaning to the emptiness in the core of the mother's being. It is not unusual to find among FDP perpetrators a constellation of borderline, antisocial, and narcissistic characterological features reflected in their interpersonal relationships and impaired empathy for the child victim as well as for others to whom she claims to be close.

FDP mothers take pride in their deception and on those rare occasions when they acknowledge their acts, they commonly express exhilaration at having duped so many important and influential people. A number of FDP mothers, upon discovery, have been heard to brag about how easy it was to deceive professional caregivers. The contempt for those who are victims of the deception is unmistakable. The contempt may extend beyond the clinical caregivers and include attorneys and other supporters or advocates who were successfully deceived.

Many mothers not only fabricate issues related to their child's illness but also may exaggerate and fabricate events that involve other areas of their lives. Deception may extend to many other relationships with authority figures, both inside and outside the family. Some mothers have expanded their cries for attention to the media or the educational or legal system. If exaggeration or fabrication is suspected within the parent-child relationship, it is important to assess if and how deception presents as a primary tool for obtaining attention, material goods, money, or other kinds of status and recognition. All of these deceptions take place within a framework of impostoring. It is not unusual to find a history of other forms of deception: financial or insurance fraud, lying, theft, or covert drug or alcohol abuse. Up to a quarter of mothers described in the literature have co-occurring diagnoses of factitious disorder.[13]

Many FDP mothers have some formal training in a health care–related discipline and have extensive knowledge about medical conditions. Some mothers may not be connected with formal or traditional health care systems but have a more informal and/or holistic medicine approach to their child's health. Mothers present as concerned and invested in their ill child's care. They have mastered the health care information specific to their child and appear competent. The nature and intensity of the parent's preoccupation is different from that of parents of genuinely ill children. The need for control over the child's medical or health-related needs is remarkably intense, and the child receives the most attention when she or he is acutely ill. Some mothers have considerable difficulty interacting with their ill children in ways that do not relate to illness.

Many mothers are unusually attentive during bouts of illness when the child is seen by health care professionals and especially when hospitalized. They are eagerly supportive of medical procedures and treatments. At times they administer or request the administration of treatments with zeal beyond that which is reasonable or necessary; their zeal may appear to outweigh their awareness of the child's pain or discomfort or even ignore reasonable assessments of risk and benefits of proposed procedures. Some mothers may be erratic about their desire to engage their child in treatment and criticize the treatment process; such unpredictable behavior appears related to the parent's need rather than the child's. Mothers are often not relieved when they hear their child is not ill. They may present as relieved initially, but there is always a "yes, but . . . " followed by a demand for further evaluation or treatment.

Mothers often have difficulty identifying their child as having feelings and needs separate from theirs. One of the most striking characteristics of the mother-child relationship, and often of extended family relationships, is that boundaries are loose. The child's needs are malleable depending upon mother's wishes rather than upon any continuity of issues or roles for the child across time. For example, at times ill children are given no choices in their environment while at other times they are asked to make adult choices about their interactions. This behavior is seen particularly in regard to choices the child is asked to make to demonstrate loyalty to mother's point of view. Loyalty is demanded and is taken by the mother as a sign of love from the child. The demand for control from the parent is powerful, while at the same time mothers present as close to their child, dutiful, committed, and all-sacrificing for their child. They often speak for their children, verbalizing that as mothers they sense or "know" how the child feels and when he or she is ill.

Denial of the factitious nature of the child's illness is central to maintaining the parent's sense of self and self-worth. So, although their actions are conscious and often meticulously planned, mothers will hold steadfastly to denial of any wrongdoing, even in the face of overwhelming evidence and potential legal consequences. Even if there is an admission of sorts, many mothers will revert to denial once the crisis or confrontation is past. A second group of mothers will side-step the issue by an admission when faced with juvenile trials or criminal proceedings, only to move on to a new part of their lives in which fabrication continues. A third group of mothers will admit to victimizing their children when confronted with criminal prosecution, especially when facing lengthy terms of incarceration and offered a reduced term or probation as part of a plea bargain.

Vigilance should be high around the time of any confrontation, be it initial identification or in permanency planning or criminal proceedings. As previously noted, an escalation of dangerous behavior has been described at these times. This behavior on the part of the women involved may be directed toward self or others. Several researchers note a history of suicide attempts by mothers, and a tendency to suicidality following confrontation and isolation from the child.[12]

Early histories of many of the women commonly but not always reflect tragedy and difficult home situations with a culmination of crises during adolescence. Some families of origin of FDP mothers were overtly abusive, with documented episodes of physical abuse, sexual abuse, and/or neglect. Others mother grew up amidst domestic violence and alcoholism. Another group of women described emotional tragedies, with an emphasis on traumatic deaths, to which they were exposed as young adolescents.

PSYCHOLOGICAL AND SOCIAL PRESENTATIONS OF THE FAMILY

Munchausen by proxy is a family system disorder,[12] and symptoms of factitious illness should be seen within the context of family dynamics that serve to maintain the perpetrating behaviors. The most common presentation of falsification or inducement of illness in additional family members is by the mother herself; she may be diagnosed with a concurrent factitious disorder. In a number of cases, attitudes about and attention to various real or factitious illnesses in the family varies, so it is important for the psychosocial evaluator to inquire about illnesses in each parent and in other family members. Attitudes toward illness and disease in the family at large are important to any psychosocial assessment for MBP.

Although mothers have been described as the "active inducers," fathers living in the home may play the role of the reinforcer or enabler; in single-parent families this may be the mother's boyfriend, or in lesbian couples her same sex partner. There have been situations in which parents were believed to actively collude in MBP perpetration. Fathers have been described in the literature as being on the periphery or altogether absent, abdicating medical care and decision making to the mother. Even in families in which fathers are involved in some aspects of their children's lives, they characteristically let their wives handle the medical issues with the sick child. Other fathers may actively participate in carrying out medical interventions induced by the mother—for example a father might go to the store to buy medicine or might collect daily specimens.

A second characteristic of fathers is their strong ability to avoid recognition or acknowledgment of uncomfortable portions of reality that are too conflicted or threatening to them. They often actively deny the possibility that their child's illness is factitious, even when there is mounting evidence of it. In this way, they resemble mothers in incestuous families who manage to ignore or minimize indications of ongoing incest between father and child. In most intact marriages, fathers side with mothers and refuse to believe the allegations of MBP.

In situations in which fathers are estranged or divorced from the mothers, there is more of a tendency to acknowledge the child's victimization. In several cases, fathers raised the issue or pursued it once it was brought to their attention. Several fathers who left intact marriages after having strongly supporting their wives' innocence reported that they had felt compelled to agree with the wife's account of events. Several fathers stated that they "just repeated her stories" and "pretended not to know differently." All described the psychological and in some cases physical danger in confronting their wife with issues at variance with her views.

Many fathers in MBP families have histories of domestic violence and a significant minority have drug and/or alcohol histories. A subgroup of men in these families have had difficulty holding down a job or have spent a good deal of time changing not only places of employment but career goals; others, however, were successful in the working world. Personality disorders are commonplace in men in intact couples and most often include narcissistic, compulsive, and dependent traits.

In two-parent MBP families, the marital interaction can have a compelling effect on the family system. One common dysfunctional dynamic is the projection of problems onto people and institutions outside the family. Often the perceived attack from "outside" provides the family, which usually interacts in steeped hostile dependency, a cause around which to feel close and to unite.

When feasible, psychosocial assessments should include interviewing parents and siblings of women with FDP. In a number of cases, maternal grandmothers' relationships with their daughters were found to be cold, controlling, covertly sabotaging, and rejecting, despite a façade of graciousness and caring. Maternal grandfathers were more caring but often passive and dependent upon their wives for decision making. In some families the rigid control by maternal grandmothers over extended members was powerful and needed careful evaluation before allowing them contact with the child. These dynamics can make placement with extended family difficult. Family loyalty to the imposturing is at times so powerful that extended family will either take the mother's side and eliminate themselves from being able to protect the child or will be so ostracized by the mother and extended family that the relative who takes the child (and believes the abuse occurred) is not only excluded from extended family interactions but is often actively persecuted. For these reasons, consideration of family dynamics is a key element in both initial and long-term placement of the child.

Many families demand strict devotion of their members to the rules and beliefs of the dominant adults. Although the dominant adult is often the mother, in a number of cases extended maternal families play a powerful role and maternal grandmothers hold a tight grasp on daughters and their families. In these situations the mother's role as "consummate mom" is reinforced in a passively hostile and rigid dependency relationship with the maternal grandmother.

MUNCHAUSEN BY PROXY AND ITS PROFESSIONAL PARTICIPANTS

As a core component of their psychological disorder, mothers with factitious disorder by proxy develop "perverse" relationships[16] with helping professionals, most commonly but not exclusively doctors. The masquerade as a "good mother" requires interpersonal interaction. It cannot be done without an audience, an audience that is selected for its powerful position relative to the child and its vulnerability to deception. MBP mothers have an uncanny way of seeking out health care professionals who are particularly vulnerable to "going the extra mile" for the committed parent with the chronically ill child. However, no professional is immune from deception. Even when suspicions of MBP arise, many mothers see the increased surveillance and structure initiated by the suspicious health care provider as a challenge to their superiority in executing the masquerade.

Helping professionals as a group are vulnerable to such deception. We are trained, not to suspect parents who present with sick children, but to diagnose and treat the children and work with the parents to achieve these goals. Because medical diagnosis in large part depends upon accurate history taking, vulnerability to deception by an FDP parent is considerable. This is also true for the mental health professional evaluating the mother and family. As providers begin to question the mother's veracity, she may up the ante and increase the potential harm to the child by making the symptoms more severe, in attempts to disprove the suspicions. This can lead to a cycle in which the health care providers work more and more intensively to come up with an explanation and diagnosis for the child. In the process of ordering more tests and treatments, the physician may further complicate the clinical picture over time, making it even more difficult to identify MBP.

Professionals who have been caught in this web of deceit tend to react in one of several ways. One common reaction includes guilt and shame; a second involves anger. A gastro-enterologist who treated a child for five years before putting all the pieces together said, "In hindsight I am sick every time I think of how I supported Mrs. Doe while all the while she was hurting her child. How could I have been so blind!" The success of the deceit may be one reason these children are often identified as possible victims when a new resident or medical student enters the case and is asked to review the history from a new perspective. There are cases in which a number of experienced professionals caring for the child in a variety of roles have confronted the primary physician with concerns, only to be told that their concerns were not warranted and that no attempts to assess the veracity of illness presentations would be undertaken. It is not unusual for professionals in these situations to become polarized over the issues of illness falsification. This kind of polarization can be replicated subsequently among staff in child protection, law enforcement, forensic evaluation, or intervention roles. The development of a multidisciplinary team to evaluate pediatric condition falsification is helpful in reducing such splitting and in coordinating the assessment of the child and family. Cooperation by all providers helps to assure the child's safety and the family's progress in treatment once MBP has been confirmed.

Other issues that make identifying MBP difficult for helping professionals include a dislike of detective or investigative work and a discomfort in dealing with conflict within families. The diagnosis of MBP is often seen as such a high stakes "label" that health care providers feel they need to have a standard of proof beyond that ordinarily used for reporting either physical or sexual abuse. This often delays interventions such as imposing monitoring or structure that might actually help clarify the nature of the child's difficulty.

THE ROLE OF PSYCHOSOCIAL ASSESSMENT IN THE IDENTIFICATION OF MUNCHAUSEN BY PROXY

The initial concern in potential MBP cases is to diagnose and report the presence of child abuse in the child in the form of pediatric condition falsification. If the child's symptoms are physical, then pediatric specialists are likely to play a primary role in this portion of the evaluation. If the symptoms are psychological, the mental health clinician will play a central role in the child abuse diagnosis of the child and the mother.

Regardless of whether the suspected condition falsification is physical, psychological, or educational, it is important that the child have psychological assessment and support throughout the identification process. Optimally this includes assessment of the mother and her interchange with the child. As a member of the multidisciplinary MBP team, the mental health professional is often assigned as an advocate for the child and given the responsibility for adequate mental health planning. Such individuals may also be designated as liaisons between protective services and the medical team.

Assessment of the parents should begin right away, if possible, and should include information about the family dynamics and its potential impact on the child. If different mental health professionals are asked to see various family members, there should be open communication among them and with the rest of the team, including the pediatric evaluators. All psychological assessments should be done with an eye to the physical findings in the child; each evaluator must have access to the larger body of information in the case and understand the implications of the information. Deliberately blind psychological evaluations of either children or parents in these situations are not only potentially invalid but can be considered unethical, since they rely upon a foundation that is inadequate for forming a responsible opinion regarding MBP.

The diagnosis of factitious disorder by proxy in the perpetrating parent offers understanding of the motivation for the victimization and some insight into treatment and prognosis for the parents. The issue of motivation is important to the planning for immediate and long-term disposition. There is a high recidivism rate in FDP. Both issues of child safety and treatment planning for the family hinge upon an accurate and detailed assessment of motivation of the parent, in conjunction with the extent, lethality, and chronicity of the abuse to the child. Motivational issues are of considerable use to the courts hearing child protection cases and, as importantly, to juries in criminal cases, for they help explain what would compel a mother to perform acts that appear to make no sense, from the view of a layperson unfamiliar with MBP.

Psychiatric consultants should have experience with diagnosis of MBP and the parental component of factitious disorder by proxy. If there is not an expert available, then consultation is imperative to avoid false accusations as well as missed MBP cases. In a hospital or clinic setting, the victimization of the child may be established and a report filed with child protective services before a conclusive psychiatric diagnosis is obtained or completed.

Often, an extended mental health assessment or forensic evaluation is requested through the juvenile or family court after the preliminary or "show cause" hearing in that court. A single evaluator or a team of court-appointed evaluators will assess the family in greater depth from a neutral perspective with a focus on the child's best interests. A forensic evaluation to address issues of parenting capacity and the best interests of the child in light of a differential diagnosis of Munchausen by proxy is a complex process. The critical focus of the forensic evaluation is the interactional patterns between caregivers and each child, as well as their individual histories and psychosocial functioning. Evaluators appointed by the court specifically to do a forensic assessment for MBP may fulfill several roles. If the documentation of illness exaggeration, fabrication, or inducement is adequate, then the primary role of the evaluator may be a psychological one. The diagnosis of FDP in the parent is often assessed through such an evaluation, as is the psychological and health status of the child. These two issues are intertwined because of the interactional nature of this disorder. Evaluations should be done in coordination one with the other.

Evaluations of this nature are very time consuming and include a series of clinical interviews with both the adults and the children and, often, comprehensive psychological testing of the adults and older children and corroboration of the essential elements of personal and medical history. Careful psychological testing has been helpful in identifying patterns of thinking and perceptual issues as well as characterological dimensions of the personalities of the suspected perpetrators and enablers.

The mental health evaluators should avoid dual roles if at all possible. This means that the clinical assessment team at the hospital or medical facility and the treatment providers should not serve as forensic evaluators. Once a treatment team is developed for the family this rule applies to them as well.

CONCLUSION

Munchausen by proxy is both a pediatric and a psychiatric disorder and its identification and treatment are complicated by the many interactions involved—mother and child; mother, child, and family members; mother and health care providers; and the various child protection, legal, and medical systems that may become involved. These complications suggest a team approach for both child and family and a coordinated effort by assessors and treatment as well as forensic personnel. These roles will be detailed in the following three chapters.

REFERENCES

1. Alexander R, Smith W, Stevenson R. Serial Munchausen syndrome by proxy. *Pediatrics* 1990;86:581–585.
2. American Psychiatric Association. *Diagnostic and statistical manual of mental disorders,* 4th ed. Washington, DC: American Psychiatric Press. 1994.
3. Ayoub C. Paper presented at the American Academy of Child and Adolescent Psychiatry annual meeting, October 1996.
4. Ayoub C, Alexander R, Beck D, et al. Definitional issues in Munchausen by proxy. *APSAC Advisor* 1998;11:1,7–10.
5. Kaufman K, Coury D, Pickrell E, McCleary J. Munchausen syndrome by proxy: A survey of professionals' knowledge. *Child Abuse Negl* 1998;13:141–147.
6. Leeder E. Supermom or child abuse? Treatment of the Munchausen mother. *Women Ther* 1990;9:69–88.
7. Levin AV, Sheridan MS. *Munchausen syndrome by proxy: Issues in diagnosis and treatment.* New York: Lexington Books. 1995.
8. Libow J. Munchausen by proxy syndrome victims in adulthood: A first look. *Child Abuse Negl* 1995;9:1131–1142.
9. McClure RJ, Davis PM, Meadow SR, Sibert JB. Epidemiology of Munchausen syndrome by proxy on accidental suffocation. *Arch Dis Child* 1996;75:57–61.
10. McGuire T, Feldman KW. Psychologic morbidity of children subjected to Munchausen by proxy. *Pediatrics* 1989;83:289–292.
11. Meadow R. False allegations of abuse and Munchausen syndrome by proxy. *Arch Dis Child* 1993;68:444–447.
12. Mehl A, Coble L, Johnson S. Munchausen syndrome by proxy: A family affair. *Child Abuse Negl* 1990;14:577–585.
13. Rosenberg DA. Web of deceit: A literature review of Munchausen syndrome by proxy. *Child Abuse Negl* 1987;11:547–63.
14. Schreier HA. Factitious presentation of psychiatric disorder by proxy. *Child Psychol Psychiatry Rev* 1997;2:108–115.
15. Schreier HA. Repeated false allegations of sexual abuse presenting to sheriffs: When is it Munchausen by proxy? *Child Abuse Negl* 1996;20:985–991.
16. Schreier HA, Libow JA. *Hurting for love: Munchausen by proxy syndrome.* New York: Guilford Press. 1993.
17. Southall DP, Plunkett MCB, Banks MW, Falkov AF, Samuels MP. Covert video recordings of life-threatening child abuse: Lessons for child protection. *Pediatrics* 1997;100:735–760.
18. Waller D. Obstacles to the treatment of Munchausen by proxy syndrome. *J Am Acad Child Adolesc Psychiatry* 1983;22:80–85.

Chapter 17

Psychosocial Management Issues in Munchausen by Proxy

Catherine C. Ayoub, R.N., M.N., Ed.D.,
Robin M. Deutsch, Ph.D., and
Robert Kinscherff, J.D., Ph.D.

Safety is the first and primary management issue for the MBP child victim, which often means removing the child from the home and permitting no contact or, at most, closely supervised contact with the perpetrating parent. Placement with another family member may be appropriate if the relative appreciates the meaning and seriousness of the MBP diagnosis. Many children recover dramatically from their physical illnesses when they are separated from the perpetrating parent, usually the mother. Long-term management should include monitoring, team-based treatment, and care oversight by the court. Treatment does not appear to be effective with perpetrating mothers who minimize the MBP perpetration. Reunification of parent and child should not be considered unless the mother has made treatment progress, acknowledging and reducing harmful behaviors and developing alternative strategies of childrearing.

GENERAL CONSIDERATONS

Management of Munchausen by proxy (MBP) becomes necessary when allegations have been made that the child may be a victim of MBP and state child protective authorities have begun an investigation and filed protective orders with a local juvenile or family court. In this phase a temporary structure is established, preceding the final ruling on whether child abuse by illness falsification has occurred and before the motivation has been clarified through psychological assessment.

The simultaneous needs to protect children, have parent-child observations, and fairly gather information require difficult balancing. Children need to know that they are safe. Careful assessment of placement of the child cannot be overemphasized. This may mean no contact or at best closely supervised contact with parents and any relatives who are not able to acknowledge the child's victimization and commit to stop its recurrence. Initial placement outside the home is often the most difficult, especially if there is not a court finding. Although our stance is to err on the side of protecting the child, placement in foster care or with relatives should be done thoughtfully, with attention to possible long-term placement options in any outside arrangement.

Danger to children escalates as confrontation occurs, because of the threat to parental imposturing that is the core of the personality organizational structure that underlies MBP. A parent who has FDP may feel pressed to "prove" that the child is ill. As a result, factitious presentations of the child's illness may become more bizarre or extreme. Professionals or the child may be accused directly. For example, it is not uncommon for the mother to accuse the hospital staff of fabricating illness at the time when she is being confronted about the true nature of the child's problems.

The primary goal of case management in this phase is to protect the child while the investigation of the allegations of MBP perpetration proceeds. At the same time, further assessment of the alleged MBP is conducted in order to

- determine whether pediatric condition falsification has occurred;
- document alleged MBP for state child protection proceedings;
- assess medical, psychiatric, and psychosocial risks to the child;
- assess the child's need for protective measures as well as legitimate medical or other needs;
- determine what, if any, interventions are likely to reduce risk to the child; and
- develop a long-term management plan in the event that the child is found in need of state child protection.

If there are siblings in the household it is also important to attend to any risks posed to them, particularly if there are allegations or documentation of a history of their involvement in MBP behaviors or a history of unexplained or suspicious deaths among siblings. Removal pending further evaluation should be considered for siblings who may be particularly vulnerable to MBP perpetration, such as preverbal children or those with genuinely existing significant medical conditions.

PLACEMENT ISSUES

Placement decisions must first consider the safety and protection of the child. In the short-term management phase, the rights of the parents and the attachment of the child are weighed against the real risk of injury or death. A protective structure is required that attends to

- collection of information to confidently establish the presence of pediatric condition falsification and factitious disorder by proxy;
- the potential lethality or injury to the child as a result of further perpetration if parents retain physical custody or have inadequately supervised contact with the child;
- placement needs of the child following the initial suspicion and allegations by medical care providers; and
- any contact or visitation between the child and parents or family pending completion of child protection investigations or court proceedings.

During the evaluation stage, separation of mother and child is recommended. At times this can be done through a prolonged hospital stay. However, with increased limits on hospitalizations and with the need to promote a health-oriented rather than an illness-oriented environment for the child, alternative out of home placement is often recommended. Many of these children begin to recover dramatically from their physical illnesses when removed from the home.

Although there may be family members willing and eager to have the child placed with them, family members often do not accept the diagnosis of MBP or fail to appreciate the risks of this disorder. Family members who do not believe that MBP may have occurred often cannot be relied upon to set firm limits on access. On the other hand, if there are family members who appreciate the potential risks to the child and are willing and able to protect the child from further abuse by the perpetrating parent, placement in their care can be beneficial. However, if a family member was the reporting party or has aligned with those who suspect MBP, the polarization between that family member and the alleged perpetrator may affect the child's sense of emotional safety and make that person's home not a good placement option.

Sometimes the child will be placed with the separately domiciled spouse or partner of the alleged perpetrator, with the understanding that the spouse or partner will enforce court orders or other conditions of placement. Although this may work when the perpetrating parent and the partner have been separated or divorced for a period of time, it is still important to assess the willingness and ability of the partner to acknowledge the seriousness of the allegations and to protect the child. It can be risky to place the child with an allegedly nonperpetrating parent when the parents or partners separate at the time the allegations arise. In these cases, it cannot easily be determined whether the separation is primarily or exclusively to mollify authorities so that the child will remain placed within the family.

In some cases, state protective or court authorities sometimes choose to leave the child in the physical custody of the alleged perpetrating parent. This is not ordinarily recommended, and it is strongly recommended against in cases where serious medical or psychiatric symptoms are fabricated or actually induced. When continued placement with a suspected perpetrator does occur, it is very important that the family notify legal or child protective authorities before presenting the child for further medical or psychological evaluation or treatment. Intensive medical monitoring should be ongoing to reduce the risk of injury or death to the child.

VISITATION ISSUES

Children who have been victims of MBP are likely to experience a sense of helplessness and apathy. These children have endured conflicting and unpredictable senses of who they are and what their bodily vulnerabilities are, as a result of fabrication or inducement of symptoms or unwarranted invasive medical procedures. To regain a sense of control, they need predictability—regularity and consistency of routine, including a schedule for visits; alteration of visitation schedules, locations, and processes should be minimized, and manipulation of them by parents should not be allowed. If the child is removed from the care of the alleged perpetrating parent while a diagnosis of MBP is being considered, very carefully structured and supervised parent-child visits are generally recommended. Visits should be regular and scheduled to minimize disruption in the child's regular routine. It is important for the child to know in advance when visits are scheduled to occur. Younger children, in particular, need predictable, consistent visits. Younger children have a tendency to blame themselves for any missed visit, so cancellations should be minimized.

Visitation between child and alleged perpetrating parent should be closely supervised pending completion of assessments, particularly where an extreme pattern of MBP is alleged. In these cases, visitation contacts should occur only in closely supervised settings. Visitation supervisors should be carefully chosen professionals—rather than friends or family members—and trained so that they can be alert to potential risk situations such as exchange of food or drink or any unmonitored contact. They should be fully informed about the specifics of the allegations of pediatric conditions falsification. Special attention and caution should be exercised at times when the usual supervisors are on vacation or otherwise unavailable.

Most visitation guidelines exclude the exchange of food or beverages and limit the number of gifts brought to the child. Excessive gift giving is a significant issue in many of these cases. Parents should be admonished to avoid discussion of the child's health or welfare. The desire of these parents to obtain and control information about their children is a powerful force and tends to present repeatedly as intrusiveness and demands for information and conformity. Boundaries are often violated if visits are not closely monitored by experienced professional supervisors who have the skills and authority to intervene if necessary to protect the child from both psychological and physical harm.

THE ROLE OF MULTIDISCIPLINARY TEAMS IN ASSESSMENT AND TREATMENT OF MBP

The very nature of the credible deception that is part of MBP makes it critical to use multidisciplinary teams to assist in the identification and management of MBP. Teams should, at a minimum, have one expert in MBP. In some hospitals, there are teams of MBP experts that can address both the pediatric and psychiatric components of the disorder. In acute care settings, these teams work closely with the attending medical and nursing staff. In addition, a number of hospitals have convened pediatric ethics review groups to assist with decision making in suspected or identified MBP cases. Both of these mechanisms offer health care providers and the systems within which they work additional input to contribute to the decision-making process. The MBP team serves not only to improve the accuracy of the diagnosis but also as a clinical and legal risk management mechanism.

After identification, professionals providing medical and psychological services to the child and family form a team and work together to share information and coordinate treatment goals. It is an error to attempt medical, child protection, mental health, and risk management measures without close coordination. This treatment team is most effective when organized under the consultation and coordination of a court-appointed MBP expert; the consultant can also serve as the liaison for reporting to the juvenile or family court. The fragmentation of treatment goals is a frequent danger if there is no communication mechanism for providers.

The treatment provider team is made up of direct providers, and its purpose is to plan, coordinate, and evaluate treatment for the child, any at-risk siblings, the custodial parent or guardian, and the parents. The family provider team sets clinical goals and provides and coordinates services for the family. The team typically consists of all active providers of physical, emotional, and educational treatment for the child and family members, representatives of child protective services, court-appointed assessors, and court-appointed advocates for the child. A court-appointed expert in MBP serves as a consultant and leader of the integrated team; the designated professional from the mandated child protection agency and/or the guardian ad litem often coordinates the team process. The team consultant is often appointed by the court to bring the group together and to act as a liaison between and consultant expert for the members. If the perpetrating parent persists in seeking serial opinions to debunk the finding of MBP, such subsequent evaluators should be examined carefully before being included in the process, where information about the children is openly shared.

The court plays an important role in defining the scope of treatment based on findings of child maltreatment in the children and in attributing its cause to the perpetrator's persistent exaggeration, fabrication, and/or inducement of physical or psychological illness in the child. Without such legal finding, it is extremely difficult to proceed with treatment of the MBP perpetrator. The MBP parent and her supporters typically initiate repeated reevaluation of the diagnostic issues rather than focusing on a treatment regimen.

A second role of the treatment team led by a court-appointed expert in MBP is to provide integrated professional information to the court on the progress of the principal adults and the child(ren). Although the court may always choose to hear from providers individually, the court-appointed expert is in a position to provide testimony regarding the strategic case goals and case management or interventioner in each case. It is the responsibility of this court-appointed team leader to provide the court with reports on a regular basis. These reports should never preclude independent reports from the mandated agency or from the guardian ad litem.

In order to coordinate and integrate services for the child and family, the team works on setting clinical goals and coordinating clinical service interventions, relying upon the holistic knowledge of the family treatment plan and the input of each therapist and health care provider in order to assure the child's adequate safety and care. Although team members may work with different family members as clients, the central purpose of the team is to assure that the child's best interests are being served. However, this does not negate a team member's obligation to represent the interests and interactions that will best serve his or her client/patient.

In cases of MBP, communications among persons can become complicated and inefficient. Professional boundaries within the team should be clear and the confidentiality shared by the team respected by all members. The purpose of therapy is a clarifying and integrative one for the family. The team serves as the model for the integration that must occur within the family if the reunification is to be considered as an option. Services delivered without full knowledge of the information and without the benefit of the perspective of each of the parties increase fragmentation and reduce the likelihood of successful intervention. This is a serious impediment to successful treatment as well as to the protection of the child in cases in which MBP is being considered. All evaluators and treating providers should have access to detailed information about the child(ren) and the parents. It is imperative that isolated evaluations of the parents or children not be performed. Particular care should be used to define and clarify roles; dual role relationships should be avoided.

LONG-TERM MANAGEMENT ISSUES

After diagnosis, a management plan must be developed. A number of factors need to be considered, and coordination is necessary among medical, child protective, therapeutic, and any legal systems that are involved, in order to limit the child's exposure to risk of harm. A process of monitoring, team-based treatment, and care oversight by the court on a long-term basis is recommended. This process is intended either to move the child toward safe reunification with the parent or to assess the appropriateness of termination of parental rights. In MBP, steps toward reunification should only be undertaken if there is a team of health care providers, mental health providers, child protective services personnel, and a court liaison who can work together to assure safety and evaluate the steps made toward reunification. If this process is not acceptable to all parties, then termination of rights is recommended.

When a diagnosis of MBP is made, risk to children depends on their developmental status and the nature and severity of the abuse. All cases of factitious disorder by proxy are of a serious nature, by virtue of the definition of the diagnosis. Developmentally, preverbal children are most at risk. Children who have suffered severe abuse such as suffocation or poisoning are at greatest physical risk. Other risk factors include characteristics of the perpetrating mother, such as

- an absence of understanding or acknowledgment of the perpetrating behavior
- diagnosis of Munchausen syndrome
- substance abuse
- ongoing fabrication after confrontation

In addition to medical risks, the psychological risks to the child are considerable and are closely associated with the extent of time the child has been exposed to the dysfunctional relationship with the perpetrating parent. Older children are at serious risk of being victimized into adulthood. Therefore, it is important to assemble a comprehensive history of the MBP case.

Gathering medical records is important, and it can be a massive task, as the parent has often moved from doctor to doctor and hospital to hospital. Careful review of medical records will provide data about the scope of illness, injury, and medical procedures. Subsequent documentation of the child's use of medical services and health status while out of the care of the alleged abuser provides a comparison of the child's medical needs in the parent's care and during a period of separation. To make this benchmark of assessment useful, it is essential that there be no unsupervised contact between the child and the alleged abuser or family members. If the child's use of medical intervention—doctor's visits, medications, need for devices, and hospitalizations—decreases significantly during separation from the alleged abuser, the child might require interventions to prepare for return to the care of the abusing parent.

The range of degree of this disorder, which can go from intermittent abuse to chronic, ongoing abuse, is of concern. For cases of intermittent abuse, a parent may be able to abstain from the abusive invasive behaviors during the course of an evaluation. While in some cases the parent appears to be driven to cause or falsify illness in the child, in other cases parents refrain from abuse while they are being investigated or monitored.

MEDICAL CARE ISSUES

Coordination of medical and psychological care in cases of MBP is essential. (Medical management is discussed in further detail in chapter 18.) If there is more than one health care provider, they should routinely communicate with each other and be familiar with the history of the child and the findings from any evaluations relevant to factitious disorder by proxy. Most importantly, the primary physician must accept the diagnosis of MBP when it has been established, or, during a period of investigation, accept the real possibility of the diagnosis of MBP and appreciate the risks involved. The primary physician should

- coordinate all care for the affected child
- monitor the child's health
- make referrals to other providers if necessary
- assess the child's ongoing growth and development

Ongoing monitoring of the child's physical status while out of the care of the perpetrator of MBP will ultimately establish the child's actual medical needs.

PSYCHOTHERAPEUTIC TREATMENT ISSUES FOR THE CHILD

The child who is at least 3 years old needs psychotherapeutic treatment. Preschool children often blame themselves for being removed from a parent. The egocentricity of this age results in magical thinking, and these children's understanding is related to physical proximity. Children this age need help understanding that removal from their parent was for their protection and not the result of something they did. Some MBP victims have accommodated to invasive procedures or serious illness, evolving an identity as a "sick child" and adopting a compliant and helpless stance. The therapeutic task is to help the child experience autonomy, accept health, seek competence, and contribute to positive identity formation.

School-aged children older than about 7 tend to align closely with the perpetrating parent. They maintain a controlled and enmeshed relationship that is not easily disrupted by either removal or psychotherapy. One explanation for this alliance is that typically the child has been deprived of normal activities and contacts central to normal development. Instead of mastering play, school, peer, and social activities, they have been involved in their parent's fabrications or induction of illness. Although free to regain health in a safe setting, these children remain acutely aware of the loyalty conflicts. Demands for secrecy, loyalty, and deception are often reinforced during parent-child encounters.

Developmentally, adolescents are supposed to be working on the tasks of separation and identity development. These tasks are frequently compromised in adolescents who have been victims of MBP. Often the parent-child relationship is characterized by extreme alliance and dependence. The parent and child may even share a folie á deux, a commitment to the same delusional beliefs. The development of the core self, particularly autonomy and independence, is jeopardized, replaced instead by an identification as a medically impaired person and a sense of helplessness, depression, and apathy.

As contact between child and parent changes, it is imperative that the child have access to a person seen as his or her own confidant and therapist. Monitoring changes in the child's behavior and affect is a critical job of the therapist. The centrality of the therapist's role to the child emphasizes the need for the therapist to remain focused primarily on the child and not attempt to be primary treatment provider to other family members as well.

TREATMENT OF PARENTS AND REUNIFICATION ISSUES

Studies of psychotherapeutic treatment on MBP mothers show little efficacy. McGuire and Feldman[2] reported that in their cases "treatment had been attempted for significant periods of time and appeared to have little effect on either the behavior of the mother or on development of insight into her condition"; Kinscherff and Famularo[1] concur with this finding, indicating that the limited data that do exist on the treatment of MBP perpetrators do not support effectiveness of psychotherapy and in fact suggest that "classic" and "extreme" perpetrators will continue to perpetrate MBP during and even after courses of psychotherapy. Successful treatment is rare, but possible; it is not usually recommended in cases where inducement of illness is a factor. There is limited published literature that recommends psychotherapeutic intervention with the perpetrating parent and eventual reunification. Reunification is only recommended when a course of treatment has ensued in which the following conditions have been met:

- there is acknowledgement of MBP by mother and other involved family members;
- the perpetrator has completed a significant course of long-term individual treatment with therapists who have experience in treating MBP; and
- family members, including fathers, have engaged in treatment (imperative if parents are still a couple and wish to remain so), understand the nature and dynamics of MBP, and have consistently taken appropriate action to protect and support the child(ren).

Treatment of perpetrating adults and enabling adults by experienced clinicians familiar with MBP treatment and willing to work with the treatment team and the court is a key element of the treatment process. In the absence of this expertise by treating professionals, close consultation with an expert acceptable to the court, the mandated agency, and the treatment team is highly recommended.

In MBP cases where FDP is a diagnosis held by the mother, treatment is ordinarily difficult and the prognosis guarded even in the case of aggressive psychiatric intervention. However, there are some mothers and families who have taken steps toward safe reunification. Sanders describes successful reunification with a mother who fabricated illness but did not induce symptoms. She describes a process which begins with acknowledgment of victimization and a willingness to enter treatment. The therapeutic process is a lengthy one and includes the co-construction of an alternative life narrative concerning issues of illness and health. The treatment process also entails significant work on parent-child interactions and demands carefully structured therapeutic goals.[3,4] The children's safety is closely monitored and parents must agree to work with medical, child protective, and mental health teams. A balance between the child's safety—both physical and emotional—and the optimal possibility of safe reunification is often difficult to assess, even in the most hopeful of cases. The soundest advice is to assess carefully each step of the process and move forward carefully, with input from the treatment team, to avoid failure for both mother and child. Sanders points out that another important aspect of the treatment process is for the mother's providers to assess the situation from outside the mother's perspective in order to stay grounded in the real risks to the child and avoid the biases that can occur.

Progress in therapy would consist of acknowledgement of the harmful behaviors, reduction or abolition of those behaviors, and alternative strategies to cope with feelings of abandonment and deprivation. Marital therapy can be used to build systems of support and to reduce the sense of isolation and deprivation. Family therapy should be considered only with great care. It may be helpful for adults and children remaining in the home as long as it does not perpetuate the secretive control often exacted over younger or weaker family members. Children should only be included in family therapy in MBP cases if they have the freedom to maintain their own identities and competence. This may mean that the target child only participates with his or her therapist present.

Fathers also should receive treatment with an experienced MBP clinician. Fathers, especially those who remain in the marital relationship, are frequently enablers of Munchausen behavior. Assessment and treatment of fathers is a critical variable in reunification. Fathers who are separated or divorced at the time of exposure of MBP are more likely to acknowledge their children's victimization. Such fathers often require extended support in order to maintain a position of advocacy for their children, particularly in the face of denial by the perpetrating parent.

Reunification of the child and parent is dependent upon both the risks to the child and the parent's progress in psychotherapy. In general the more lethal the abuse, the greater the ongoing and future risk to the child despite efforts at psychiatric intervention. In cases of extreme MBP, where there is a high risk of death or permanent injury to the child, prompt termination of parental rights may need to be considered.[1] Reunification is a slow and extended process in any successful reunification situation and should be approached with extreme caution. These mothers require extended therapy to develop alternatives to MBP behaviors. Additional considerations with regard to maternal mental health and stability should be carefully considered as well. On average, treatment takes five or more years of intensive work.

Monitoring over a period of years (often until the child reaches adulthood) may be necessary in cases of MBP. This often means that court oversight will be lengthy as well. Fragmentation of long-term care is likely if court-appointed team coordinators and active team participants are unable to continue for the duration of treatment.

CONCLUSION

Continuing psychosocial management of children who are victimized by MBP requires the involvement of a therapist who is focused on the child's interests and welfare. The primary and continuing goal of case management of these children is to protect them from further harm and for the children to know they are safe. This usually means placement outside the home. Placement decisions must consider the risks of awarding custody to other family members, who may not understand or accept the MBP diagnosis. Visitation with the offending parent must be closely supervised by a qualified professional who is aware of the dangers of reabuse, and reunification should be attempted only if the parent has made sufficient progress to assure no risk to the child. Reunification with the perpetrating parent is a difficult process, fraught with risk. It must be conditioned upon adequate compliance with interventions, and it may not be possible where MBP has been chronic or has involved potentially injurious or lethal medical symptoms. Every step in the process must be considered extremely carefully with the interests of the child always the primary consideration.

R E F E R E N C E S

1. Kinscherff R, Famularo R. Extreme Munchausen syndrome by proxy: The case for termination of parental rights. *Juvenile Fam Court J* 1991;42(4):41–53.

2. McGuire T, Feldman K. Psychologic morbidity of children subjected to Munchausen by proxy. *Pediatrics* 1989;83:289–292.

3. Parnell T, Day D. *Munchausen by proxy syndrome: Misunderstood child abuse.* Thousand Oaks, CA: Sage Publications. 1998.

4. Sanders M. Narrative family treatment of Munchausen by proxy: A successful case. *Fam Sys Med* 1996;14:315–328.

Chapter 18

Medical Treatment of Munchausen Syndrome by Proxy

Randell C. Alexander, M.D., Ph.D.

For medical professionals, MBP cases are among the most complex, frustrating, and time-consuming examples of child abuse or any other medical condition they will treat. Because of the manipulation practiced by the MBP perpetrator, medical providers can become unwitting pawns in the case. There is need for expert consultation whenever MBP is suspected. A comprehensive review of past medical records of the child and mother can help support the case for MBP. Early diagnosis of this disorder can prevent the high morbidity and mortality that is associated with it. Medical management considerations include hospitalization, outpatient treatment, protection of siblings, and psychotherapeutic treatment of the perpetrator, usually the mother.

GENERAL CONSIDERATIONS

Early diagnosis is the key to limiting the high morbidity and mortality currently seen in many cases of Munchausen by proxy. Strategies to treat or prevent MBP include efforts that may also enhance the early identification of cases. The use of such techniques is presently in the formative stages, although there has been some selected experience with certain high-risk populations.

Once there is a suspicion of MBP, extensive review of previous medical records and other documentation is imperative.[3] Particular attention should be given to reviewing the suspected perpetrator's own medical records. A timeline is critical for

- organizing the extensive data,
- identifying apparent gaps in treatment which may indicate that the child was seen elsewhere, and
- establishing relationships between events.

For example, the mother rarely is hospitalized herself at the same time as the child. Nearly always, only one child is the focus of medical treatment, even if eventually more than one child is victimized in the family.[1] The role of the father in the family constellation should

236

be established to determine his understanding of the child's condition and his possible involvement with the induction or simulation of illness.

A review of insurance records and reviews of visits to medical clinics known to be havens for MBP mothers, such as clinics that evaluate apnea, seizures, or gastrointestinal disorders, may aid in investigating the suspicion that the child is a victim of MBP.

MEDICAL MANAGEMENT CONSIDERATIONS

Once the initial diagnosis is either made or strongly suspected, intensive efforts are often necessary to further refine the diagnosis, protect the child, evaluate the rest of the family, and address medical, psychosocial, and legal concerns. During the entire process, the health and safety of the child are paramount. The diagnosis of MBP itself not only characterizes what has occurred but is also a predictor of future risk. Thus, further diagnostic, treatment, and medical-legal interventions should be pursued so as not to put the child at further risk.

Hospitalization

The advantages and disadvantages of putting the child in the hospital should be carefully considered. Although further evidence of MBP can sometimes be gathered in this more controlled setting, it is not without consequences. If the diagnosis has already been suspected strongly or has been established, hospitalization is unnecessary and substitute care should be considered instead.

Video Surveillance

Videotaping is sometimes considered for hospitalized children who have been alleged to have frequent episodic events such as apnea, seizures, fevers, or vomiting and diarrhea. The intent is to document the inducement of symptoms and signs. However, this tactic may not be helpful in diagnosing the many forms of MBP in which episodes are infrequent and might not be seen during a period of hospital surveillance. It also would not be considered for forms of MBP in which only a simulation of illness took place and there was absence of an actual inflicted condition, unless the purpose is to show that the child was normal during a time when abnormality was alleged.

The advantage of videotape surveillance is obtaining a visual demonstration of abuse, which is felt to be more convincing than the written documentation in the medical record. However, there are many problems with this approach. These include all the usual disadvantages of hospitalization, exposure of the child to a known potentially dangerous situation, the need for constant videomonitoring of the room by trained personnel to detect any possible adverse act, questions about privacy of the monitoring if covert, and liability concerns. Consultation with a hospital attorney should be undertaken before embarking upon such a procedure.

Perhaps the largest drawback of videotaping is that, if the taping reveals no acts of abuse during the surveillance period, the diagnosis can be called erroneous. Too much emphasis on the videotape as the litmus test for MBP may make it the only standard by which the diagnosis of MBP is proved. No other form of child abuse or any other crime has such a standard. In practice, videotaping may on occasion be supportive, but it is attempted in a minority of cases. The argument has been made that if a suspicion of MBP is strong enough to prompt videotape surveillance, then the diagnosis can be made without the need for taping.[4]

Hospital and Outpatient Protocols

Once the diagnosis has been made, a consistent approach to treatment helps ensure that critical steps are not overlooked. For a low-incidence problem like MBP, the approach is usually unfamiliar to the medical staff and the opportunities for significant omissions or other treatment errors are correspondingly high. Although each case may have some unique circumstances, protocols should be used as guidelines.

The safety of the child is the highest priority. Additional interventions intended to confirm or supplement the diagnosis of MBP may be important, but they are secondary to the child's immediate and continuing health and safety. The diagnosis of MBP itself may be a life-saving step in protecting the child.

Expertise is essential in MBP cases, as placement and court considerations will inevitably arise. A thorough background investigation may illuminate other concerns. If old enough, the child must be psychologically supported through all of the ensuing investigations and legal circumstances (see chapter 17). Because these cases are so complex and convoluted for the triers of fact in court, errors occur frequently. Even when the MBP children are safely placed initially, they are often returned home when social service and court personnel mistakenly conclude that the child's medical condition can be monitored there and safety assured. When this occurs, quick medical intervention to reduce or stop the implementation of further unnecessary medical procedures or the use of needless medical devices (apnea monitors, gastrostomy tubes, central intravenous lines, medications, special diets) may achieve at least some increased safety for the child.

The perpetrator in MBP cases is almost always the mother. Investigation of her medical and psychological history may further define the nature and extent of the dysfunction. Her medical records may show a pattern of behavior characteristic of Munchausen syndrome. In such cases, an increased risk for suicide has been observed, and emergency psychological or psychiatric support for the mother may be warranted. Psychological evaluation of the mother cannot determine whether MBP has occurred, nor is it a good predictor of future risk of abuse; however, it is helpful in continuing work with the family.

In addition to individual considerations for the child and the perpetrator, a series of other actions is necessary to address the MBP itself and limit possible further abuse. As with any form of child abuse, it is necessary to work with social services and legal authorities to carefully document what has occurred. Because MBP is uncommon and involves differentiating the presenting signs and symptoms from a wide variety of complex medical conditions, considerable assistance may be necessary from the medical evaluation team. Since no treatment approach is known to correct MBP behavior, foster care placement is often the only viable option for protecting the child from the offender. Siblings may also need protection, as it is the perpetrator who poses the risk for children, not some personal characteristic inherent in one child that precipitates the abusive behavior. Medical responsibility includes making the diagnosis of MBP, after ruling out possibilities of rare disease states, and the ensuing process of adjudication and follow-up.

PROFESSIONAL RESPONSE TO THE MBP DIAGNOSIS

For the medical professional, MBP cases are among the most complex, frustrating, and time-consuming examples of child abuse or any other condition. Understandably, physicians are upset when they discover that they have been unwitting pawns of the perpetrator of MBP and have committed medical injury to the child. This is in direct contradiction to their self-perception of delivering necessary medical care to their patients and practicing in a humanitarian fashion. When challenged with the possibility of MBP, a physician or any other medical provider may react with anger and denial or an uncharacteristic support of the perpetrator that may approach blind advocacy. One's investment in a long-held diagnosis and even one's professional reputation can be tested in such circumstances.

Nowhere in the field of medical diagnosis, even in the field of child abuse, is the collection of medical and social service evidence more critical than in the diagnosis of MBP. The following approach is offered to assure the best possible assembling of facts, medical diagnosis and treatment, and the most effective legal case by which to protect the child from further harm.[2]

The Hospital Team

At the first suspicion of MBP, the staff who are responsible for the care of the child should be called into conference to discuss the problem. Each of the staff should be allowed to express feelings about the proposed diagnosis, so that any strong doubts can be given serious consideration before proceeding. Often, perpetrators of MBP are quite adept at "splitting" the staff, forming strong alliances with some who are more comfortable with a supportive and empathic role. Because it is imperative that all team members be working to gather unbiased evidence, they must avoid being co-opted into alliances with the suspected perpetrator. Education of the staff about the elements of MBP and why the current case fits into the description of the syndrome must be done, to combat sabotaging of the effort to collect unbiased data.

Medical consultants from appropriate disciplines need to be included in the deliberations of the team, so that they can lend their expertise to the medical diagnosis. For example, if polymicrobial bacteremia is present, it is necessary to have the infectious disease consultant help everyone understand why the infection is not due to natural disease; a gastroenterologist can assure that there is no identifiable site of rectal bleeding; a hematologist can assure that bleeding or clotting disorders are not responsible for recurrent blood loss.

Inclusion of a psychiatrist and psychologist on the team is necessary, not only for their insights about the syndrome, but also to give support to the staff and to detect possible dysfunctional group dynamics among team members.

Professionals from child protective services, the district attorney's office, and law enforcement must be included early in the deliberations, to avoid delays that could be costly to the child's health. They should be consulted before an official report is made, since the evidence is being collected to make a report that can be substantiated and acted upon quickly.

The team should gather daily for sign-out conferences. These may take only a few minutes or much longer, depending on the stage of the case.

It is desirable that one or two members of the staff be assigned to be supportive of the suspected perpetrator, so that she is not sequestered and alienated.

Assembling the Medical Record

The requirements for accurate and detailed charting of all events, large and small, should be made clear from the outset. Summary sheets for each day should iterate the significant events of the day in terms of diagnostic procedures, the demeanor and affect of the suspected perpetrator, and the reactions of the child.

All of the child's past medical records should be requested and reviewed as soon as possible. This may require going to other institutions and actually reading the records on site.

The medical records of the siblings and the parents should also be reviewed. In the case of the siblings, this is necessary to determine similar problems in their past and also to determine whether there have been other cases of child abuse or child death. In the case of the parents, it is to determine if there are elements in their past medical history suggesting psychopathology or Munchausen syndrome.

Disposition

Out-of-home placement should be recommended if the diagnosis is strongly suspected. Such placement could be in a pediatric convalescent or rehabilitation facility. If this is done, it is important that the staff of the new facility understand the diagnosis and that parental visitation is either prohibited or sharply delineated.

Safety of the siblings must be ensured. This can be done by out-of-home placement for them or by careful surveillance by child protective services, with the children all receiving medical evaluations by the hospital team. Follow-up medical care for the index child should also be carried out by the hospital team.

CONCLUSION

Both complex and uncommon, cases of MBP pose unusual and difficult challenges for medical practitioners, who are often involved not only with medical issues but with the ensuing cascade of psychological and legal events that attend a case of MBP. Because the diagnosis of MBP not only characterizes events that have occurred to date but also predicts future events, diagnostic and treatment interventions will play an important role in preventing further risk or injury to the child, and perhaps to siblings as well. It is recommended that, whenever possible, medical management of MBP be carried out by experienced professionals with an understanding of the disorder.

REFERENCES

1. Alexander R, Smith W, Stevenson R. Serial Munchausen syndrome by proxy. *Pediatrics* 1990;86(4):581–585.

2. Reece RM. *The medical manifestations of child abuse: A curriculum.* Boston: Institute for Professional Education, Massachusetts Society for the Prevention of Cruelty to Children. 1994.

3. Rosenberg DA. Web of deceit: A literature review of Munchausen syndrome by proxy. *Child Abuse Negl* 1987;11:547–563.

4. Yorker BC. Covert video surveillance of Munchausen syndrome by proxy: The exigent circumstances exception. *Health Matrix* 1995; 5:325–346.

Chapter 19

Legal Aspects of Munchausen by Proxy

Robert Kinscherff, J.D., Ph.D., and
Catherine C. Ayoub, R.N., M.N., Ed.D.

The conduct associated with Munchausen by proxy has a wide range of legal implications, and the legal challenges can match the medical and psychosocial challenges. Attorneys and courts must deal with MBP cases in criminal prosecutions, child protection proceedings, and divorce actions. Health care providers working with suspected MBP cases should be aware of the legal considerations that arise when MBP is suspected. Not only are the means by which health care professionals detect and document an alleged case of MBP crucial to legal proceedings, but the practitioners' conduct is also subject to scrutiny on issues including professional standards of care for diagnosis and treatment, informed consent for covert video surveillance or medical diagnostic procedures, and compliance with mandated reporting of child abuse. Both the child and family are best served if medical, mental health, social service, and legal personnel are knowledgeable. Construction of a national database of MBP cases is recommended as an aid to earlier diagnosis and better understanding and disposition of these difficult cases.

GENERAL CONSIDERATIONS

The conduct involved in the perpetration of Munchausen by proxy (MBP) can range from the fabrication or exaggeration of reported medical history or symptoms to the mimicry or induction of medical, psychiatric, educational, or other symptoms through a variety of methods. MBP is now incorporated in the DSM-IV[1] as a factitious disorder by proxy (FDP). Its designation as a "Factitious Disorder Not Otherwise Specified" in the DSM-IV highlights the volitional and intentional nature of the perpetrator's actions, properly focuses upon the misconduct of the perpetrator in the maltreatment of the victim, and eliminates the legally complicated term *syndrome*. The use of the term *factitious disorder by proxy* clarifies that the diagnosis properly belongs to the perpetrator rather than to the victim and underscores that the perpetrator has falsely caused the victim to be seen by others as ill or impaired.

Controversy continues about the best terminology to use to describe MBP behaviors and their variants. In this chapter, we will use the name Munchausen by proxy, partly because of the familiarity of the name Munchausen and its links to the adult form of the factitious disorder, but also because the DSM-IV description does not yet adequately capture the variants of deceptive or exaggerated presentations of illness and impairment in children.

The term *syndrome* is eliminated because recent research increasingly distinguishes among the variants of factitious illness presentation among child victims and because the focus must be upon the specific conduct of the perpetrator rather than a cluster of nonspecific perpetrator characteristics, such as history of training in health related fields, maternal relationship to the victim, or evidence of personality dysfunction. More importantly, *syndrome* has different meanings and ramifications when used in clinical and in legal settings. Dropping the word *syndrome* forces clinicians to focus more precisely upon the specific perpetrating behaviors and psychological characteristics of perpetrator and victim in each case. It also accommodates the requirement that legal decision makers focus upon specific acts of misconduct, as reflected in the discomfort many courts show in relying upon syndrome characteristics that may be too general to use in making decisions in individual cases. Focusing clinicians upon specific conduct rather than syndrome characteristics works to the benefit of detection, clinical management, child protection, and assessment of risks and prognosis for interventions. Finally, dropping *syndrome* serves to eliminate a psychiatric mystique that may lead clinicians and courts to improperly or too quickly conclude that the perpetrator is suffering from a major mental illness that implies legally significant impairments in the perpetrator's capacity to form intent, recognize the wrongfulness of the perpetrating behavior, or refrain from the abusive misconduct.

The most detailed literature about MBP describes factitious presentation of medical signs or symptoms. However, even in cases of medical MBP there may be the concurrent false presentation of psychiatric, educational, or social impairments. The medical outcome for the child may range from an immediate detection of the deception, through a continuum of unnecessary medical examinations and procedures, to significant injury or death of the child as a direct result of the perpetration or the medical response to the presumed illness. Other variants of MBP without false medical symptom production can result in other forms of unnecessary and intrusive evaluation and intervention. These can include special educational placement, sexual abuse evaluations, or child custody evaluations in divorce cases that are based on factitious presentation of emotional or behavioral disturbance of the child that is ascribed to the other parent.

Whatever its manifestation in a particular case, however, the hallmark of MBP is that the perpetrator factitiously establishes a "sick role" through the child that is primarily motivated by

1. an intense need to seek attention and recognition from helping professionals who are seen as powerful;
2. the gratification associated with the subsequent sadistic deception and manipulation of the caregivers; and
3. the adoption of the sick role for herself and her instrument of recognition, the child.

Schreier and Libow[2] have characterized the dynamics of perpetration and deception as a form of perversion in which the child is used as an object to create and maintain a highly disturbed but gratifying relationship with clinical caregivers and others perceived as wielding power who have the capacity to endow the perpetrator with recognition and efficacy.

The dynamics of deception and manipulation of powerful figures may also include lawyers, judges, child protection or law enforcement personnel, school staff, and others who may play a role in the case. Schreier and Libow[3] have held that MBP perpetrators are able to prey upon the narcissistic sense of certainty and self-confidence of physicians who are deceived and discount evidence of the MBP. This dynamic is undoubtedly the same when the deception focuses upon lawyers, judges, child protection authorities, therapists, family members, and others who remain convinced of the innocence of the perpetrator despite increasingly compelling evidence to the contrary.

Cases in which a child is falsely presented as ill or impaired primarily to achieve economic gain, to win child custody by engineering a false abuse complaint, or to exact revenge upon another person who loves the child should not be characterized as MBP. Neither should cases in which an overly anxious parent of a genuinely ill child may exaggerate symptom reports out of that anxiety, resulting in a greater degree of medical scrutiny than might be absolutely necessary. As discussed below, clarity regarding the nature and motivations for the perpetration is important in distinguishing MBP cases from others that may share some features of MBP. Specificity is also critical in

- assessing risks to the child, since some kinds of MBP perpetrators reportedly have a high recidivism rate even after court intervention or psychiatric treatment;
- assessing the suitability of immediate and long-term management, intervention, and disposition strategies; and
- making clear to courts and others the kinds of motivations that might prompt this form of child maltreatment

LEGAL DIMENSIONS OF MBP

A wide variety of legal issues may be implicated by MBP. Some of these stem from the perpetrating behaviors themselves, particularly if they involve induction of symptoms by poisoning, suffocation, or other highly risky and intrusive acts. Others arise from the duties of health care providers to maintain the standards of clinical care in the assessment and treatment of medical or other conditions, or the duty of health care professionals to make mandated child protection reports when a child is at risk of abuse or neglect.

Actions by MBP perpetrators may result in criminal prosecution or civil child protection proceedings filed by state child protection authorities. MBP allegations also may arise in child custody disputes between parents in divorce actions before probate and family courts. However, whatever the specific legal issue that is involved when alleged MBP cases come before courts, the means by which health care professionals have detected and documented an alleged case of MBP are crucial to these legal proceedings.[4] When a case involving MBP comes before a court, it is not only the alleged perpetrator who will be examined closely. The conduct of health care professionals and medical centers who become involved in MBP cases also are subject to scrutiny on issues including the methods by which the MBP was detected and documented, professional standards of care for diagnosis and treatment, informed consent for covert video surveillance or medical diagnostic procedures, and compliance with mandated reporting of child abuse.

Depending upon jurisdiction, courts have shown considerable variability in handling MBP cases. In many jurisdictions, if brought forward at all, MBP allegations tend to be treated as civil child protection cases rather than criminal prosecutions of serious child abuse, except in cases where children have been seriously injured or died. Juvenile and family courts hearing them as child protection cases have shown wide variability in judicial management, some courts rapidly imposing orders for "no contact" or "supervised visitation only" pending further investigation while others have been slow to respond to the potential lethality of MBP and reluctant to place the child outside the custody of the mother or family members while the case proceeds.

There has been significant variation in the relevance and weight assigned to medical evidence or expert testimony regarding MBP. Lack of familiarity with MBP, lack of funds to pursue the prerequisite detailed and complex investigation, and difficulty believing that an apparently "model" mother would maltreat her child in such a systematic, bizarre, and premeditated manner all contribute to the variability with which such cases are pursued in civil or criminal courts.

On the other hand, some persons accused of MBP and their supporters assert that false allegations have been made and "confirmed" in legal proceedings that are characterized by lurid fascination with the unusual diagnosis and apparently incredible allegations, and the distortions or errors of overzealous or poorly informed clinicians, investigators, attorneys, and judges.[5] Both of us and other clinicians with interests in MBP have been involved with cases in which careful investigation ultimately determined that these were not cases of MBP.

This can occur most commonly in cases where a child has a genuine chronic illness and is being cared for by a parent who anxiously overreports medical signs and symptoms in an effort to secure care or find explanations for the child's illness. In some cases, a parent may even begin to fabricate false symptoms in a way that does not risk injury to the child, in a desperate effort to be validated in her anxiety by medical staff. While clearly the parent's MBP-like behavior has to be halted and the case closely managed, in these kinds of cases it would be incorrect to understand either the dynamics of the parent's behavior or the risks to the child as representing MBP.

The stakes are high for all parties in possible cases of MBP. Legal consequences for the parent can include loss of custody of a child or incarceration. It is essential that a balanced and sophisticated approach be maintained by clinical, child protection, and legal professionals involved in the investigation and management of these cases.

There are two areas in particular with which pediatricians and other health care providers often struggle in cases of suspected MBP. First, because it is often difficult to make a confident diagnosis of MBP prior to the separation of the perpetrator from the child, clinical professionals are often reluctant to make mandated child protection reports. We are aware of multiple cases in which medical personnel had very strong suspicions of potentially lethal MBP but did not contact state child protection authorities or even tell other medical caregivers of the child of their suspicions, for fear of being wrong. This reluctance is compounded in situations where medical care providers have previously made mandated child protection reports based upon their strong suspicions and preliminary evidence, only to have state child protection authorities fail to respond adequately or at all.

Second, some clinical professionals have aversions to entering legal proceedings and may even actively disdain an investigator role in gathering legally useful data. However, in cases involving possible MBP, it is critical that helping professionals be prepared to be involved in child protection investigations or legal proceedings, including by becoming familiar with basic legal principles for informing and documenting their clinical work. Schreier and Libow[6] note three particularly important areas of law with which medical and mental health professionals should have some familiarity as they begin assessment of any potential MBP case:

- the importance and admissibility of indirect or circumstantial evidence,
- the use of professional opinions as evidence, and
- legal considerations regarding the use of surreptitious videotape or other surveillance and monitoring in suspected MBP cases.

This is not a call for health care professionals to become detectives or attorneys. It is a call to recognize that the information developed by clinical professionals becomes the information upon which courts must rely in making most-serious and far-reaching decisions for a child and family. Clinical professionals must be familiar with the kinds of legal and evidentiary issues that can arise in criminal or civil proceedings where MBP is alleged. However, once familiar with these issues, rather than second-guessing the needs of the legal system, clinical professionals should attend to the *clinical* needs of the child, including the need to be protected from further perpetration.

Because involvement of the legal system is often necessary to protect a child victim of MBP, clinical professionals should generate very detailed written documentation of the clinical observations giving rise to the suspicions of MBP, written as soon as possible upon the emergence of suspicion of MBP, and written in a manner that is as objective, descriptive, and devoid of judgmental statements and assumptions as possible. Detailed and contemporaneous medical records containing observations and rationales for clinical decision making also can provide protection should professional license complaints or malpractice claims subsequently be filed.

The adequacy of child protection and clinical intervention in MBP cases is closely tied to the specific nature of the legal actions taken and the subsequent response of the parties and the courts. Most MBP cases that go to court will be in civil child protection proceedings, although there may sometimes also be parallel criminal or divorce proceedings. Where courts are involved in child protection proceedings, or where MBP has become central to divorce or child custody proceedings, experience has taught that these cases require consistently assertive judicial management in the courtroom, as well as frequent and direct judicial oversight of the child protection and clinical intervention aspects of the case through at least the adjudication of the MBP allegations. If there are going to be efforts at intervention and parent-child reunification after MBP perpetration is established, it is most helpful for the court to continue to assert direct oversight of the case until reunification is accomplished or parental rights terminated.

Given the complex clinical and legal issues that tend to characterize alleged MBP cases when they come before courts, it serves the interests of all parties to involve independent clinical professionals who are skilled and knowledgeable about MBP, working under the direct and neutral authority of the court. Both the child and the family are best served by well-informed judges, attorneys, pediatricians and other health care providers, mental health providers, forensic evaluators, guardians ad litem, and child protection and law enforcement personnel. Exaggerated or erroneous allegations are more likely to be distinguished from true MBP cases when there is an experienced team of professionals involved in the case. At the very least, an independent expert consultant should be available to the court, the parties to the case, and persons providing social service and clinical investigation or intervention during the pendency of the case.

This is readily accomplished through court appointment of an independent expert in MBP who can serve as a liaison and consultant to the treatment team and the court. In jurisdictions where this is permissible, designation of this independent expert as a guardian ad litem (GAL) allows oversight of the intervention process and integrated management of the treatment of the child and family, while freeing direct care providers from the potential tensions that can arise when clinical care providers must routinely make reports directly to the court. Additionally, this court-appointed GAL can maintain a focus upon the child's best interests, inform and educate clinical, child protection, and legal professionals who do not have prior experience with such cases, help contain the fragmentation of services and polarization of views that so often come to characterize MBP cases, and maintain a balanced neutrality of the intervention process under the ultimate scrutiny of the court. In jurisdictions where the GAL statute is restrictive, consideration might be given to appointing the consultant as a court-appointed special advocate (CASA) operating under a direct order of the court.

CRIMINAL AND CIVIL CASES INVOLVING MBP

Many of the acts associated with MBP perpetration can be charged as violations of criminal law. Poisoning or other direct induction of symptoms resulting in injury can often be charged under general criminal statutes such as battery or attempted murder. Some states have specific felony child abuse statutes that can be invoked in MBP cases. Nonetheless, to date there have not been many criminal prosecutions of MBP behavior. As clinical professionals become more familiar with MBP and more cases are identified and reported to child protection and/or law enforcement authorities who are themselves are more informed about MBP, it is likely that more criminal prosecutions will occur.

Because MBP perpetration constitutes a form of child maltreatment, child protection proceedings pursued by state authorities in civil rather than criminal courts may also be initiated, and in some cases they may run simultaneously with criminal prosecutions for the same misconduct. Divorce actions are proceedings brought by the two parents without the state's being a party to the action; they are heard in civil sessions of court. Child custody disputes involving MBP may also run simultaneously with child protection proceedings or criminal prosecutions.

Regardless of the kind of case that is initiated, two important issues typically arise and interact in legal proceedings involving allegations of MBP: (1) establishing the MBP perpetration according to the rules of evidence, and (2) making decisions about whether or how to demonstrate to the court the mental state, motive, and intent of the MBP perpetrator at the time of perpetration.

Direct and Circumstantial Evidence in MBP Cases

Direct evidence allows for resolution of the issue in dispute without the fact finder having to draw inferences from the information, although the fact finder may assess the credibility of the information. Examples of direct evidence in MBP cases include testimony by persons who directly observed the misconduct, videotapes of misconduct, and confessions by defendants.[7] Covert video surveillance is discussed in a separate section below.

Circumstantial evidence is indirect in the sense that the judge or jury must draw inferences from the information in order to establish a fact that is in dispute. For example, in a homicide case the presence of the defendant's fingerprints on the handle of a firearm permits the inference that the defendant has held that gun. Splatters of a victim's blood on the shoes of the defendant permit the inference that the defendant has been in the presence of the victim's bleeding body. An inference that the defendant fired the fatal shots could be drawn from witness reports that they observed the defendant entering the room where the victim was alone, heard the defendant and victim arguing immediately before the firing of gunshots, then saw the defendant exiting the room of the victim. That it could not have been anybody else who fired the shots could be inferred from witness reports that they immediately ran into the room where the victim was slumped and observed nobody else in the room or fleeing from the room. Taken together, these bits of circumstantial evidence might well result in the conviction of the defendant even though nobody actually saw the defendant shoot the victim.

Perhaps the most common form of circumstantial evidence in MBP cases is the child's rapid medical stabilization or recovery upon physical separation from the suspected MBP perpetrator.[8] Strong circumstantial evidence in MBP cases can also include discovery of toxic substances in the possession of the perpetrator that are the same as those detected in laboratory tests on the child, evidence of tampering with feeding or other lines, or failure of medical staff to observe medical signs and symptoms that are routinely reported by the perpetrator but seem to occur only in her presence.

Courts are likely to be most reluctant to rely upon nonspecific "syndrome" evidence, such as the fit of the alleged MBP perpetrator with characteristics commonly found among MBP perpetrators. Without more compelling evidence, courts will give little weight to "profile" characteristics such as being the mother of the alleged victim, having a background with medical training, or having a history of "doctor shopping."

In order to prosecute under criminal law, prosecutors must establish both that the perpetrator engaged in the alleged acts (*actus reus*) and had the prerequisite mental state and intent (*mens reus*) to harm the child. This must be established "beyond a reasonable doubt," the highest standard of proof. The high standard of proof can make criminal prosecution of MBP cases difficult, since the kind of conduct most likely to result in criminal charges (symptom inductions that injure the child, rather than offering false or exaggerated medical history) is typically done secretively, and courts must often rely upon circumstantial rather than direct evidence of the misconduct of the MBP perpetrator.[9]

Criminal courts are most likely to convict in cases in which direct evidence or very strong circumstantial evidence links the defendant to the induction of symptoms resulting in physical injury or the death of the child. For example, in *Commonwealth v. Robinson*[10] (see summaries of cases in appendix following this text), circumstantial evidence in this involuntary manslaughter conviction of the mother included massive sodium poisoning as her infant's cause of death, discovery of a syringe in her possession, and detection of her fingerprints on salt packets. In most cases, merely showing that the child clinically deteriorated or died during a period of contact with a defendant or improved after enforced separation from the defendant is unlikely to result in criminal conviction unless there is other very strong circumstantial evidence. Even when there is apparently strong circumstantial evidence, however, prosecutors should seek to obtain expert consultation regarding possible alternative explanations for the child's clinical course and the available medical evidence.[11]

Despite the evidentiary difficulties, however, prosecutors have shown a greater willingness to proceed with criminal cases than to defer to civil courts, which would hear the case as a child protection matter. Prosecutors are most likely to proceed where there is direct evidence or extremely strong circumstantial evidence of the MBP. They may be deterred when prosecution would involve a costly and time-consuming presentation of complicated medical opinion testimony or if the alleged conduct is so extreme or bizarre that it seems the perpetrator "must be crazy."

Despite the complications of proceeding in MBP cases, prosecutors should be thought-

Hearsay evidence is ordinarily excluded, because it is not possible to test the credibility or truthfulness of the statements that are conveyed through a witness. However, there are numerous exceptions to the hearsay rule. Most of these exceptions rely on events or circumstances that are deemed sufficiently reliable to warrant consideration as evidence. For example, the law regards as more likely to be reliable the statements of persons who blurt something out when excited, information given to doctors by patients for the purpose of treatment, or the recording of information in routine business records. These exceptions are not introduced to prove a matter that is in dispute. For example, a courtroom statement by a doctor that a mother had told him that the child had already been diagnosed with a rare gastrointestinal syndrome could not be introduced to show that the child *did* have that syndrome. It could not be introduced to prove that some other physician had *actually* told the mother that the child had this rare syndrome. However, it could be introduced to show that the testifying doctor *believed* at the time care was given that the child had been diagnosed previously with the syndrome. Should the doctor who allegedly had offered this diagnosis later deny ever having done so, the mother's statement to the doctor testifying in court could be introduced to show that there was a contradiction between these two claims of what had happened.

Several hearsay exceptions might be helpful in bringing information before the court.[16] One exception is statements made to medical professionals for the purpose of obtaining medical diagnosis or treatment. This exception has been used to introduce statements from victims about the circumstances of rape, childhood sexual abuse, or assault. Another exception allows statements purportedly made by a defendant to be introduced to help characterize the defendant's state of mind. This exception was used in the child protection case *In the Matter of Jessica Z.*[17] to permit a nurse to testify about the mother's verbatim statements about a laxative found in the child's formula.

A third hearsay exception allows introduction of statements found in records made in the ordinary course of business. This includes statements found in medical records that are recorded as part of a contemporaneous and routine clinical record. Of course, if the statements are viewed as privileged professional communications, then this issue would have to be addressed separately. Arguably, a videotape or other electronic record made for diagnostic purposes as part of a medical record would be admissible as a medical record. In some cases the business records exception might be applicable to correspondence between MBP perpetrators and political figures, charity groups, or donors to medical funds. (Hearsay exceptions in child abuse cases are discussed further in chapter 23.)

Yorker[18] describes the value of invoking exceptions to the rule ordinarily barring evidence of prior crimes. Evidence of prior crimes or bad acts is ordinarily barred in criminal cases, since it may be highly prejudicial and not necessarily relevant to the specific allegations being prosecuted. However, such evidence may be introduced if it shows a common plan or scheme, or a modus operandi. Yorker cites MBP cases in which information regarding prior sibling deaths or prior suspicious deaths linked to a particular babysitter was admitted in prosecutions under this exception. For example, in *United States v. Woods*[19] the appellate court hearing this successful homicide prosecution upheld the trial court's admission into evidence information that nine other children in the defendant's care had multiple episodes of cyanosis and that seven of the nine had died. The court of appeals upheld the trial court because "when the crime is one of infanticide or child abuse, evidence of repeated incidents is especially relevant because it may be the only evidence to prove the crime."

Issues Regarding Criminal Charges Brought, Mental Status Defenses, and Disposition

Criminal violations require both an illegal action (*actus reus*) and the intention to commit the criminal conduct (*mens reus*). It is the burden of the prosecution to establish beyond a reasonable doubt the prerequisite intent to commit the criminal act.

The *mens rea* required for criminal misconduct traditionally falls into three categories: general intent, specific intent, or criminal negligence. Both the severity of the charge and the potential consequences will vary with the nature of the alleged act and the degree of harm intended and/or resulting for the victim.

General intent crimes require only the voluntary commission of an act that is a violation of law. The defendant need not have intended to violate the law nor even been aware that the act was illegal. Unless otherwise shown by the defense, persons who voluntarily commit acts are presumed to have intended that act and its reasonably foreseeable consequences.

Specific intent crimes require that the defendant intended to commit some specified further illegal action or to cause some additional consequence. Unlike general intent crimes, specific intent cannot be inferred from the commission of the *actus reus,* but the proof of specific intent may be circumstantial. For example, the difference between first degree murder and second degree murder may be a specific showing that the defendant intended in a premeditated way to kill the victim.

Criminal negligence is found when a defendant acted without specific intention but with a gross or reckless disregard for the consequences of his or her conduct. For example, a death that results from a reckless disregard for the potential consequences for the victim may be charged as an involuntary manslaughter.

In MBP, directly injurious acts such as poisoning, contamination of central lines, suffocation, breaking of bones, or injections can be charged as violations of the criminal codes. Most often these acts can readily be charged as general intent crimes; in some cases they may fulfill some specific intent requirements, such as premeditation.

A careful analysis of relevant law regarding intent and criminal responsibility is useful in determining the charges and in anticipating potential defenses. Although many MBP perpetrators flatly deny their misconduct when confronted with their behavior, some MBP perpetrators do admit to acts that harmed the child but deny a specific intent to injure or harm the child. For example, one of us was involved in a case where the mother ultimately admitted suffocating her infant son in order to feign apnea but asserted that she had no intent to seriously harm or kill her son and that his death was accidental. In another case, the mother admitted she grossly neglected care of a gastrointestinal tube site until it became infected but held that she did so only to trigger further medical care for a condition that she was utterly convinced existed and without an intent to cause her child to suffer.

From a legal perspective, people are ordinarily expected to be responsible for the reasonably predictable consequences of their actions. One defense to criminal charges is to establish that the perpetrator lacked the capacity to form the legally necessary level of intent towards the victim. The defense may seek to show that the perpetrator was acting with psychiatric impairment that resulted in a "diminished capacity" to form the necessary intent or appreciation for the potential consequences of the defendant's actions. A successful showing of this kind can result in conviction on lesser charges or mitigation of penalties imposed for the criminal misconduct.

A more difficult but complete defense is to show that the defendant was legally "insane." This requires evidence that the defendant was so impaired by psychiatric symptoms or other conditions that she was unable to appreciate the wrongfulness of her acts or conform her conduct to the requirements of law. Essentially, the defendant admits the misconduct but asserts she lacked the necessary mental state or control over her conduct for the misconduct to constitute a "crime."

This "insanity defense" is rarely tried or successful in criminal cases. Even very mentally ill persons may be held criminally responsible for their acts if they were able to understand that the acts were wrong or if they were able to conform their conduct to the requirements of law. In order to assess the degree of criminal responsibility that people have for their acts, courts often look to such things as evidence of planning, efforts to hide actions or destroy evidence of actions, and the degree of predictability between the defendant's behavior and its outcome upon the victim. Where an insanity defense is successful the defendant is found "not guilty" because he or she lacked the mental state or degree of control over his or her behavior required for the commission of the crime.

In MBP cases, claiming impairments that are sufficient to constitute "diminished capacity" or legal "insanity" is greatly complicated by the persistent, highly planful, and deliberate nature of the perpetration.[20] The description of MBP in the DSM-IV[21] as a "Factitious Disorder Not Otherwise Specified" explicitly refers to the "*intentional* production or feigning of physical or psychological signs or symptoms in another person who is under the individual's care for the purpose of indirectly assuming the sick role" (emphasis added). The absence of obvious major mental illness in most MBP perpetrators also makes it difficult to pursue these defenses, as does the insistence common among MBP perpetrators that they have not committed any of the alleged misconduct.

Nonetheless, in those cases where the defendant does raise a criminal responsibility defense by pleading "not guilty by reason of insanity," it is imperative that the prosecution be prepared to respond. In *Marie Claudia Olivier v. State of Texas,*[22] the appellate court reversed and remanded for new trial the defendant's murder conviction for the strangulation and beating death of her infant. The defendant had raised a defense of insanity and provided uncontradicted expert testimony that she suffered from Munchausen's syndrome and schizoaffective disorder.

This case did not specifically involve MBP, and it is likely that the florid psychosis related to her schizoaffective illness was the most important psychiatric factor in the incident leading to her infant's death. However, the case was reversed because the prosecution had relied only upon cross-examining the defendant's experts and therefore had failed to provide a response sufficient for a jury to reject the insanity defense.

In cases that do not involve severe injury or death of a child, the issue of whether MBP is a "psychiatric illness" is less likely to play a role in formal criminal defenses than in plea bargaining or the dispositional phase after the defendant has been found guilty. The "psychiatric" nature of MBP typically has a more central role in civil child protection or divorce custody proceedings where there is some legal mandate or tradition of attempting to "rehabilitate" or to "treat" a parent.

In practice, alleged MBP perpetrators may strenuously deny misconduct until a court determines that the allegations are true. Perpetrators may then seek to cast their behavior as a form of "illness" that now requires "treatment," as an alternative to incarceration, before parental rights can be terminated or before a permanent transfer of child custody to an ex-spouse should be ordered.

The DSM-IV research criteria for factitious disorder require that "external incentives for the behavior, such as economic gain," be absent and that the behavior be "not better accounted for by another mental disorder." In reality, MBP cases commonly present with a variety of potential motives and a broad spectrum of psychiatric disturbance. Evidence of a major psychiatric disturbance such as a psychotic disorder, delusional disorder focused upon the child's illness, or major depression with psychotic features could obviously have a significant bearing on the criminal and civil proceedings and disposition. However, prosecutors and clinical care providers must look beyond mere psychiatric diagnosis in order to find evidence of what, if any, links exist between a parent's psychiatric disturbance and the intentional production or feigning of symptoms in the child.

Careful and sophisticated consideration should be given to what specific MBP conduct was involved in the case, the degree of potential risk to the child, and any comorbid psychiatric conditions with which the perpetrator may present. This information should be considered in terms of: (1) what, if any, links may exist between treatable psychiatric conditions and the MBP perpetration, (2) what specific forms of psychiatric treatment and child protection strategies might be successful; and (3) the actual prognosis for successful intervention in the current case.

The determination of prognosis[23] can play an important role in a court's disposition of the case. For example, In *State v. DeJesus*[24] the Connecticut Superior Court refused a reduction in an eight-year prison sentence imposed upon a defendant convicted of MBP perpetration, holding that testimony at trial showed that psychotherapy would be ineffective and that incarceration served the goal of protecting children. Other courts hearing criminal cases have demonstrated a similar willingness to impose terms of incarceration on defendants whose charges stem from MBP perpetration.

This analysis of risk and prognosis should be completed *before* a criminal court imposes a disposition that leaves the MBP perpetrator in the community, or *before* courts hearing child protection or divorce custody matters authorize service plans or parenting plans. Naïve referrals of a perpetrating parent for generic "counseling" or "treatment," or treatment of a potentially noncontributory psychiatric problem such as depression or alcohol abuse may leave a child at substantial risk while creating the misperception that the parent is participating in rehabilitative treatments likely to be effective. On the other hand, highly specialized intervention with carefully selected MBP perpetrators may result in lowering the risk to the child and in more adequate functioning on the part of the parents.[25]

The DSM-IV diagnosis of factitious disorder not otherwise specified excludes cases of factitious illness production where it is done for external gains, such as financial enrichment. The DSM-IV stipulation that MBP "behavior is not better accounted for by another mental disorder" requires awareness that the diagnosis does not always capture the range of potential psychopathologies and intentions of the MBP perpetrator. In actual cases, there may be evidence of multiple motivations for the MBP perpetration, including gaining attention and support by factitiously adopting the sick role, access to financial resources, special treatment by organizations or facilities, or access to public figures and the media. Of course, where factitious illness production is motivated primarily (although perhaps not exclusively) by external factors such as financial gain, clinicians should be reluctant to conceptualize the case as MBP and courts should handle the legal actions as if they were more common forms of child exploitation.

In order to assess the nature of the perpetration, the potential motives for the perpetration, the risks of renewed perpetration, and the prognosis for various forms of intervention, clinicians and child protection authorities should specifically and descriptively document the following kinds of information from the first moment that MBP suspicions are raised or allegations made:

- perpetrating behaviors, the impact of perpetration upon the child, risks to the child
- statements by the suspected perpetrator confirming or refuting medical history
- information relevant to the capacities, motives, and intentions of the MBP perpetrator
- information that may go to one or more possible motives for the perpetration
- evidence of ability to hide, delay or mislead others about incidents of perpetration
- evidence of presenting distorted or incorrect information to others about the child's case
- suspected perpetrator's capacity to appreciate the impact upon the child

MBP in Child Protection and Divorce Custody Proceedings

Juvenile and family courts have ranged widely in their response to MBP. Some courts have difficulty finding MBP in the absence of direct or physical evidence,[26] or even clearly holding that MBP itself qualifies as a form of child abuse.[27] However, courts are increasingly willing to consider MBP a form of child abuse. Perhaps because it has become more familiar to medical and legal professionals, as well as having been portrayed in the mass media, courts now accept MBP more readily as something that exists and is both a form of child abuse and probative evidence of parental unfitness.

Courts have cited MBP alone or as part of a broader pattern of factors[28] to find grounds for state child protection or transfer of custody from one parent to another.[29] Courts are more likely to act when there is direct evidence or very strong circumstantial evidence, but at least one court, in New York, invoked a statute embodying the doctrine of *res ipsa loquitur* ("the thing speaks for itself") in finding circumstantial evidence of MBP when a child clinically improved upon physical separation from the mother.[30]

Juvenile and family courts have also ranged widely in their disposition of child protection and divorce child custody cases. Even in cases in which there were legal findings of child abuse due to MBP behaviors, it is difficult to determine what distinguishes cases in which the court returned the child to the parent[31] from those in which the child was placed in substitute care.[32] The variance may be due to many factors, including

- differences in statutory schemes among the states
- emphasis each state places on reunification efforts
- specific facts of each case
- adequacy of available clinical testimony or expert testimony regarding MBP
- the age, developmental stage, and specific strengths and vulnerabilities of the child
- availability of adequate psychiatric or foster care resources
- variations in the reluctance of courts to disrupt extended family relationships
- variations in the reluctance of courts to expose the child to the uncertainties of foster care
- a high degree of discretion traditionally reserved to trial courts for crafting dispositions

A similar disparity of outcome is found in cases involving siblings of a suspected MBP victim. This may reflect differences in the facts of each case, as well as differences in the ways individual courts assessed the risks posed to siblings. In the *Matter of Aaron S.*,[33] the trial court was upheld on appeal in finding Aaron to be a victim of MBP by feigned apnea, then declared his three siblings in need of state protection, with the comment that courts should not "await a broken bone or shattered psyche" before moving to protect siblings. In a Massachusetts case known to us, the juvenile court judge who heard a child protection case based on MBP allegations ordered permanent transfer of custody of the child from the mother. When he subsequently heard by chance that the mother had given birth to another child, he ordered the state child protection services to conduct an investigation, although the case regarding the first child was no longer before the court. However, in *Matter of M.A.V.,*[34] a Georgia appellate court overturned a trial court's termination of parental rights to an older sibling of an MBP victim. This sibling did not live with the mother, had been raised by grandparents, and there was no evidence that the mother intended to become a primary caretaker for that child.

In recent years, some states have responded to federal legislation by imposing limits on how long a parent may take to become "fit" following a finding of parental unfitness in a child protection proceeding. The time limits typically range from 15 to 24 months. Particularly in these states, the effectiveness and required duration of interventions in MBP cases become critical, because failure to be restored to parental "fitness" within the allotted time frame presumptively triggers proceedings for the termination of parental rights. While some commentators[35] have argued for swift termination of parental rights in cases involving extreme cases of MBP, courts have generally been reluctant to terminate parental rights except in cases where the physical harm to the child has been substantial and the parents can be shown to have resisted rehabilitative efforts or to be exhibiting significant parenting problems in addition to the MBP.

In divorce child custody proceedings, courts have considered MBP as a factor in determining child custody and pattern of visitation contact with the noncustodial parent. For example, in *Place v. Place,*[36] the appeals court upheld the trial court's decision to grant physical custody of two daughters to the father, finding that the mother could not accept that the older daughter was healthy and could be expected to subject her to unnecessary medical care if the child was left in her physical custody.

As indicated above, experience has shown that active judicial management in the courtroom and oversight of the case is often essential to preserving the rights of the parties and prevents evolution of an unproductively contentious and litigious atmosphere, strains upon the court's docket and resources, and loss of focus upon the central issues of the case.

COVERT VIDEOTAPE OR OTHER ELECTRONIC SURVEILLANCE

Videotaping in suspected MBP cases can be a very powerful diagnostic tool during hospitalization and can constitute direct evidence of MBP perpetration in the courtroom. The use of videotaping for diagnostic purposes when it is preceded by an adequate informed consent procedure is ordinarily not going to create legal difficulties. For example, on pediatric neurology units it is not uncommon to secure parental permission for telemonitoring that includes videotaping in order to identify and monitor possible seizure activity.

In contrast, the use of covert videotaping or other electronic surveillance methods is controversial[37] and can raise a variety of legal and clinical issues because of the intrusion into privacy that surreptitious electronic monitoring represents. Covert videotaping cannot always be relied upon for diagnostic certainty, since it can readily be evaded if the suspected MBP perpetrator becomes suspicious, is likely to be used only in hospital settings, and even in hospital settings will capture only what occurs "on camera." Additionally, it would inevitably be used by the defense in cases that are ultimately determined not to constitute MBP, thereby threatening the hospital's treatment alliance with the parents of a genuinely ill child. The potential legal and clinical consequences have resulted in a lively debate about the use of covert video surveillance, despite its demonstrated utility in clearly documenting some instances of MBP behavior.

The Fourth Amendment of the Constitution protects citizens from "unreasonable searches and seizures" by the state. It does not provide protection from intrusive searches or seizures by "private parties," persons who are not acting as state authorities or in concert with them. Additionally, persons are constitutionally protected only where they have a "reasonable expectation of privacy." Generally speaking, the more public the area, the less of an expectation of protected privacy an individual may assert.

Law enforcement personnel must be very cautious about utilizing covert videotaping that they arrange themselves or in concert with hospital personnel as part of a criminal investigation. Such covert surveillance by police would ordinarily require a search warrant based on probable cause to suspect that a crime was being committed and that evidence of this crime would be found. Some commentators hold that covert videotaping without a warrant might be justified under the "exigent circumstances" exception to the rule barring illegally obtained evidence from admission at trial. The crux of this argument is that the high risk to the child from the MBP perpetrator may justify warrantless covert videotaping. However, to date no court of which we are aware has accepted this argument, and it would be difficult to argue that police could not have obtained a warrant on an urgent basis, and that the danger to the child was so immediate and extreme as to justify warrantless videotaping yet still manageable enough to allow exposing the child to the MBP perpetrator in order to record the dangerous behavior.

A stronger argument might be that a parent does not have a reasonable expectation of privacy in a hospital room. In her review of the issue, Yorker[38] cites cases in which courts have held that there is not an expectation of privacy in hospital parking lots, open and accessible areas in places of employment, or in hospital emergency rooms where there is a constant flow of staff. She notes that a court has yet to make a specific determination of whether a person has a reasonable expectation of privacy in a hospital room, but she observes that modern hospital rooms commonly are very busy places, with a flow of medical staff and routine use of electronic monitoring equipment.

Yorker[39] also observes that courts have held that some intrusions into the body of a defendant do not violate the constitutional protection against self-incrimination. The law against self-incrimination focuses primarily upon the improper eliciting of the defendant's own words, so when the information does not require the defendant to literally speak against himself the consent of the defendant may not be required before "searching." These bodily intrusions by law enforcement have been permitted because they do not involve coercing the defendant to make self-incriminating statements. For example, courts have admitted laboratory evidence of blood alcohol levels and have even compelled defendants to provide hair and other samples of body tissue for DNA testing and other laboratory comparisons. There is ordinarily no bar to admitting videotapes from security surveillance cameras in businesses, even if the defendant was unaware of the videotaping.

Yorker extends this argument, holding that in suspected MBP cases a covert electronic surveillance arranged by clinical personnel can constitute a medically necessary "diagnostic" procedure *for the child* that does not intrude directly upon the parent nor improperly elicit self-incriminating statements. Informed consent by the parent may not be necessary in this unusual situation, in which notification of the parent would defeat the purpose of the diagnostic procedure. Seen in this way, covert electronic recording of MBP perpetration might be admissible or even support obtaining further medical evidence over the objection of the parents.

Still, the best practice for law enforcement personnel is to obtain a warrant before engaging in covert video or electronic surveillance. Other government personnel, whether or not they are law enforcement authorities, have also been held to be constrained by the Fourth Amendment. Government employees who staff state and federal medical facilities should consider themselves more akin to law enforcement staff than to private citizens for purposes of this analysis. Similarly, state child protection personnel should consider whether their actions are constrained by the Fourth Amendment and should seek specific legal advice before initiating covert videotaping as part of a child abuse investigation.

Medical staff in private facilities have been held to be "private parties" and therefore not subject to the constraints of the Fourth Amendment proscription of unreasonable search and seizure. Medical staff who are "private parties" and engaged in covert video-taping for purposes of diagnosis or insuring patient safety will not ordinarily implicate Fourth Amendment considerations. However, this assumes that the covert videotaping is not part of a state investigation in any way. "Private party" medical staff may still be sanctioned for intrusive searches, covert videotaping, or unauthorized diagnostic procedures by complaints to state licensing boards or in lawsuits claiming professional malpractice.

State law varies as to whether evidence obtained through unconsented searches conducted by private parties is admissible in a criminal trial. In order to avoid undue liability to themselves and the hospital, and to limit inadvertent compromise of a criminal prosecution or child protection action, medical staff in private hospitals should secure a specific legal opinion regarding their obligations and liabilities prior to engaging in covert video-taping or covert staff surveillance.

The best approach to managing the perils of surveillance is likely to be a combination of obtaining adequate informed consent for videotaping and electronic monitoring at the outset of hospitalizations and having an established hospital protocol on how to proceed when MBP is suspected. Ideally, informed consent for permission to videotape for diagnostic, medical, and educational purposes would be part of the standard protocol for admission to hospital or, at the very least, for those units or clinical services most likely to come into contact with MBP cases.

An adequate informed consent for covert and open videotaping might be included in the informed consent statements that parents must sign upon a child's admission to hospital, particularly where the informed consent statement indicates that television or video-taped monitoring might be used for clinical or educational purposes as part of routine hospital case management. Signing an informed consent statement that includes reference to telemonitoring methods waives expectations of privacy that the parent might otherwise assert. Where the covert surveillance or videotaping has been done by hospital staff for diagnostic purposes—and not in concert with police—prosecutors will still have to proceed according to the law in their jurisdiction regarding any testimonial privilege[40] that might be claimed, since such a "diagnostic" surveillance or other interactions with parents would be part of the medical record of the child and/or parent.

HOSPITAL PROTOCOLS FOR SUSPECTED MBP CASES

The hospital protocol in cases of suspected MBP should include

1. prompt case consultation with relevant medical specialties and a consultant knowledgeable about MBP
2. prompt notification and consultation with hospital legal staff familiar with the protocol and state child protection and criminal law procedure
3. provisions for ensuring the safety of the child, including
   a. intensive monitoring or temporary suspension of parent-child contact pending more definitive diagnosis and/or the involvement of child protection authorities
   b. a procedure by which a preemptive court order barring removal of the child by parents might be secured prior to informing parents of the allegations of MBP
   c. a protocol permitted under state law by which a physician might place a "hold" upon discharge pending notification of the court
4. statements of conditions under which covert staff or electronic surveillance would be initiated as a routine element of the protocol, as well as specification of who has the authority to initiate covert staff or electronic surveillance
5. description of how the mandated reporting requirement will be accomplished, including designation of a specific person to make the mandated report and the content of the report to be made to state child protection authorities
6. indication of the steps to be followed in the event a parent attempts to remove a child against medical advice, including the role to be played by hospital security
7. provision for designation of a single source of information to whom the family or others with an interest in the case can turn for reliable information regarding the situation and the condition of the child
8. designation of persons responsible for assessing the reactions of hospital staff, including the need for staff meetings to resolve differences regarding case management or involvement of child protection authorities

(See also chapter 18.)

Optimally, the MBP protocol pulls together a team for clinical management that has access to consultation from professionals capable of offering recommendations regarding clinical care, child protection, documentation, and legal case management. Hospital child maltreatment or psychiatric consultation-liaison teams should receive specific training regarding MBP and be promptly contacted when medical or psychiatric units have concerns about a case.

Having an MBP hospital protocol reduces the likelihood that individuals or units will make legal errors in managing suspected cases and provides documentation of parental informed consent, execution of mandated legal duties, and evidence of a process of thoughtful "professional judgment" that is the best defense in the event of formal complaints against professional licenses or malpractice lawsuit. Following a protocol is also more likely to identify genuine MBP cases and accurately assess the level of clinical risk to the child. This, in turn, makes it more likely that cases requiring a response from state authorities for effective management will result in the temporary placement of the child in state custody or the appointment of a guardian to make medical decisions pending the outcome of further investigation.

CONCLUSION

The conduct associated with MBP may implicate an extraordinary range of legal issues. The clinical challenges posed by MBP for clinical care providers are paralleled by the legal challenges posed to attorneys and courts who must deal with MBP cases in child protection proceedings, criminal prosecutions, or divorce actions. As more clinical care providers identify suspected MBP, more cases will come before the courts and appear in the news and entertainment media. We concur with those who fear that the potential exists for a backlash response to this kind of case, just as there has been with sexual abuse cases.

The best way to avoid a backlash is also the best way to balance the extraordinarily important and sensitive interests that arise when state and citizen, child and parent, clinical caregiver and patient may come into conflict: thoughtful and sophisticated clinical work devoid of zealotry on the part of clinical care providers, along with well-informed, careful consideration of the legal and dignitary interests of children and parents by child protection and legal professionals.

Public health and legal policy is best informed where there is research upon which medical decision making or developments in statutory and case law can be made. A national case bank of MBP cases maintained by a government agency or jointly by agencies responsible for tracking child maltreatment and/or medical illness would be helpful in keeping track of identified MBP cases. Although MBP is arguably not a "disease" at all, factitious illness presentations are likely to be costly both in terms of dollars for unnecessary medical care and in the consequences of this form of child maltreatment. Keeping data through a national center may also allow for assessing the costs of MBP, earlier identification of suspected MBP cases, and tracking of suspected or known cases of MBP across jurisdictions.

Just as with sexual offender registries commonly found in the states, privacy rights might be protected through a system of not providing individually identifying information to the national center unless there has been a finding in a criminal court or civil child protection proceeding that the allegations of MBP were correct.

Gathering information through a national data bank for clinical and legal decision making might include follow-up of cases of children returned by courts to their parents after a legal finding of MBP. Because the available research literature regarding morbidity and mortality in MBP cases has been so ominous, information regarding clinical, psychiatric, and child protection services should be included in each case reported. Also included in initial reports and subsequent follow-up reports should be reports of morbidity and deaths among siblings of the children identified as a targets of MBP, as well as among the identified targets of MBP who are returned to the custody of their parents by courts or child protection authorities. It is important to know if courts and child protection authorities are generally successful in balancing legal and protective interests through effective utilization of supervision and intervention plans, or if the children of parents who perpetrate MBP continue to be maltreated through MBP or in other ways.

APPENDIX: SUMMARIES OF CASES

Civil Cases (Child Protection, Termination of Parental Rights)

Geringer v. Iowa Department of Human Services, 521 N.W.2d 730, 730–31 (1994)

Mother was a resident of Arizona who had taken the child for inpatient medical care to Iowa, where after nine days the infant was declared a victim of MBP. The case was transferred to the state child protective authorities in Arizona since that was where the parents lived.

The Arizona authorities had another doctor review the case. This doctor concluded that mother did not have MBP, finding instead that the "extraordinary anxiety and concern of [the child's] mother likely exacerbated the already complex medical condition of her child."

However, the doctor also stated that to completely rule out MBP would require consultation with each physician that child had seen over the prior year and that he was not able to carry out this extensive review. Based upon his review, Arizona returned the child to mother's care.

The case captioned above was mother's action to have the child abuse report in Iowa expunged, but this request was denied by the court.

In the Interest of B.B., 500 N.W.2d. 9, 10–12 (1993)

The trial court had found the child to be in need of assistance and ordered continued foster placement and placed restrictions on parental visitation. The appellate court overturned this decision and ordered the child to be placed back with the parents, but the Supreme Court of Iowa affirmed the trial court. In this case the parents persistently refused to send the boy to school on grounds he was too ill, particularly with stomach problems and vomiting, even after doctors had declared him healthy. Following initial placement in foster care, mother made unsubstantiated claims that the child was "drugged, hypnotized, and brainwashed by his social workers and foster parents," and also sexually abused by the foster parents.

In its opinion, the Iowa Supreme Court found "two themes have pervaded this entire litigation: [Mother's] obsession with [the child's] health and her resulting failure to send him to school despite repeated opportunities and court orders to do so. We refuse to abandon [the child] to her irrationality." The court footnoted that at trial a physician had testified that mother "is a Munchausen syndrome by proxy type person," and the court specifically cited mother's actions during a visit during which she had persistently asked the child if his stomach hurt until he stated that it did.

Among the restrictions on visitation upheld by the Iowa Supreme Court was a provision forbidding both parents from originating "any discussion of vomiting or stomach problems, with all other inquiries about [the child's] health being limited to general inquiries which are positive in focus."

In the Matter of M.A.V., 206 Ga. App. 299, 300–301 (1992)

In this case an appellate court found that state child protection authorities had failed to prove parental unfitness and overturned a lower court decision to terminate parental rights based upon mother's MBP.

There were two children involved in this case. A younger child had been the target of the MBP and removed from mother's care on that basis. However, the appellate court held this was insufficient to warrant termination of mother's parental rights regarding the older child, who did not live with the mother and had been raised by grandparents. Evidence at trial indicated a verbal child would not be as vulnerable to MBP, and there was no evidence that mother intended to become primary caretaker for the older child.

In the Matter of Aaron S., 163 Misc.2d 967, 971 (1993)

Following dental surgery, the child, Aaron, was held for observation in order to assess a history of central apnea. A tracheotomy was considered to help link Aaron to a breathing machine, but physicians wanted a medically trained person to witness an attack before it would be ordered, as well as an arterial line to monitor his blood gases while sleeping. Mother refused and 24-hour nursing observation was ordered, resulting in sudden cessation of the apnea episodes. Physicians concluded that Aaron did not have apnea and the case was taken to court.

The court held that mother had neglected Aaron by "subjecting him to [a] continuous course of medical treatment for apnea, which he does not have, as a result of Munchausen Syndrome by Proxy." The court also then relied upon the neglect of Aaron to consider whether his three siblings were also neglected. The court declared the siblings neglected children for the purpose of placing them in the custody of state child protection authorities, noting that "in order to meaningfully protect the rights of siblings to remain free from harm a court cannot and should not 'await [a] broken bone or shattered psyche.' "

Mother appealed the judgment of neglect, claiming that her conduct towards Aaron for a nonexistent central apnea did not constitute neglect. The appellate court affirmed the trial court's decision regarding Aaron and his siblings, noting that courts can find neglect based on "parental acts of a serious nature requiring the aid of the court."

In the Matter of Jessica Z., 515 N.Y.S.2d 370 (1987)

In a case characterized by conflicting medical and psychiatric expert testimony and mother's denial of MBP, the court relied upon circumstantial evidence, including laboratory findings, the timing of the child's symptoms and mother's behavior, and cessation of symptoms upon removal of mother. The court's opinion also cited classic literature regarding MBP, characterizing the disorder and the conduct of the perpetrators.

Significantly, the court explicitly applied the legal doctrine of *res ipsa loquitur* (the thing speaks for itself). This doctrine allows the court to draw inferences when the event or injury at issue does not ordinarily occur without negligence or wrongdoing, the defendant was exclusively responsible for the negligence or wrongdoing resulting in the event or injury, and the injured party did not voluntarily contribute to the event or injury in any way. As Yorker (1996) has commented, this doctrine is very useful in cases involving MBP and "is exemplified by the miraculous recovery of a very ill child once removed from the exclusive control of the alleged perpetrator."

In the Matter of Tucker, 578 N.E.2d 774, 777 (1991)

This appellate decision upheld a trial court's determination to terminate the parental rights of the mother. The child's mother was variably diagnosed with "schizophrenic symptoms with strong paranoia," personality disorder, and possible MBP.

She had claimed she could not control the child. During home visits, child protection authorities had observed "frequent medica[tion] and in bed at odd times of the day," and that the mother administered medications despite no signs of illness. Mother also had taken an overdose of Dilantin prescribed for seizures. On one occasion, she had taken the boy to child protection authorities demanding they care for him, and the boy began "biting himself, beating his head against the floor, and beating his face with his knees." Noting the child's improvement after placement in foster care, the court found sufficient cause to terminate parental rights.

In Re S.R., 157 Vt. 417, 419–420 (1991)

Following determination of MBP on the part of mother, state child protection authorities offered services for over three years in an effort to keep the family together. The court determined that the father abused alcohol and the mother had seizures and engaged in MBP towards the child. The court noted provision of services by state authorities had included "counseling for the mother, family counseling, parent education for [the parents], supervised home visits, and one period of home placement during which S. R. sustained several injuries." The court terminated parental rights after finding that the parents had failed to make adequate use of the services offered by state authorities and failed to acknowledge mother's MBP. In terminating the parental rights of father, the court noted his alcohol abuse but also pointed to the danger to the child posed by father's denial of mother's MBP.

Straten v. Orange County Department of Social Services, 628 N.Y.S.2d 818 (A.D. Dept. 1995)

State child protection authorities had removed a child after discovering a history of chronic illness that a number of doctors had failed to treat and after mother refused to hospitalize the child for psychological evaluation. A court awarded temporary custody to the state after hearing argument that mother had MBP. Despite hospitalization and treatment over the next year, the child failed to improve. Parents then brought suit claiming medical malpractice and false imprisonment. The court dismissed these charges.

Criminal Cases

Commonwealth v. Robinson, 565 N.E.2d 1229 (1991)

The appellate courts upheld the conviction of mother on a count of involuntary manslaughter for poisoning her infant child while hospitalized. The trial court had ruled that the prosecution could not introduce evidence regarding MBP but convicted the mother on circumstantial evidence. Further rulings stemming from this case included the suppression of information based upon mother's contact with a child psychiatrist provided by the hospital for psychiatric support shortly following the child's death. The court held that the trial court erred in permitting testimony by the psychiatrist, since a protected doctor-patient relationship had been established when the psychiatrist held herself out for professional support, however briefly.

Kansas v. Lumbrera, **845 P.2d 609, 612 (1992)**

This Supreme Court of Kansas decision reviewed the conviction of a mother prosecuted for murdering her child after she had brought him to the emergency room. Police interviewed mother after doctors determined the child had been asphyxiated and mother replied that "it wasn't with a pillow" when police asked her if she had smothered the child with a pillow. Medical records of the mother and subsequent investigation indicated that all of her five other children had died unattended at a young age.

During the opening statement, the prosecution mentioned the possibility that mother suffered from MBP and that a desire for attention and sympathy may have motivated the conduct leading to the death of the child. However, because there was no expert opinion offered during trial that mother herself suffered from MBP, the trial court ordered all references to MBP stricken from the record.

Mother was convicted of the murder of the one child. The state Supreme Court reversed the conviction on appeal and remanded for retrial because of prejudicial trial errors. However, the Supreme Court indicated the trial court had acted sufficiently when instructing the jury to ignore references to MBP in the absence of expert testimony.

People v. Phillips, **122 Cal. App.3d 69 (1981)**

A California appellate court rejected the appeal of a mother convicted of murder of one child and willful endangerment of the life of a second child. Despite mother's persistent denial and the absence of eyewitness testimony, the trial court convicted the mother by relying upon circumstantial evidence including laboratory tests, detection of excessive salt in the feeding formula prepared by mother, improvement in the child's condition in the absence of mother, and failure to detect a genuine medical condition. The court also noted the similar clinical presentations between the children.

Commentators have described this case as an important legal precedent, since the court was permitted to rely upon circumstantial evidence and because the appellate court specifically affirmed that the expert witness could present an opinion that mother had MBP without directly examining her or having a history of treating MBP (Yorker, 1996; Searle, 1993).

Marie Claudia Olivier v. State of Texas, **850 S.W.2d 742 (1993)**

The conviction of a mother in the death of her infant was reversed and remanded for new trial. The prosecution had failed to produce a sufficient response to testimony by defense experts that she suffered from Munchausen's Syndrome and Schizoaffective Disorder that rendered her "not guilty by reason of insanity" for the death of the child. While the case facts indicate that mother's florid paranoid psychosis at the time of the killing of the infant was probably the most important factor, and while mother was not viewed as engaging "by proxy" with the child in Munchausen behavior, it is a reminder that cross-examination of defense witnesses alone may be legally insufficient to overcome a criminal responsibility defense.

Tanya Thaxton Reid v. State of Texas, 964 S.W.2d 723 (1998)

The murder conviction in the death of her son by asphyxiation intended to feign apnea was upheld on appeal. The appellate court held that: (1) the trial court had properly admitted expert testimony regarding MBP after finding it had a sufficiently reliable scientific basis; (2) MBP testimony could be admitted as relevant to the motive of the defendant; (3) MBP testimony regarding a pattern of conduct on the part of the defendant did not invade the jury's right to determine guilt; and (4) it was permissible to allow testimony showing that another child of the defendant's had, until removal from the mother, experienced the same symptoms as had the dead child.

N O T E S

1. American Psychiatric Association, *Diagnostic and statistical manual of mental disorders,* 4th ed. [DSM-IV] (Washington, DC: American Psychiatric Press, 1994).

2. H Schreier and J Libow, *Hurting for love: Munchausen by proxy* (New York: Guilford, 1993).

3. Ibid.

4. Ibid.

5. There are now internet websites where parents can seek support for what they maintain are false allegations of MBP, share information about their cases and potentially helpful sources of expert testimony, and describe the legal proceedings in which they find themselves.

6. Schreier and Libow, *Hurting for love.*

7. BC Yorker, Legal issues in factitious disorder by proxy. In M Feldman and S Eisendrath, eds., *The spectrum of factitious disorders* (Washington, DC: American Psychiatric Press, 1996). Yorker cites *United States v. Welch,* 36 F.3d 1098 (SD Ohio 1973), in which a mother challenged the admissibility of her secretly videotaped confession to smothering her three children, resulting in the deaths of two of them. The mother had been told by police that her presence at the interview was voluntary, that she could refuse to answer any questions, and that she could leave at any time. She was not offered her Miranda rights nor cautioned that anything she said could be used against her. The Sixth Circuit Court of Appeals rejected her effort to have her confession suppressed, holding that the confession had been validly obtained although she was not given her Miranda rights until after she had made incriminating statements, the two-hour interview had been secretly videotaped, and the police officer had "acted like a therapist" and falsely asserted that a new DNA test showed her other children could not have died of SIDS.

8. Yorker, Legal issues in FDP.

9. T Vollaro, Note: Munchausen syndrome by proxy and its evidentiary problems, *22 Hofstra Law Review 495* (winter 1993).

10. *Commonwealth v. Robinson,* 565 N.E.2d 1229 (Ma. App. Ct. 1991).

11. M Flannery, Munchausen syndrome by proxy: Broadening the scope of child abuse. *28 U. Richmond Law Review 1175* (December 1994). This article reports on the case of Ryan Stallings, who died in childhood of apparent ethylene glycol poisoning believed to have been induced by his mother, Patricia Stallings. Five months after her arrest on charges of first degree murder, she gave birth while incarcerated to a child who subsequently died of similar symptoms while hospitalized. Patricia Stallings was nonetheless convicted for the murder of Ryan and sentenced to life without parole in January 1991. Subsequent retesting of Ryan's frozen lab samples resulted in a determination that the first tests had been incorrect, and that he had actually died from a rare genetic disorder in which the

metabolism of amino acids produces a toxic compound that is easily confused with ethylene glycol. Prosecutors dismissed the case against Patricia Stallings after she had served fourteen months of her life sentence.

12. *People v. Phillips,* 175 Cal. Rptr. 703 (Ct. App. 1981).

13. *Tanya Thaxton Reid v. State of Texas,* 964 S.W.2d 723 (1998).

14. *Commonwealth v. Robinson.*

15. *Kansas v. Lumbrera,* 845 P.2d 609 (1992).

16. Yorker, Legal issues in FDP.

17. *In the Matter of Jessica Z.,* 515 N.Y.S.2d 370, 135 Misc. 2d 520 (Fam. Ct. 1987).

18. Yorker, Legal issues in FDP.

19. *United States v. Woods,* 484 F.2d 127 (4th Cir. 1973).

20. See *People v. Phillips.* The defendant in this case did not claim a defense based upon her mental state, but the prosecution survived an appellate challenge to admission of expert testimony regarding MBP, despite the fact that she had not put her mental state at issue.

21. DSM-IV.

22. *Marie Claudia Olivier v. State of Texas,* 850 S.W.2d 742 (1993).

23. For a review of literature on the prognosis for psychiatric intervention in MBP cases, see R Kinscherff and RA Famularo, Extreme Munchausen syndrome by proxy: The case for termination of parental rights, *Juvenile Fam Court J* (November 1991); Schreier and Libow, *Hurting for love;* R Nicol and M Eccles, Psychotherapy for Munchausen syndrome by proxy, *Arch Dis Child* 1995; 60:344–348.

24. *State v. DeJesus,* No. CR92-73269, 1993 WL 171866 (Conn. Super. Ct., April 27, 1993).

25. Personal communication regarding MBP perpetrator selection criteria and intervention protocol devised by David Jones and Gerry Byrne at Park Hospital for Children, Oxford, England (August 1996).

26. See Flannery, Munchausen syndrome, reporting the case of *In Re Bowers,* No. 1490, 1992 WL 2870 (Ohio Ct. App., January 2, 1992), in which the trial court heard conflicting testimony from physicians and, troubled by the lack of physical evidence of MBP, concluded that the state had failed to demonstrate MBP by the applicable standard of "clear and convincing" evidence. In upholding the trial court, the appellate court noted that in "this very real and dangerous condition, there may still be reluctance on the part of some courts to accept this as a bona fide mental illness." The appellate court also noted criticism of courts "because of the skepticism with which those cases are approached" but refused to characterize MBP as child abuse as a matter of law, stating, "[W]e adopt no hard rule, or litmus test, for determining neglect or dependency whenever there is a diagnosis of Munchausen Syndrome by Proxy."

27. Ibid.

28. For discussion of MBP as part of an evidentiary pattern reflecting parental unfitness, see Vollaro, Note (see n. 9 above).

29. *Place v. Place,* 525 A.2d 704 (N.H. 1987), in which a court in a divorce action regarding child custody awarded custody to the father following a showing that the mother had MBP and was psychologically unstable.

30. *In the Matter of Jessica Z.,* in which the court relied upon Section 1046(a)(ii) of the New York Family Court Act, which states: "Proof of injuries sustained by a child or of the condition of a child of such a nature as would not ordinarily be sustained or exist except by reason of the acts or omission of the parent or other person responsible for the care of such child shall be prima facie evidence of child abuse or neglect, as the case may be, of the parent or other person legally responsible."

31. Yorker, Legal issues in FDP, citing *Geringer v. Iowa Department of Human Services,* 521 N.W.2d 730 (Ia. 1994), in which the Iowa Supreme Court upheld a juvenile court finding of child abuse and decision to return the child to custody of the mother despite finding evidence of the mother's "staging baseless vomiting and bleeding incidents" in the child; *In the Matter of Jessica Z.,* in which a child was returned to custody of her mother following determination by the court that the mother had poisoned her 18-month-old daughter with laxatives; *In Re Colin R.,* 493 A.2d 1083

(Md. App. 1985), in which the court returned to parental custody with a supervision plan a 3-year-old child who had been found "in need of assistance" because his mother had injected him with a powerful diuretic.

32. *In the Interest of BB.*, 500 N.W.2d 9 (Ia. 1993), in which the Iowa Supreme Court affirmed a juvenile court decision to place the child in foster care; unpublished Massachusetts Juvenile Trial Court decisions in which: (1) one child was found in need of care and protection due to the extreme MBP conduct of her mother and placed with her nonperpetrating divorced father; (2) a child was placed with the sister of the unmarried biological father following a finding of MBP on the part of the mother during efforts to effect interventions towards reunification of mother and child.

33. *In the Matter of Aaron S.*, 163 Misc.2d 967 (1993).

34. *In the Matter of M.A.V.*, 206 Ga. App. 299 (1992).

35. Kinscherff and Famularo, Extreme MBP.

36. *Place v. Place.* The authors are also aware of several unpublished trial court decisions in divorce/child custody proceedings in which physical custody was awarded to a nonperpetrating parent following a determination by the court that the custodial parent was engaging in MBP conduct and that the best interests of the child warranted transfer of at least physical custody.

37. See T Thomas, Covert video surveillance, *New Law Journal* 1994; 44:966–967, including arguments that covert video surveillance may actually endanger children; K Greenfield, Cameras in teddy bears: Electronic visual surveillance and the Fourth Amendment, *58 University of Chicago Law Review 1045 (1991),* holding that the unregulated use of electronic visual surveillance results in extreme infringements upon the right to privacy. Compare B Yorker, Covert video surveillance of Munchausen syndrome by proxy: The exigent circumstances exception, *Health Matrix: Journal of Law and Medicine* 1995;5:325–346, reviewing legal issues and privacy concerns but arguing for the utility of covert video surveillance and proposing an avenue for the admissibility for videotapes obtained without warrant; M Samuels et al., Fourteen cases of imposed upper airway obstruction, *Archives of Disease in Childhood* 1992;67:77–79, presenting justifications for the use of covert surveillance in MBP cases.

38. Ibid.

39. Ibid.

40. For a discussion of privilege issues in MBP cases, see Flannery, Munchausen syndrome (see n. 11 above). See also *Commonwealth v. Robinson* (see n. 10), in which conversations between a mother and a child psychiatrist who had been sent to meet with her following the death of her child were deemed privileged and inadmissible at trial.

PART V

Multiple Traumatization

Chapter 20

Treatment of Multiply Traumatized Abused Children

Mark Chaffin, Ph.D., and
Rochelle F. Hanson, Ph.D.

Some children are multiply abused and experience trauma as a chronic part of their lives. It is difficult to determine how many children experience more than one type of victimization, but there is no doubt that severe and ongoing abuse can affect core parts of personality and well-being. The multiply abused child must not only deal with the abuse that has occurred but also face the ongoing threat of more abuse. It is unfortunately true that the more trauma a child has experienced, the more trauma that is likely to be forthcoming. These children exhibit a wide range of symptoms, including aggression, externalizing behavior problems, poor social competence, affective symptoms, developmental delays, and cognitive-neuropsychological deficits. New classifications that incorporate the complexities of these cases, for example, variations of posttraumatic stress disorder, might be needed to describe the disorders these children suffer. Cognitive behavior therapy shows promise in treatment, but adaptations must be made to consider the special needs of children who suffer multiple and ongoing traumatization.

GENERAL CONSIDERATIONS

Generally, we think of trauma as acute and sudden, but for some abused children trauma is a chronic and all too repetitive part of their lives. However, much of the scientific literature on childhood emotional trauma has focused on the acute variety, and examined posttraumatic stress disorder (PTSD) reactions to events such as sniper attacks, kidnapping, witnessing homicide, and burns.[51] One of the key elements of acute trauma is that the traumatic event is experienced as shocking, coming out of the blue, and overwhelms the individual's ability to cope or process the event. Three core features thought to characterize traumatic abuse of children are lack of controllability, perception of the event as negative, and suddenness.[11]

However, many childhood traumas are qualitatively different from these sorts of abrupt events and involve emotional or psychological blows that are, unfortunately, a routine part

271

of the child's life. Chronic and repetitive interpersonal trauma requires circumstances of captivity or dependency, which may involve hostage situations or institutionalization, but may also apply to some family environments.[39] Because of their dependent status, children may be especially vulnerable to repeated abuse and trauma. Often, trauma becomes chronic and repetitive because it occurs at the hands of the child's parent or caretaker in the form of sexual, physical, and psychological abuse.

Not all child abuse is traumatic. Many forms of abuse may not be experienced by the child as terrifying, shocking, or highly upsetting at the time. For example, some forms of physical abuse may be accepted as normal or expected discipline. Nonviolent sexual fondling of a young preschooler might lack meaning at the time of the event, although it might be reinterpreted as significant later in life. And simply because an event is potentially traumatic does not mean that trauma will be the result. Events widely agreed to hold traumatic potential, such as natural disasters or sexual abuse, do not automatically result in PTSD or PTSD symptoms in all or even most survivors.[44,51,67]

Finally, abuse need not involve trauma in order to have other nontraumatic but nonetheless significant effects. Trauma-based diagnoses (such as PTSD) fail to address many important abuse sequelae, such as stigmatization or feelings of betrayal,[30] or the impact of many factors thought to mediate between presumably traumatic events and outcomes, such as family and community environment[15] or abuse-related attributions and coping strategies.[13,50,58] In other words, abuse is neither a necessary nor a sufficient condition for trauma, and conceptualizing abuse as trauma is likewise not sufficient to understand all abuse effects. Nonetheless, the data do support a PTSD or modified PTSD conceptualization in a high percentage of cases of multiple or chronic abuse.

This chapter considers treatment of children who have been repeatedly traumatized by abuse, often in addition to experiencing other traumatic life events, and whose problems loosely fit a PTSD or expanded PTSD model. We will not explore the larger theoretical or scientific questions involved in this topic—for example, how *trauma* can be defined or operationalized, what the mechanism is by which traumatic events result in trauma, or how diversity of outcomes can be explained. (For a discussion of these issues, see Carlson, Furby, Armstrong, and Shlaes, 1997). Nor will we undertake a critical analysis of the existing literature. We will explore the prevalence of multiple traumas, examine some selected research and thinking on its effects, and then discuss how cognitive behavioral treatment approaches can be applied to these cases.

PREVALENCE OF REPETITIVE CHILD VICTIMIZATION AND TRAUMA

It is extremely difficult to determine how many children are affected by multiple and repetitive types of trauma or victimization experiences (i.e., physical abuse, sexual abuse, witnessing violence). Most of the research on each type of abuse has been conducted separately, with physical abuse, sexual abuse, and domestic violence researchers working relatively independently of each other. To date, most of the attention has focused on sexual abuse in childhood; less research attention has been paid to other types of victimization experiences. Because of this independence of focus within the field, it is difficult to determine how many children experience more than one type of victimization.

Studies using clinical samples[25,49] suggest that there may be a high rate of co-occurrence among sexual abuse, physical abuse, witnessing of violence, and other trauma. One study[12] reported that children who had been both sexually and physically abused experienced an average of ten other separate types of potentially traumatic events during their childhood (e.g., criminal victimization, assaults, suicide of a family member, early separation from a caretaker), compared to less than three such events for nonabused children. A telephone survey of 2,000 children aged 10–16[32] asked questions concerning a variety of victimization experiences, including attempted or completed sexual assault, physical assault, kidnapping, violence to genitals, and corporal punishment, and found that one type of victimization increased the likelihood of another victimization experience. For example, children who reported a sexual assault were 2.67 times more likely than other children to have experienced an additional form of victimization. Children who had experienced an attempted kidnapping or act of genital violence were the most likely to experience additional victimizations.

A slippery slope logic seems to apply when it comes to childhood trauma—the more trauma experienced, the more trauma likely to be forthcoming. Revictimization of abused or traumatized children is a commonly noted occurrence and a presumed abuse sequela. Previously sexually victimized children are at increased risk to be abused or victimized again, either as children or in adulthood.[6,65] Even more perniciously, children who have been both physically and sexually abused appear to be at additionally increased risk for subsequent victimization than children who have experienced sexual abuse but not further physical abuse.[16]

PSYCHOSOCIAL EFFECTS OF PHYSICAL OR SEXUAL ABUSE

No single symptom or collection of symptoms uniquely characterizes abused children. Instead, there are a wide range and a broad array of outcomes associated with childhood victimization, some clearly trauma related (e.g., PTSD) and some that may result whether or not the abuse was traumatic. Studies examining the sequelae of physical abuse report associations with

- aggression
- externalizing behavior problems[62]
- poor social competence[42]
- affective symptoms such as fear, anxiety, PTSD[25,29,45]
- developmental delays[22,41,54]
- deficits in relationship skills
- cognitive/neuropsychological deficits[10,64]

Retrospective data from clinical[60] and community samples[27,56] indicate that child physical abuse is associated with an increased risk for substance abuse, major depression, and PTSD in adulthood.

The sequelae associated with child sexual abuse include the entire array of mental health, emotional, familial, and social problems,[1,2] including

- depression
- inappropriate sexual behaviors

- aggression
- anxiety
- dissociation
- posttraumatic stress disorder

Of interest are the findings that not all sexually abused children appear to develop symptoms, at least not at the time of assessment. One review of the research[44] noted that between one-quarter and one-half of children were asymptomatic at the time of assessment. The authors point out that these findings may be due to the use of insensitive measures or to the fact that abuse-related symptoms are gradual or delayed. However, the results do suggest that abuse is not inevitably pathogenic, and many abuse victims have limited sequelae.

PSYCHOSOCIAL EFFECTS OF COMBINED PHYSICAL AND SEXUAL ABUSE AND MULTIPLE TRAUMAS

Because available data primarily examine the effects of physical and sexual abuse separately, drawing conclusions about the cumulative or combined effects of multiple types of abuse on child functioning is difficult. However, not unexpectedly, the data that are available consistently point to worse and more traumatic outcomes as the numbers and types of traumas accumulate. Posttraumatic stress disorder and other trauma-related symptoms (e.g., dissociation) have generally been lowest among those surviving only one type of abuse (physical or sexual) and highest among those surviving combined abuse. In a national study of 4,008 adults, results indicated that victims of both childhood physical and sexual assault evidenced higher rates of PTSD and major depression than victims of either type of assault alone.[38] Another study found vastly higher scores on measures of dissociation among clinical patients reporting both physical and sexual abuse.[14] Among children who have been both physically and sexually abused, rates of PTSD range from 71 percent to 82 percent.[12,45]

Finally, as noted earlier, a history of abuse is associated with an increased risk for additional sexual or other revictimization during both childhood and adult life. In addition to increasing the risk for additional abuse, prior abuse also appears to increase the risk that subsequent traumatic events will result in PTSD. A childhood abuse history has been found to be associated with an increased risk for subsequent combat-related PTSD, even when controlling for level of combat exposure.[7,68] Prior victimization has also been found to increase the level of children's posttraumatic stress symptoms in response to a revictimization episode, even after controlling for demographic variables and victimization characteristics.[6] Thus, rather than hardening or acclimating its victims, repetitive abuse appears to weaken their resistance and increase their vulnerability.

POSSIBLE SEVERE AND CHRONIC ABUSE SYNDROMES

Severe and prolonged child abuse, whether physical or sexual, is a complex trauma that can affect core aspects of personality and emotional well-being. It is intrinsically interpersonal, may involve purposeful violence, and often occurs in the context of relationships that are complicated by affection, identification, ambivalence, dominance, or dependency. Moreover, because it occurs during childhood, chronic child abuse has the potential to alter critical developmental tasks, such as identity, affect regulation, temperament, interpersonal styles, expectations of others, and other basic cognitive schemata.

The subjective experience of prolonged repetitive abuse trauma has been described as distinct from that of the acute blow. Rather than abrupt and unexpected, chronic traumas come to be anticipated and dreaded, perhaps even acquiring an aura of inevitability. While survivors of acute trauma cope retrospectively with a past event, children living with chronic abuse also must cope prospectively with events that have not yet happened but are grimly awaited. Rather than asking "Why did it happen?" they may more likely ask "Will it happen again tonight?" Some of these children may have been anally or vaginally sexually assaulted on literally hundreds of occasions and beaten or hurled against walls on many more occasions.

A comparison of child victims of ongoing versus single-event abuse[45] found that ongoing abuse was associated with greater depression, somatic features, and wider-ranging symptoms. Another comparison of abused children with acute versus chronic PTSD[29] noted a number of symptom differences between the groups. Acute PTSD children displayed more hyperarousal symptoms, for example, hypervigilance, exaggerated startle, generalized anxiety. Chronic PTSD children were found to have more-diminished interest in usual activities, restricted range of affect, dissociative features (dissociative symptoms, imaginary playmates, odd behavior, daydreaming), dysphoria, and feelings that their lives would be short and hard.

Although PTSD anxiety features are common among multiply abused children, it has been suggested that the PTSD syndrome as currently described fails to capture many of these important variations in trauma-related symptoms seen when repeated chronic abuse trauma is involved. Terr,[61] for example, suggests dividing trauma-stress conditions of childhood into two rough categories, Type I and Type II, the former resulting from sudden blows and the latter from longstanding and repeated ordeals. Type II presentations would include features reflecting children's long-term adaptation to trauma, such as psychic numbing, dissociation, self-hypnosis, and chronic rage. Herman[39,40] similarly describes multiple trauma as resulting in "complex PTSD," which is characterized by a multiplicity of symptoms, including psychoticism, somatic symptoms, withdrawal, depression, changes in relatedness to others, identity disturbances, revictimization, and dissociation. Many of these features have been subsumed under the proposed diagnostic category of "Disorders of Extreme Stress Not Otherwise Specified," or DESNOS.[40] DESNOS encompasses a wide variety of symptoms not directly included in PTSD, such as distrust, despair, hopelessness, and self-destructiveness, which have been supported by empirical studies of abuse survivors.[20] However, it is not clear that DESNOS is, in fact, sufficiently distinct from PTSD to warrant a separate diagnostic category.

Although borderline personality disorder (BPD) is a diagnosis most directly applicable to adults and older adolescents, many DESNOS, Type II, or complex PTSD symptoms are similar to those of BPD. These include self-destructiveness, intense anger, affective instability, dysphoria, chronic feelings of emptiness, and identity disturbance. Histories of chronic and severe abuse have been reported to be common among patients presenting with BPD,[9] and BPD symptoms are reported to be positively associated with both physical and, especially, sexual abuse as well as neglect.[37,53] A dose-effect relationship with abuse trauma has also been reported with both the duration and the severity of sexual abuse positively associated with BPD symptoms.[57] Briere[8] suggests that chronic and extreme abuse, particularly sexual abuse, is probably sufficient to produce BPD symptoms in some individuals, especially when vulnerability has been increased by previous traumas that affect early childhood attachment, such as abandonment, neglect, or prior maltreatment.

However, we should not infer that simply experiencing multiple traumatic events inevitably results in some or any of these syndromes or diagnoses. There is no clear consensus on the validity of these diagnostic formulations for abused children. However, clinicians working with multiply traumatized children should be aware that these children are at risk to suffer from a variety of problems related to core personality features, affect regulation, and identity, in addition to the fear and anxiety symptoms commonly seen in response to abrupt trauma. In the following section, we review the general outline of cognitive-behavioral treatments for PTSD or PTSD symptoms and suggest treatment modifications that may be required for multiply traumatized children with these additional problems.

COGNITIVE-BEHAVIORAL TREATMENT

Although there is a variety of approaches to the treatment of abused children, there have been few controlled treatment outcome studies that support the efficacy of one particular type of intervention over another. However, the treatment outcome literature does provide some limited support for the use of trauma or abuse-specific therapy. A direct focus on the traumatic event(s) and symptomatology seems to provide the most beneficial treatment results, at least for some sorts of symptoms.[17,31,34]

Cognitive-behavioral therapy (CBT) has been widely used and studied with adult victims of trauma as well as with sexually abused children and their nonoffending parents[18,24,26,59] and with physically abused children.[46] (For application of CBT to sexually abused children and physically abused children, see chapters 2 and 10, respectively.) We begin this section by discussing the theoretical model that underlies our approach to treatment. The model provides a rationale and explanation for both the treatment goals and the specific interventions.

The CBT Treatment Model:
The Three-Channel Explanation of Fear and Anxiety Symptoms

The three-channel model provides a rationale that guides our approach to the treatment of multiply traumatized children. This model has been adapted from work done with adult victims of traumatic events that have included rape, other types of sexual assault, physical assault, and natural disasters. According to this model, children, like adults, react to any kind of fearful situation in three different ways: physically, mentally, and behaviorally. These types of response correspond to our Feeling, Thinking, and Doing Channels.

Physical Reaction (The Feeling Channel)

Physical reactions are *automatic;* nothing has to be done on a conscious or intentional basis. When faced with danger—or anything interpreted as dangerous—our bodies automatically respond. Children may say that their stomach hurts or that they had butterflies in the stomach or that their heart felt like it was going to come out of their chest. These physical reactions occur first at the time of the trauma itself and may occur later when something reminds the child of the assault(s). A child may try to avoid certain places, situations, or people (including the therapist) because these stimuli remind the child of the abuse and trigger the physical response. Even if it has been weeks or months since the trauma, these reminders may cause the physical fear reaction.

Mental Reaction (The Thinking Channel)

Even with children, fear may be experienced in the mind, the mental or thinking channel. That is, thoughts sometimes trigger or stimulate fear. For example, it is not unusual for the child to wonder if his assailant will come back and harm him again, or to distrust others. Sometimes certain people, places, things, or circumstances will trigger these thoughts (e.g., the dark or a person who looks like the assailant). At other times, the thoughts may simply enter the child's mind, with no apparent stimuli. For example, some children may see pictures of the abuse in their mind, even though no person, place, thing, or situation has triggered the thought. Some children experience these thoughts involuntarily and despite efforts to suppress them. The experience may feel uncontrollable at times and can impair concentration or participation in day-to-day activities. This adds to a child's feelings of having no control over his or her life. Younger children may have difficulty understanding these thoughts and lack the verbal ability to communicate these fears to others.

Many children also have nightmares about the trauma they have experienced. Again, limited cognitive and verbal abilities in young children may make it particularly difficult for them to convey these fears to others. At times, they may also experience night terrors, in which they wake up crying out but cannot recall what they were dreaming about. This is distressing for caretakers, who may not know how to help their child. It is very important to help both child and caretaker understand that these reactions are not abnormal and that very stressful, traumatic events such as physical or sexual abuse commonly lead to these kinds of reactions.

Behavioral Reaction (The Doing Channel)

A third way children may respond to fear and anxiety associated with traumatic events is on the behavioral level, commonly exhibiting behaviors that attempt to control or avoid the fear response itself or the intense discomfort associated with the physical and mental aspects of fear and anxiety. For example, children may avoid things that trigger or stimulate the fear response. They may try to avoid persons, places, things, or situations that remind them of the assault. However, because multiply traumatized children may be unable to avoid persons related to their abuse (e.g., parents), they may have to resort to more extreme approaches to managing fear and anxiety. As a consequence, they may become depressed, withdrawn, numb, or dissociated, or, conversely, become hyperactive and agitated, and as a result be labeled behavior problems.

Again, it is important to emphasize that these kinds of reactions—physical, mental, and behavioral—while not expressed by every child surviving trauma and while sometimes related to preexisting coping or defensive styles or constitutional diatheses, are understandable reactions to chronic trauma.

Interactions

The physical, mental, and behavioral responses or reactions to fear and anxiety may occur separately. Most often, however, they occur all at once and influence or interact with each other. For example, thoughts, flashbacks, or even dreams (mental reactions) about the traumatic events usually trigger or stimulate physical reactions, such as rapid breathing, increased heart rate, and muscle tension. These reactions, in turn, may lead to behaviors or coping mechanisms that help to avoid the stimuli that trigger the mental and physical reactions.

Here is an example to illustrate the interactive relationship of responses to fear. A girl may see a man on the street who reminds her of her abusive stepfather. Just seeing this man may trigger a fear response both mentally (she thinks about the abuse) and physically (her heart starts to pound, she feels sick to her stomach, her palms become sweaty). As a result, she cries when she has to leave the house and becomes very demanding and attention-seeking towards her mother (behavioral reaction) or becomes detached and withdrawn (coping reaction).

TREATMENT GOALS

The fundamental goal of CBT is to target the physical, mental, and behavioral reactions to the abuse incidents and reduce the child's symptoms. This requires a complete assessment of the child's behavioral and emotional status prior to beginning treatment. Although a full discussion of assessment is beyond the scope of this chapter, it is important to note that assessment should target both general and abuse-specific symptoms, use multiple sources for information, and be sensitive to the child's developmental level (see chapters 1, 6, 12, and 16).

Treatment goals directly follow from assessment and the CBT model. For example, instruction in relaxation and anxiety management might be used to help the child cope with physical reactions such as fear or anxiety. It is not possible to relax and feel anxious at the same time. Teaching the child incompatible autonomic responses (e.g., desensitization, coping skills, stress inoculation) can reduce the physiologic symptoms. Psychoeducation, cognitive reframing, and cognitive processing are examples of interventions directed towards the child's thoughts about the events (the mental channel). These help to reduce intrusive thoughts, maladaptive self-statements, and misinformation that the abuser(s) may have given to the child. Gradual exposure[23] is an intervention used to target the behavioral channel, specifically symptoms of avoidance. It involves gradual direct exposure to the actual feared stimulus or symbolic representations of it. Directing a child away from detachment, numbing, or dissociation and encouraging more adaptive responses targets previously functional but currently dysfunctional coping strategies.

IMPLEMENTING A CBT TREATMENT PROGRAM

Prioritizing Treatment

It may be difficult to make decisions about the focus of treatment for a child who has been the victim of multiple types and incidents of abuse. Should the initial focus be on the sexual abuse or the physical abuse? Should the focus be on the individual child or the whole family? Should treatment include the offending parent(s)? As has been argued elsewhere, treatment of a multiply traumatized child needs to include the entire family, but the entry point into treatment is the abused child. Before making any decisions concerning specific treatment components, the first priorities must be:

- making the child safe from harm
- stabilizing emotional crises in the child
- establishing a working relationship with the child
- securing environmental support for the child

Safety is the first order of business. If the child still lives with the offender or the offender has unsupervised contact with the child, it will be virtually impossible to obtain any benefits from treatment. There is a high risk for further abuse as well as recantation by the child. Direct interaction with the child protection caseworker will be needed to find ways to provide and maintain safety for the child and other family members. If the family has not yet become involved with child protection services, this may be the first priority of treatment.

The second early step in treatment is crisis stabilization. Trauma-specific treatment cannot begin if a child is severely depressed, experiencing acute panic, actively suicidal, homicidal, or psychotic. Instead, the treatment must focus specifically on reducing the crisis symptoms at hand. We assume that children are better able to deal with abuse-related material when they feel stronger and when acute distress has been relieved, rather than assuming that uncovering and processing abuse-related materials is the vehicle to reducing acute crisis symptoms. Obtaining relief may involve use of psychotropic medications, brief hospitalization, or providing increased support, both within and outside the therapy setting. It is critical that acutely distressed children come to associate therapy with the experience of symptom relief, in order to mitigate the intrinsic association between coming to therapy and the cuing of distressing abuse-related memories and emotions.

As with any treatment approach, CBT requires a working relationship in which the child feels accepted, comfortable, understood, and safe. CBT does not share some of the highly expressive or cathartic elements of other treatments, and favors mastering and coping with overwhelming or frightening emotions rather than ventilating them or recovering hidden affect presumably attached to trauma. CBT is also highly structured, especially initially. Consequently, CBT may be less threatening than more emotive or unstructured approaches, and this can expedite formation of a positive working relationship between child and therapist. Highly structured treatments have been found to perform better for some groups of highly traumatized children.[55] With a chronically abused child, expectations of exploitation, patterns of intense and unstable relationships, or withdrawal from others may make relationship building complicated at best. This process, with its many ups and downs, may traverse the length of therapy. Safe feelings with the therapist can be fostered through stability, predictability, and a friendly but not overly solicitous attitude that maintains clear boundaries. Making the therapy setting predictable (e.g., same office, same appointment time and day, similar structure to the session) will help increase a child's feelings of safety and create the basis for a strong therapeutic relationship.

Finally, it is important that the child have adequate social support, especially from his or her nonabusive primary caregiver. If the nonoffending caretaker is unable to believe the child's allegations of abuse and/or provide needed support, this needs to be an early focus of treatment. It should be noted that many nonabusive parents may be in the midst of processing the abrupt trauma of abuse disclosure or may have been traumatized themselves. These parents may need extra attention while they process the events, before they are able to focus on their child's needs. Parental ambivalence and confusion are common and are not necessarily signs that the parent is malignant or uncaring. However, if nonabusive caretakers are violent or brutally hostile toward the child, it may be necessary to consider placement with another caretaker (e.g., foster parent, relative, family friend), who can provide the needed support. If the nonoffending parent is cooperative, collateral work can be conducted in tandem with the child's treatment.

Physical Channel Interventions: Relaxation and Anxiety Management Skills

To cope with the physiological manifestations of fear and anxiety, children are taught relaxation and anxiety management skills. These skills are particularly useful for children who are experiencing extreme anxiety when faced with any reminders or memories of their trauma experiences, including when they are asked to discuss their abuse experiences. Children can be taught skills such as breathing retraining,[21] deep muscle relaxation,[52] or guided imagery[5] at the onset of treatment. Use of these skills during treatment will enable the child to discuss the abuse and process the experience. Processing the experience means that the child has the opportunity to feel his or her feelings concerning the victimization. The anxiety management strategies enable the child to discuss trauma-related thoughts and feelings without becoming overwhelmed.

It is important to present these skills in a manner consistent with the developmental level of the child. For young children, it is helpful to provide simple models and analogies. For example, in teaching muscle relaxation exercises, the therapist can instruct the child to "act like a tin soldier" to demonstrate muscle tension, and to "act like a wet noodle" to illustrate the relaxation component of the exercise. The use of an inflated and deflated balloon serves as a visual aid for instruction in the inhalation and exhalation components of controlled diaphragmatic breathing. These types of anxiety management techniques are taught at the initial stages of therapy to cope with symptoms of fear, anxiety, and posttraumatic stress. The child is then instructed to use these skills during further processing of the trauma. In working with multiply traumatized children, it is important to be alert to dissociative or self-hypnotic coping responses, which can mimic some of these anxiety management techniques. The goal of anxiety management techniques is for the child to be able to experience memories, thoughts, and stimuli reminiscent of the abuse without the associated negative emotions, whereas the goal of dissociation or self-hypnosis is to escape these stimuli entirely. When children begin to stare blankly or become unresponsive, it is important to gently and calmly redirect them to the material at hand and reinforce positive coping. If anxiety management techniques appear to be leading to increased detachment or dissociative coping, it may be wise to discontinue them until a more opportune time.

Mental Channel Interventions

The key component of interventions geared towards the mental channel is to target mistaken or dysfunctional beliefs the child may have acquired concerning the abuse, including justifications for the abuse used by the abuser(s), depressive cognitions, or unrealistic schema involving self and others. Cognitive approaches are used to challenge faulty beliefs and, where appropriate, to replace these beliefs with more adaptive cognitions. Techniques such as cognitive restructuring, thought-stopping, and guided self-dialogue may be used.[26] For example, children experiencing significant feelings of self-blame regarding the abuse may benefit from identifying the source of these beliefs and assimilating information that helps reduce the feelings. Children—especially children whose cognitive development allows them to reason logically—can be encouraged to routinely challenge irrational or maladaptive beliefs, and therapy may include practice sessions in which the child learns to respond to a problematic cognition with a more adaptive one. For example, the child might practice challenging the idea "you can't trust anyone" with the associated idea "no, you can't trust *some* people, but not all people are bad."

Another way to target faulty or maladaptive beliefs is through education. Psychoeducation helps to normalize thoughts and feelings about the abuse experience(s). Psychoeducation efforts with multiply traumatized children need to include information regarding both sexual and physical abuse, sex education, and risk reduction. Children should be informed about the various types of sexual abuse, why abuse occurs, who perpetrates the abuse, how abused children feel, and why children often do not disclose their abuse. The therapist might explain, for example, that sexual abuse often happens because abusers have sexual feelings for children which most people don't have, that they deliberately choose to do it even though they know that it is wrong, and that they may use tricks or fear to get what they want from children. For physical abuse, children may need to differentiate appropriate from inappropriate parental discipline and understand how psychological abuse (e.g., berating) is commonly a part of physically abusive behavior rather than an indication of the child's worth as a person. Instruction in nonviolent behavioral management techniques may need to be explained to both parent and child. Children who have witnessed violence between their parents need information about such behavior, to keep or stop them from blaming themselves for their parent's difficulties and to teach them that violence is not an appropriate way to handle disagreements. It may be necessary to emphasize that most people can disagree or even get angry without becoming violent. After any type of traumatic event experience, it is important to provide the victim information concerning "normal" emotional reactions and associated cognitions.

The focus of sex education should be on healthy sexuality.[23] Sex education should help to clarify misinformation children may have received from others or a lack of information concerning healthy sexuality, body awareness, and health-related issues, such as sexually transmitted diseases. It is important to obtain caretakers' permission before beginning sex education, and preferable to enlist their participation in the education process. Information should be geared towards the child's current developmental level. Basic information should be combined with exercises that provide children the opportunity to explore their feelings about sexuality.[23]

The third psychoeducational issue is risk reduction. Children should be taught

- how to identify "red flags" that may indicate a high-risk situation
- how to develop a safety plan in response to a violent or abusive situation
- that they have the right to say "no"
- the difference between appropriate and inappropriate touch
- development of skills to respond to inappropriate sexual touch

Multiply traumatized children who may manifest aspects of learned helplessness[43] need to practice and be encouraged in active and confident responses to potential life challenges, including situations of potential revictimization, in order to foster both appropriate self-protective behaviors and the child's sense of efficacy.

Although the educative and cognitive components are critical to CBT, some multiply traumatized children have such strong negative affect attached to these topics that they may be unable to discuss them without experiencing undue anxiety, detachment, or avoidance. In these cases, be sure that the physical and behavioral channel targets have been sufficiently addressed before initiating the more cognitive components of CBT.

Behavioral Channel Interventions: Gradual Exposure

Gradual exposure is a key aspect of CBT and is used to help the child confront fears and prevent avoidance. (See also chapter 3.) Avoidance, very broadly, may be thought of as the symptomatic behavior that is being targeted. The rationale behind gradual exposure is that anxiety results from the pairing of an unconditional stimulus, such as physical or sexual abuse, which automatically elicits fear, with a previously neutral or even reinforcing stimulus such as a parent, a room, an area of the house, the smell of beer. Because of this association, the previously neutral stimulus acquires the capacity to elicit fear. When confronted with this stimulus, or any reminders of it, the child experiences symptoms of fear and anxiety. One way children cope with these symptoms is to avoid any thoughts or reminders of the abuse. Thus, the avoidance response becomes reinforced. Unfortunately, avoidance does not give the child the opportunity to process his or her experiences, making it likely that symptoms will intensify and/or continue occurring longer into the future. Although avoidant coping may produce some short-term relief, it runs the risk of causing long-term problems.[13, 48]

Gradual exposure techniques encourage the child to face the fear-producing stimuli, breaking the association between these negative feelings and the abuse-related cues.[23] The goal of gradual exposure is for the child to be able to discuss trauma experiences in detail without experiencing undue distress, avoidance, numbing, or detachment. As with systematic desensitization, the child first begins with stimuli that provoke low levels of anxiety (e.g., where they were or what they were wearing) and then gradually moves on to increasingly distressing stimuli. As treatment progresses, the child is asked to talk about specific sights, sounds, smells, and bodily sensations remembered from the events. Relaxation and anxiety management techniques taught earlier in treatment are used to help the child deal with any symptoms of distress. The exposure sessions are repeated until the memories no longer elicit the fear or avoidance response. Clinically, achievement of this goal may serve as an indication that the therapy is approaching a successful conclusion.

CBT focuses on gradually discussing progressively distressing elements of the trauma and mastering the associated affect and cognitions at each step. Although this is invariably an emotional process, catharsis, abreaction, or implosion is not encouraged within this framework. If affective distress becomes overwhelming, children are encouraged to slow down, master the distress, and process the associated cognitions before proceeding.

Children who have experienced multiple incidents and types of abuse may have difficulty remembering specific details or discrete events. The therapist can help the child by providing cues and anchor points to trigger memories of specific events. For example, the therapist can ask about the first and last episodes and episodes associated with special occasions, such as holidays, birthdays, vacations, or school events. Since the child may be unable to remember specific details about multiple events, it is up to the clinician to decide how far to pursue the exposure. A general rule is to have the child recapitulate any memories that cause distress. These memories should be processed until they no longer elicit significant fear symptoms or avoidance. When ordering or sequencing events, it is generally preferable to let the child have input, keeping in mind that it is best to begin with events that cause lower levels of anxiety and move gradually towards more anxiety producing stimuli. In order to facilitate the exposure sessions, a variety of mediums, such as talking, drawing, the use of puppets or dolls, or even singing, can be used. The selection of the particular mode will vary, depending on the child's developmental level and choice.

It is often difficult to convince children, and particularly caretakers, of the benefits of exposure, given the initial high rates of anxiety experienced by the child. Because of this anxiety, a child may try to avoid attending treatment. Predicting this response in both the child and parent and preparing them for it helps increase the likelihood of compliance. It is also helpful to provide a rationale before beginning the exposure sessions. For example, Deblinger and Heflin[23] explain to children that exposure sessions are "like getting into a cold swimming pool." At first, "it feels like an iceberg . . . but after a few minutes . . . the water feels great." It is explained to the child that getting used to talking about the abuse is like getting used to that cold pool. As with any behavioral approach, specific positive praise should follow the desired behaviors, or approximations of them, and the therapist should point out and reinforce successes and accomplishments along the way. It is particularly important to note symptomatic improvements and to link them with the child's efforts in therapy. For example, we might tell children, "see, you've done such a great job learning to relax that now the dark doesn't make you so afraid anymore."

TRAUMA-RELATED BEHAVIORAL PROBLEMS

A number of behavioral problems, including aggression and inappropriate sexual behaviors, are sometimes seen among multiply traumatized children[19,36] and often must be additional treatment targets. In our opinion, CBT would not assume that these behaviors will disappear once their presumably underlying elements of trauma have been resolved, but rather assumes that the behaviors need to be a focus of treatment in their own right. CBT for sexual problems typically involves setting up systematic reinforcement schedules for appropriate behavior that is incompatible with sexual behavior problems (e.g., reinforcing children for "keeping your hands to yourself"), learning sexual behavior rules, and teaching self-control procedures.[3,55] Although sexual behavior problems can sometimes be persistent, our experience has been that most preadolescent children respond rapidly to behavior modification programs directly targeting these behaviors. (See chapter 3 for further discussion of using CBT for problems related to sexual abuse.)

COLLATERAL TREATMENT WITH THE NONOFFENDING PARENT(S) OR CARETAKER(S)

In response to abuse, parents and caretakers themselves may experience significant symptoms of distress, which can hinder the child's recovery. The parent's ability to provide support can have a profound impact on the child's recovery.[28,68] Researchers in the area of child sexual abuse have just begun to examine the effects of including nonoffending parents in the treatment process, but preliminary findings indicate that inclusion of a nonoffending parent in treatment results in parent-reported decreases in child behavior problems and increases in effective parenting skills.[18,24,59] Treatment with the nonoffending parent is thus an integral component of the child's recovery process. This treatment should involve three components:[23]

- coping skills training, to assist parents in coping effectively with their own thoughts and emotions

- gradual exposure of the parent's experiences, to enable them to assist their child in exposure sessions
- behavioral management skills training, to reduce abuse-related behavioral problems and increase effective parenting

CBT techniques can be used to help caretakers cope with their own distress, facilitating their ability to deal with their child's distress. Caretakers may also have misinformation concerning child development, trauma outcomes, child abuse dynamics, healthy sexuality, and discipline. Psychoeducation with the parent or caretaker is used to correct faulty beliefs and provide important information. Gradual exposure is used to reduce abuse-related symptoms and to help the parent or caretaker assist the child during exposure sessions. Instruction in behavior management skills teaches parents how to model and reinforce appropriate behaviors. Parents also may be taught effective child behavior management techniques, such as parent-child interaction therapy.[63]

EXTENDED-TREATMENT ISSUES

CBT is typically a short- to moderate-term treatment (around 10 to 20 sessions), and for many or most children this term can provide sufficient benefit. However, some symptoms may persist past this time, and some children remain symptomatic after moderate-term CBT.[4] Children experiencing more severe traumatic sequelae such as psychotic-like symptoms, identity problems, or attachment problems, may require longer-term treatment; and other symptoms, such as dissociation or intense anger, also have been reported to change less rapidly in therapy.[47] The decision to extend therapy needs to be based upon a careful assessment of ongoing symptoms and treatment potential. Within this treatment model, the need for extended treatment is determined by (1) the ongoing presence of identifiable symptoms that (2) cause significant distress or impairment and that (3) can reasonably be expected to respond to further treatment. Treatment is not extended simply on the basis of "unresolved issues" in the absence of distressing symptoms or impairment.

Where extended treatment is needed, CBT can serve as an excellent springboard by providing initial relief and stabilization, fostering positive expectations about therapy, and initiating a trusting relationship in which the abuse can be openly discussed. Longer-term cognitive therapy for dissociative problems, psychotic-like features, and identity or attachment disturbances often involves less-structured approaches and fewer clear-cut goals, because the problems themselves may be difficult to define precisely or operationalize.[35] Extended sessions may focus on more elaborate cognitive processing of basic attitudes towards self and others and may use feelings and behaviors that arise in the client-therapist relationship as basic data for exploration. Regardless of focus, the same general techniques of CBT apply (i.e., normalizing and conceptualizing responses to trauma, gradual exposure, cognitive processing, education, use of behavioral practice, encouraging and reinforcing positive behavior change, etc.). This lends continuity to the treatment. Although extended treatment may have a modified focus, it is important that the approach remain consistent and follow the general CBT model. We believe that good therapy, regardless of the particular model, should be based upon a sound theoretical and empirical framework, and not mix techniques from potentially incompatible models.

For other children, short- to moderate-term CBT may produce sufficient gains, but they may continue to need some degree of support. Abuse trauma seldom ends abruptly, and children may be exposed to ongoing stressors, such as court involvement or changes in family structure and composition. Ongoing supportive group therapy may be useful, as well as periodic follow-up or booster sessions in maintaining and consolidating gains, as well as mastering ongoing stresses related to the abuse. Again, in considering referral for concomitant or follow-up supportive group therapy, it is important that the treatment model be compatible with CBT.

CONCLUSION

Treatment of the multiply abused child presents an ongoing therapeutic challenge. While their problems may loosely fit a PTSD model, these children require personalized treatment plans that recognize the special needs of a child who may have spent much of his or her life anticipating, if not experiencing, abuse. Cognitive behavioral therapy has been found to be a useful treatment tool, addressing physical, mental, and behavioral pathways, but for some children the short to moderate term of conventional CBT may not sufficiently address their problems. Continuing therapy should be consistent with a CBT framework, to provide the child with familiar and compatible approaches.

R E F E R E N C E S

1. Beitchman J, Zucker K, Hood J, daCosta G, Akman D. A review of the short-term effects of child sexual abuse. *Child Abuse Negl* 1991;15:537–556.
2. Beitchman J, Zucker K, Hood J, daCosta G, Akman D, Cassavia E. A review of the long-term effects of child sexual abuse. *Child Abuse Negl* 1992;16:101–118.
3. Berliner L, Rawlings L. *A treatment manual: Children with sexual behavior problems.* Washington State Department of Community Development. 1991.
4. Berliner L, Saunders B. Treating fear and anxiety in sexually abused children: Results of a controlled 2-year follow-up study. *Child Maltreat* 1996;1:294–309.
5. Berliner L, Wheeler R. Treating the effects of sexual abuse on children. *J Interpers Viol* 1987;2:415–434.
6. Boney-McCoy S, Finkelhor D. Prior victimization: A risk factor for child sexual abuse and for PTSD-related symptomatology among sexually abused youth. *Child Abuse Negl* 1995;19:1401–1422.
7. Bremner J, Southwick S, Johnson D, Yehuda R, Charney D. Childhood physical abuse and combat-related posttraumatic stress disorder in Vietnam veterans. *Am J Psychiatry* 1993;150:235–239.
8. Briere J. *Child abuse trauma: Theory and treatment of the lasting effects.* Newbury Park, CA: Sage. 1992.
9. Briere J, Zaidi L. Sexual abuse histories and sequelae in female psychiatric emergency room patients. *Am J Psychiatry* 1989;146:1602–1606.
10. Burke AE, Crenshaw DA, Green J, Schlosser MA, Strocchia-Rivera L. Influence of verbal ability on the expression of aggression in physically abused children. *J Am Acad Child Adolesc Psychiatry* 1989;28:215–218.
11. Carlson E, Furby L, Armstrong J, Shlaes J. A conceptual framework for the long-term psychological effects of traumatic child abuse. *Child Maltreat* 1997;2:272–295.
12. Chaffin M. Working with multiply traumatized children. Paper presented at the San Diego Conference on Responding to Child Maltreatment, APSAC Advanced Training Seminars. January 1995.
13. Chaffin M, Wherry J, Dykman R. School-age childrens' coping with sexual abuse: Abuse stressors and symptoms associated with four coping strategies. *Child Abuse Negl* 1997;21:227–240.

14. Chu JA, Dill DL. Dissociative symptoms in relation to childhood physical and sexual abuse. *Am J Psychiatry* 1990;147:887–892.

15. Cicchetti D, Rizley R. Developmental perspectives on the etiology, intergenerational transmission, and sequelae of child maltreatment. *New Dir Child Dev: Development Perspectives on Child Maltreatment* 1981;11:31–56.

16. Cloitre M, Tardiff K, Marzuk P, Leon A, Portera L. Childhood abuse and subsequent sexual assault among female inpatients. *J Trauma Stress* 1996;9:473–482.

17. Cohen J, Mannarino AP. Interventions for sexually abused children: Initial treatment outcome findings. *Child Maltreat* 1998;3:17–26.

18. Cohen J, Mannarino AP. A treatment outcome study for sexually abused preschoolers: Initial findings. *J Am Acad Child Adolesc Psychiatry* 1996;35:42–50.

19. Conaway LP, Hansen DJ. Social behavior of physically abused and neglected children: A critical review. *Clin Psychol Rev* 1989;9:627–652.

20. Corwin D. Sexually abused children's symptoms and disorders of extreme stress not otherwise specified: Does this proposed psychiatric diagnosis fit? In Burgess A (ed.), *Child trauma I: Issues and research,* 87–115. New York: Garland. 1992.

21. Craske MG, Barlow DH. Panic disorder and agoraphobia. In Barlow DH (ed.), *Clinical handbook of psychological disorders: A step-by-step treatment manual,* 2nd ed., 1–47. New York: Guilford Press. 1993.

22. Crittendon PM, Ainsworth M. Child maltreatment and attachment theory. In Cicchetti D, Carlson V (eds.), *Child maltreatment: Theory and research on the causes and consequences of child abuse and neglect,* 432–463. New York: Cambridge University Press. 1989.

23. Deblinger E, Heflin AH. *Treating sexually abused children and their nonoffending parents.* Newbury Park, CA: Sage. 1996.

24. Deblinger E, Lippmann J, Steer R. Sexually abused children suffering posttraumatic stress symptoms: Initial treatment outcome findings. *Child Maltreat* 1996;1:310–321.

25. Deblinger E, McLeer SV, Atkins MS, Ralphe D, Foa E. Post-traumatic stress in sexually abused, physically abused, and nonabused children. *Child Abuse Negl* 1989;13:403–408.

26. Deblinger E, McLeer S, Henry D. Cognitive behavioral treatment for sexually abused children suffering post-traumatic stress disorder: Preliminary findings. *J Am Acad Child Adolesc Psychiatry* 1990;29:747–752.

27. Duncan RD, Saunders BE, Kilpatrick DG, Hanson RF, Resnick HS. Childhood physical assault as a risk factor for PTSD, depression, and substance abuse: Findings from a national survey. *Am J Orthopsychiatry* 1996;66:437–448.

28. Everson MD, Hunter WM, Runyon DK, Edelsohn GA, Coulter ML. Maternal support following disclosure of incest. *Am J Orthopsychiatry* 1989;59:197–207.

29. Famularo R, Kinscherff R, Fenton T. Symptom differences in acute and chronic presentation of childhood post-traumatic stress disorder. *Child Abuse Negl* 1990;14:439–444.

30. Finkelhor D. The trauma of child sexual abuse: Two models. In Wyatt GE, Powell GJ (eds), *Lasting effects of child sexual abuse,* 61–82. Newbury Park, CA: Sage. 1988.

31. Finkelhor D, Berliner L. Research on the treatment of sexually abused children: A review and recommendations. *J Am Acad Child Adolesc Psychiatry* 1995;34:1408–1423.

32. Finkelhor D, Dzuiba-Leatherman J. Children as victims of violence: A national survey. *Pediatrics* 1994;84:413–420.

33. Foa EB, Meadows EA. Psychosocial treatments for posttraumatic stress disorder: A critical review. *Annu Rev Psychol* 1997;48:449–480.

34. Freidrich W. Clinical considerations of empirical treatment studies of abused children. *Child Maltreat* 1996;1:343–347.

35. Freidrich W. Managing disorders of self-regulation in sexually abused boys. In Hunter M (ed.) *Child survivors and perpetrators of sexual abuse: Treatment innovations,* 3–23. Newbury Park, CA: Sage. 1995.

36. Freidrich W. Sexual victimization and sexual behavior in children: A review of recent literature. *Child Abuse Negl* 1993;17:59–66.

37. Guzder J, Paris J, Zelkowitz P, Marchessault K. Risk factors for borderline pathology in children. *J Am Acad Child Adolesc Psychiatry* 1996;35:26–33.

38. Hanson RF, Saunders BE, Smith DW, et al. The impact of childhood physical and sexual assault on adult mental health. Paper presented at the Conference on Responding to Child Maltreatment, San Diego, CA, January 1993.

39. Herman J. Complex PTSD: A syndrome in survivors of prolonged and repeated trauma. In Everly G, Lating J (eds.), *Psychotraumatology: Key papers and core concepts in post-traumatic stress,* 87–102. New York: Plenum. 1995.

40. Herman J. Sequelae of prolonged and repeated trauma: Evidence for a complex posttraumatic syndrome (DESNOS). In Davidson J, Foa E (eds.), *Posttraumatic stress disorder: DSM-IV and beyond,* 213–228. Washington, DC: American Psychiatric Press. 1992.

41. Herrenkohl RC, Herrenkohl EC, Egolf B, Wu P. The developmental consequences of child abuse: The Lehigh Longitudinal Study. In Starr RH, Wolfe DA (eds.), *The effects of child abuse and neglect: Issues and research,* 57–81. New York: Guilford Press. 1991.

42. Kaufman J, Cicchetti D. Effects of maltreatment on school-age children's socioemotional development: Assessments in a day-camp setting. *Dev Psychol* 1989;25:516–524.

43. Kelley S. Learned helplessness in the sexually abused child. *Issues Compr Pediatr Nurs* 1986;9:193–207.

44. Kendall-Tackett KA, Williams LM, Finkelhor D. The impact of sexual abuse on children: A review and synthesis of recent empirical studies. *Psychol Bull* 1993;113:164–180.

45. Kiser LJ, Heston J, Millsap PA, Pruitt DB. Physical and sexual abuse in childhood: Relationship with post-traumatic stress disorder. *J Am Acad Child Adolesc Psychiatry* 1991;30:776–783.

46. Kolko DJ. Individual cognitive behavioral treatment and family therapy for physically abused children and their offending parents: A comparison of clinical outcomes. *Child Maltreat* 1996; 1:322–342.

47. Lanktree C, Briere J. Outcome of therapy for sexually abused children: A repeated measures study. *Child Abuse Negl* 1995;19:1145–1156.

48. Leitenberg H, Greenwald E, Cado S. A retrospective study of long-term methods of coping with having been sexually abused during childhood. *Child Abuse Negl* 1992;16:399–407.

49. Lewis DO, Lovely R, Yeager C, della Femina D. Toward a theory of the genesis of violence: A follow-up study of delinquents. *J Am Academy Child Adolesc Psychiatry* 1989;28:431–436.

50. Mannarino A, Cohen J. A follow-up study of factors that mediate the development of psychological symptomatology in sexually abused girls. *Child Maltreat* 1996;1:246–260.

51. McNally R. Stressors that produce posttraumatic stress disorder in children. In Davidson J, Foa E (eds.), *Posttraumatic stress disorder: DSM-IV and beyond,* 57–74. Washington, DC: American Psychiatric Press. 1992.

52. Ollendick TH, Cerny JA. Clinical behavior therapy with children. New York: Plenum. 1981.

53. Paris J, Zweig-Frank H, Guzder J. Psychological risk factors for borderline personality disorder in female patients. *Compr Psychiatry* 1994;35:301–305.

54. Pianta R, Egeland B, Erickson MF. The antecedents of maltreatment: Results of the mother-child interaction. In Cicchetti D, Carlson V (eds.), *Child maltreatment: Theory and research on the causes and consequences of child abuse and neglect,* 203–253. New York: Cambridge University Press. 1989.

55. Pithers WD, Gray A, Busconi A, Houchens P. Children with sexual behavior problems: Five distinct child types and related treatment considerations. *Child Maltreat* 1998;3:384–406.

56. Pollock VE, Briere J, Schneider L, Knop J, et al. Childhood antecedents of antisocial behavior: Parental alcoholism and physical abusiveness. *Am J Psychiatry* 1990;147:1290–1293.

57. Silk K, Lee S, Hill E, Lohr N. Borderline personality disorder symptoms and severity of sexual abuse. *Am J Psychiatry* 1995;152:1059–1064.

58. Spaccarelli, S. Stress appraisal and coping in child sexual abuse: A theoretical and empirical review. *Pychol Bull* 1994;116:340–362.

59. Stauffer LB, Deblinger E. Cognitive behavioral groups for nonoffending mothers and their

young sexually abused children: A preliminary treatment outcome study. *Child Maltreat* 1996; 1:65–76.

60. Surrey J, Swett C, Michaels AI, Levin S. Reported history of physical and sexual abuse and severity of symptomatology in women psychiatric outpatients. *Am J Orthopsychiatry* 1990; 60:412–417.

61. Terr LC. Childhood traumas: An outline and overview. In Everly G, Lating J (eds.), *Psychotraumatology: Key papers and core concepts in post-traumatic stress,* 301–320. New York: Plenum. 1995.

62. Trickett P, McBride-Chang C. The developmental impact of different forms of child abuse and neglect. *Dev Rev* 1995;15:311–337.

63. Urquiza A, McNeil C. Parent-child interaction therapy: An intensive dyadic intervention for physically abusive families. *Child Maltreatment* 1996;1:134–144.

64. Vondra JI, Barnett D, Cicchetti D. Self-concept, motivation, and competence among pre-schoolers from maltreating and comparison families. *Child Abuse Negl* 1990:14:525–540.

65. Wyatt G, Guthrie D, Notgrass C. Differential effects of women's child sexual abuse and subsequent sexual revictimization. *J Coun Clin Psychol* 1992;60:167–173.

66. Wyatt G, Mickey M. Support by parents and others as it mediates the effect of child sexual abuse: An exploratory study. In Wyatt G, Powell G (eds.), *The lasting effects of child sexual abuse.* Newbury Park, CA: Sage. 1988.

67. Yehuda R, McFarlane A. Conflict between current knowledge about posttraumatic stress disorder and its original conceptual basis. *Am J Psychiatry* 1995;152:1705–1713.

68. Zaidi L, Foy D. Childhood abuse experiences and combat-related PTSD. *J Trauma Stress* 1994;7:33–42.

PART VI

Disposition Issues

Chapter 21

Treatment of Offenders

David B. Doolittle, Psy.D.

There is some evidence that treatment can prevent recidivism among offenders who abuse or maltreat children. The offenders, their offenses, and their victims are so heterogenous, however, that further research is needed to determine what type of offender can be treated successfully with which form of therapeutic intervention. Treatment decisions will depend upon the age and gender of the offender and victim, their relationship, the type of offense, and the severity and chronicity of offending. Substance abuse and psychiatric disorders are also relevant factors. In general, the younger the offender when offenses began and the wider the range of deviant thoughts, the higher the likelihood of recidivism and greater the need for intensive treatment. Behavioral, cognitive-behavioral, and psychodynamic treatment modalities are used, and each can play a role, although the shorter term and quicker impact of cognitive behavioral approaches are often preferred because of the threat posed by not correcting the offender's behavior quickly. Specialized techniques have been developed for the treatment of sexual offenders but are not yet widely used. Treatment goals include the offender's acknowledging and clarifying cognitive distortions related to the abusive behavior, developing empathy for the victim, and developing the social skills and impulse control to behave nonabusively.

GENERAL CONSIDERATIONS

The treatment of offenders who abuse or maltreat children and adolescents is an extensive field, encompassing a wide variety of forms of child maltreatment and a range of populations engaged in maltreatment, with varying degrees of severity and recidivism. Treatments fall within a number of formats from a variety of theoretical perspectives, although there are common goals and objectives of offender treatment that supersede theoretical perspectives or format. This chapter discusses preliminary issues to be considered in offender treatment, the range of offenders and types of offense, and the various theoretical perspectives and treatment formats.

PRELIMINARY CONSIDERATIONS

Recidivism

One of the first issues to be considered in offender treatment is recidivism. Not many years ago, offenders against children, particularly sexual offenders, were considered so recidivistic that treatment was thought to be a poor dispositional outcome from assessment or court procedures. However, some studies of treatment outcomes [9,25] find that treated offenders are less recidivistic than untreated offenders. While this represents an endorsement of treatment activities with offenders, the generalizability of these studies is hampered by the fact that all offenders are considered in an indiscriminant fashion and the criterion for recidivism is a new convicted offense for a sexual or nonsexual crime. Another review[9] found between 11 percent and 35 percent of perpetrators reoffended for sex crimes. While lower rates of reoffense for sex crimes were found following treatment, this study makes clear that recidivism data were compromised by brief lengths of follow-up and the likelihood that new incidents of sexual offending would not be reported to police.

Differences in methodology led one research team,[23] to conclude unequivocally that offender treatment is successful while another research team,[28] raised caution whether statistical proof of the success of offender treatment has been established. It is now clear that the heterogeneity of offenders against children is so broad that recidivism studies indiscriminantly grouping all offenders together are misleading and represent an inadequate research design. Treatment outcome studies that consider separately cases representing different offense types and prior histories of offending will do a better job of demonstrating the heterogeneity of treatment response of offenders and their differential response to the treatment process.

Countertransference

Countertransference, a key treatment issue regardless of format or theoretical perspective, is the next preliminary consideration for therapists treating child abuse offenders. Evaluators and therapists inevitably experience emotional reactions of distress, anger, and outrage as histories of sexual and physical offenses against children are catalogued and understood. The need to control offending behavior leads some clinicians to want to control the offender's behavior in wide-ranging ways that run the risk of changing the clinical goal from treatment to social control. Marshall[21] comments that many clinicians have begun to perceive the offender as a monster who simply requires social and clinical control.

Marshall also refers to an opposite countertransference tendency commonly seen in offender treatment, in which clinicians identify with the needs and historical pain of the offender and perceive him or her as a victim of tragic life circumstances. This response leads to an incorrect and even dangerous underestimation of the victimization. The offender is empathized with, but the child victim's pain and the risk to society are not adequately perceived. Marshall states the obvious need for an approach that balances understanding and empathy for the offender with appreciation for the destructiveness of victimization. Only in this way can society's need for control of victimization be accomplished while responding to the offender's need for clinical intervention and treatment.

MANAGEMENT CONSIDERATIONS

Type of Offender

The range of child maltreatment offenders spans age and gender of offender, age of victim, offense type, and context of the offense, especially concerning relationship of offender to victim. In addition, severity and chronicity of offending represent important aspects of offending that significantly affect disposition and treatment-planning decisions. Becker and Quinsey[3] discuss assessment of child molesters and report that assessment of attitudes and beliefs of the offender, as well as sexual physiological assessment (i.e., phallometric, or strength of erection measures) of the offender, are critical for treatment planning. While measures of psychopathy are useful for predicting recidivism, Becker and Quinsey note that such measures have less utility in treatment planning. For sexual abuse offenders, assessments establishing that offenders have an early (i.e., adolescent) onset of sexual offenses and a wide range of deviant sexual thoughts, feelings, and behaviors (i.e., paraphilic behaviors and fantasies) are consistent with the highest likelihood of recidivism and entrenchment of the deviant sexual arousal pattern.[22] These cases will require the most intensive treatment and monitoring efforts and are thus often unsuitable for typical outpatient offender treatment programs.

The type of sexual offense against children has been the most thoroughly researched. The assessment and treatment efforts of both adolescent and adult sexual offenders (though more typically male than female offenders) have been studied. Efforts to treat perpetrators of physical abuse, domestic violence (e.g., spousal abuse), and verbal and emotional abuse are less extensively examined in the research and clinical literature. Society has thus far been more tolerant of physical than sexual maltreatment of children. As a result, research into assessment and treatment of sexual offending against children is far more developed, compared to other forms of child maltreatment.

However, there are some studies we can look to. Many domestic violence programs are focused on spousal violence and violence against women. One review of research on treatment programs for spousal and family violence[24] focuses on qualitative research and reports the degree to which programs that treat family violence offenders concentrate on values and attitudes within the cultural context. While such treatment programs have been seen as successful, the cultural context of such programs indicates they may be refocused as the values and attitudes of society change.

Research into treatment for verbal and emotional maltreatment of children is truly in its infancy. Emotional abuse and neglect of children is examined in chapter 15 of this book. Briere[5] reports this as perhaps the most common form of maltreatment of children. Societal responses to verbal and emotional abuse of children are ambivalent at best, exemplified by the lack of laws proscribing such behavior or child protection statutes indicating that such behavior represents legally reportable child abuse. What is clear is that verbal and emotional abuse often accompany physical or sexual maltreatment of children. Reported and treated cases of physical or sexual offenders should invariably consider the verbal and emotional treatment of the child as well. Chronic cases of verbal or emotional maltreatment of children and adolescents in the absence of physical or sexual abuse are likely to remain unidentified and untreated at the present time.

Age Difference

The age span between offender and victim is a critical treatment variable. In the area of sexual maltreatment of children, male adult offenders against children represent the majority of cases and have received the greatest attention in the research and clinical literature. Treatment goals for male adolescent sexual offenders differ from the treatment goals for male adult sexual offenders principally because adolescents are still in a major developmental stage. Thus, their sexual development is less entrenched and deviant sexual arousal patterns have not been as extensively reinforced. Male adolescent sexual offenders do differ, as do adult offenders, with regard to the chronicity, severity, and pervasiveness of their sexual offending, and subgroups of adolescent offenders do exist.[16] Subgroups of adult sexual offenders against children also exist, although these classifications have been a subject of debate.[9] Designation of an offender as a member of a particular subgroup based on offense type, chronicity, modus operandi, or nature of skills deficits tends to aid the treatment process, as treatment goals can be better clarified and targeted.

Female Offenders

Both adult and adolescent female sexual offenders against children differ from their male counterparts in important ways that are essential to understand in providing treatment. Because many fewer females than males sexually offend against children, our understanding of this population is inadequate, and some commentators deny the reality of their sexual offenses. In this context, clinical lore about these women and inadequate research about their offending has been common.

Female adolescent sexual offenders have now been described in a systematic way based on empirical research[8] and can be treated utilizing treatment goals common to the forms of offender treatment that are reviewed below. As with adolescent male offenders, the presence of conduct disorder symptomatology in adolescent female offenders complicates treatment goals, as the conduct disorder must be treated along with the sexual offending.

Another distinction of women sexual abusers is that many do not sexually abuse independently, but in conjunction with a male offender.[17] Many of these women have passively acquiesced to the initiative of a male offender and their treatment goals must include achieving independence and self-reliance in the world. A minority of women who sexually abuse do so in the context of invasive or harmful genital care practices of their children. Most women who sexually abuse alone have severe histories of sexual and physical abuse in childhood as well as significant substance abuse difficulty.[14] Treatment of these women is complicated by the extensive range of psychiatric and psychosocial problems they present along with the sexual offending. Reduction of risk for reoffending cannot be assured through treatment unless these problems are addressed along with the history of sexual offending.

Siblings

Siblings who abuse[33] and children who sexually abuse other children[13] have been identified in the literature and are now commonly seen as in need of treatment. Gil and Johnson's work represents an area that was in need of identification for some time. How can prepubescent children who force other children to engage in sexual behavior be conceptualized and treated? It is clear that sexual offenders are partly defined by the existence of a deviant sexual arousal pattern.[27] Such an arousal pattern does not fully develop until after pubescence, as repeated masturbation and orgasm are critical in the establishment of the deviant arousal pattern. Thus, prepubescent children cannot be thought of as offenders in the usual manner, yet they can act in sexually aggressive and forceful ways. Gil and Johnson's term *sexualized children*—or the corollary term, *sexually reactive children*—identifies that children who are sexually abusive or aggressive to other children do so in reaction to being sexualized. Clearly, treatment of the sexualizing milieu of the child as well as treatment of the child is essential in these cases. Severe forms of sexual aggression in children often indicate the need for out of home or even residential treatment. Identifying such children as sexualized places the focus on the child's response to a maladaptive or maltreating environment and clarifies that deviant sexuality has not yet been internalized, as it typically is for adolescent and adult sexual offenders.

Sibling incest, i.e., sexual abuse between siblings, has not received extensive attention in the research and clinical literature.[1] In fact, if the age span between the parties is less than two to three years, the nature of the sexual process may be very different. Smith and Monastersky[31] utilize an age difference of four years or greater to differentiate a peer sexual assault from child sexual abuse. Thus, sibling abuse may comprise a form of sexual abuse of a considerably younger sibling or a form of sexual contact, forced or mutual, between siblings close in age. The existence of a three-year age span or a significant power differential between siblings (e.g., one sibling is mentally retarded) are clinical guidelines for this differentiation.

Treatment of siblings close in age and power who engage in sexual contact typically focuses on parental neglect and emotional deprivation, as well as a sexualized family milieu and poor parental limit setting. Sibling incest where a significant age difference is present contains the elements of abuse of power and force that are universal in sexual abuse. In these cases, treatment focuses less on parental deprivation and siblings who turn to each other for succor than on anger and power needs that are frustrated in the offending sibling. Several researchers[4,26,33] have found that physical abuse is widely represented in the histories of sibling sexual offenders where a significant age span between offender and victim is present. An offender history of sexual abuse, however, was present only in a minority of cases, far less often than a history of physical abuse in the family. These findings clarify the need to focus on treatment efforts that address anger management and social skills regarding anger as well as distortions in the area of sexuality and sexual functioning. The need to treat anger and power difficulties as an integral component of the treatment is greater with sibling offenders than with adolescent offenders who abuse outside the family.

Substance Abusers

The co-incidence of substance abuse represents a common and important problem in the treatment of offenders. Again, the research and clinical literature has examined the relationship of substance abuse to sexual offending, particularly sexual offending by adults, more than to other types of offending. Clearly substance abuse is an important disinhibiting factor in offending of all forms. Finkelhor[9] includes disinhibition among the four factors he identifies to explain sexual offending. He cites a review of 13 studies conducted by Aarens and colleagues showing alcohol involvement in 30 to 40 percent of sexual abuse cases. Further, review studies[9] note that female-target pedophiles and particularly incest offenders have far higher co-incidence of alcohol abuse with sexual abuse than male-target pedophiles.

As is conventional in psychotherapeutic treatments for emotional, behavioral, and psychiatric disorders, treatment of offenders is best conducted when the offender is not in an active condition of substance abuse. Offenders should be referred for substance abuse treatment prior to beginning treatment for sexual or violent offending. The risk of recidivism for offenders in treatment who remain active substance abusers is considerable. Women who sexually offend also should be evaluated and treated with careful consideration of the possibility of a co-incidence of substance abuse with sexual offending. Green and Kaplan[14] found that substance abuse was typically a co-morbid factor in their sample of female adult offenders.

Psychiatric Disorders

Psychiatric conditions, particularly depression, have also been noted as frequently co-morbid factors with sexual offending. A study of an outpatient sample of men with paraphilic and nonparaphilic sexual disorders[15] found a high incidence of depression among these men and that the total sexual outlet (i.e., number of orgasms from any form of sexual activity), roughly related to sexual drivenness or impulsiveness, was decreased when the men were treated for depression with serotonin re-uptake inhibitor drugs (e.g., fluoxetine). Thus, for many offenders, especially sexual offenders, depression should be considered a likely co-morbid factor, and evaluation for psychopharmacologic treatment, as a component of the overall treatment approach, is indicated. Offenders with compulsive sexual impulses and indication of many prior victims may be especially likely to benefit from the reduction in sexual impulsiveness offered by treatment with antidepressants. Other forms of psychiatric disorders as co-morbid factors (e.g., schizophrenia, bipolar disorder) present infrequently in offenders.

Relationship between Offender and Victim

The relationship between offender and victim is an important treatment consideration for both case management and treatment planning. For intrafamilial (i.e., incest) sexual offenders, the presence of the offender in the home during the treatment process may not only present risks for reoffense but may also compromise treatment efforts with the victim, family, and even the offender. This is especially true in cases where the offender does not acknowledge or denies the validity of well-established allegations of sexual abuse. Violent or physical offenders will routinely be separated from their homes by means of orders of protection (i.e., restraining or noncontact orders) during the course of the treatment process. Women who sexually offend against their own children represent difficult case management issues, as the child's, and siblings', placement in the home often cannot be maintained if the female offender is removed from the home. Adolescents who sexually abuse children in their own homes require very careful assessment to determine if their reoffense risk is low enough to warrant continued placement in their homes. Adequate parental support and involvement is vital to maintaining an adolescent offender in his or her home.

Adult incest offenders have been shown to differ from extrafamilial sexual offenders in important ways. Quinsey and Lalumiere[27] note that incest offenders demonstrate less arousal to children as measured by phallometry, assessing penile tumescence (i.e., strength of penile erection) in response to pictures of male and female children, adolescents, and adults. Audiotapes of scripted interactions involving sexual contact are sometimes used instead of pictures or slides. Extrafamilial sexual offenders were found to reliably demonstrate more sexual arousal to sexual pictures or scenes of children than did adult incest offenders. This finding has important implications for treatment, as it is vital to treat the deviant sexual arousal of sexual offenders when it is present, in addition to treating distortions in the area of sexual and social functioning, as is common in most offender treatment.

In addition to important implications regarding the probable extent of deviant sexual arousal patterns in incestuous as opposed to extrafamilial sexual offenders, the nature of the relationship between the offender and victim has important implications for the meaning of the child to the offender. Predatory offenders who offend against unknown children abducted from their common environments are a minority of offenders but a dangerous minority indeed. They differ considerably from offenders who abuse children they know and care for, albeit in a distorted fashion. The confusion of love, affection, and sexuality, as well as disturbances in the recognition and acceptance of power imbalances, are nearly universal aspects of abuse and must be addressed in treatment of incestuous offenders. Predatory or overtly violent sexual offenders against children need to be carefully assessed and treated for their psychopathic, aggressive, and violent tendencies. The risk of reoffense in treating such offenders on an outpatient basis must be carefully assessed utilizing appropriate risk assessment protocols.[6] Many such offenders will not be appropriate candidates for outpatient treatment because of the risk of reoffense they pose.

TREATMENT MODALITIES

The most common theoretical perspectives currently used in treatment efforts with offenders are behavioral, cognitive behavioral, and psychodynamic. Psychodynamic and psychoanalytic theory have been concerned with perversions and "sexual aberrations"[10] since the beginning of interest in psychological methods of treatment. However, in the 1960s, disappointment with the poor results of these approaches to treatment for those who are sexually fixated on children,[9] along with concerns about the length, expense, and limited availability of psychoanalytic therapy, led to interest in behavioral methods of treatment for sexual offenders. Karl Freund was a pioneer in the development of methods to assess sexual arousal, and attempted to assess and treat homosexuality,[11] then considered a disorder by the American Psychiatric Association and the mental health professions at large.

Attention soon turned to the use of behavioral methods to assess and treat sexual deviance in men.[12] Gene Abel and Judith Becker initiated the use of measures of sexual arousal within an overall treatment program focused on reducing deviant sexual arousal patterns with behavioral methods and addressing social skills deficits and cognitive distortions concerning sexuality and relationships with cognitive behavioral treatment methods, principally applied in the context of group therapy. These latter methods have now become widespread in treatment programs for adolescent as well as adult sexual offenders. Cognitive behavioral treatment methods are also widely utilized in programs for treatment of domestic violence offenders which typically use a group approach focusing on cognitive distortions in the areas of power and gender.

While behavioral treatment methods of sexual deviance and sexual offending directly address and treat the deviant sexual arousal pattern, cognitive behavioral methods address the distorted beliefs, anticipations, and patterns of relating that characterize sexual offenders. Three specialized behavioral techniques were developed by Gene Abel and Judith Becker to diminish deviant sexual arousal and strengthen sexual arousal to age-appropriate individuals:

- masturbatory reconditioning, which associates the deviant arousal pattern (i.e., the sexually inappropriate individuals or acts) with the boring and uncomfortable activity of masturbating for lengthy periods of time following ejaculation, while masturbation to orgasm is directed to involve appropriate sexual partners and activities;
- covert sensitization, which directs the patient to associate negative outcomes and consequences with acting on the deviant arousal pattern; and
- aversive counter-conditioning, which is based on the patient's self-administering a noxious or uncomfortable stimulus when he experiences the deviant arousal pattern.

All three of these specialized techniques in behavioral treatment of offenders limit deviant arousal and strengthen appropriate arousal patterns. They are typically used as part of a treatment program that includes social skills training and treatment of distorted beliefs and attitudes about sexuality.

However, these techniques do not appear to be sufficiently utilized. Maletzky[20] decries the fact that most sexual offender treatment programs focus only on the cognitive aspects of treatment and only a minority are presently engaged in using specialized behavioral techniques such as those described above. He notes that clinicians, clinics, and institutions have avoided the messy and direct involvement with an offender's sexual life and practices that is required in behavioral treatment. Marshall[21] has focused attention on the cognitive aspects of treatment and notes the paucity of programs using direct behavioral techniques with offenders. His research indicates cognitive approaches can positively affect key treatment variables. It does seem clear that many clinicians are more at ease with the cognitive aspects of treatment, which more closely resemble therapeutic processes they are trained in, specifically verbally oriented interventions utilizing homework and a problem-solving approach.

In addition, use of behavioral techniques has been strongly associated with use of the penile plethysmograph for phallometric studies. As most clinicians and clinics will not devote the resources or staff to obtaining and operating a plethysmograph, many have assumed that behavioral techniques are beyond their reach. This is unfortunate; behavioral techniques can certainly be used in a setting where deviant arousal can only be measured by self-report and a plethysmograph is not available. Specialized training and supervision is, however, necessary to use these techniques and the fact that many clinicians are not trained in their use limits their availability. These techniques are most often used with adult male offenders demonstrating clear indications of a compulsive, deviant arousal pattern. Use with adolescents and females has been controversial and is not widely established.

A cognitive behavioral approach has been demonstrated to be effective with parents and children in situations of domestic violence as well as sexual abuse and sexual offending.[18] Among the most important goals and objectives of offender treatment, to be discussed below, are those appropriate to a cognitive behavioral approach. Establishing and increasing victim empathy, cited as the most commonly utilized treatment variable in sexual offender treatment programs,[9] is invariably approached through a cognitive behavioral treatment perspective. Likewise, relapse prevention, assessing and treating cognitive distortions in the area of sexuality, and recognition of the offender's offense cycle are all approached through a cognitive behavioral approach. Clear advantages exist in a cognitive behavioral approach to problems such as sexual offending that have a behavioral focus with behaviors supported by distorted cognitions and beliefs. The problem-solving focus of the cognitive behavioral approach also lends a pragmatic nature to the treatment. Further, many sexual offenders are not psychologically minded and relate best to a more concrete, directive, and pragmatic approach.

Psychoanalytic and psychodynamic therapies tend to focus on underlying and historical emotional conflicts rather than disordered behavior. These approaches have been criticized in treatment of offenders where the interests of the offender and society require a substantial focus on the offending behavior. Scalia,[29] however, describes an important limitation of cognitive behavioral approaches that is well addressed in psychodynamic therapies. Basing his comments on work with domestic violence offenders, he notes that those treated may positively identify with the therapist and speak the language and ideas the therapist wants to hear. The insights being voiced may not actually be internalized by the patient, and the therapist who focuses on the target cognitive or behavioral changes may not recognize that the treatment relationship is more a collusion than a collaboration. A psychodynamic approach, often focused on the relationship (i.e., transference) as well as symptomatic changes, may be more sensitive to situations where patients are superficially complying with the goals and objectives of the treatment without struggling to truly change ingrained patterns of thinking and behavior. Of course, theoretical perspective alone is no guarantee that an offender in treatment will be confronted with the extent to which he is involving himself in a compliant as opposed to committed fashion. Whatever the theoretical perspective, clinical sensitivity is necessary in treatment to ensure that offenders are challenged to go beyond behavioral requirements of the treatment process and actively work to change their lives.

Clinicians who treat offenders are invariably concerned with the protection of society from offending behavior as well as assistance to the offender to find productive and satisfying patterns of living and end the offending behavior. Clearly this differentiates offender treatment from usual practice of psychotherapy, in which the clinician's felt responsibility is to the patient alone. Another key difference between offender treatment and other psychotherapy is that many offenders are required to be in treatment in order to satisfy the stipulations of third parties such as probation, courts, or statutory child protection agencies. In such coerced treatments, the risk of offenders' engaging in treatment superficially to meet external requirements without truly engaging in the struggle to change is clearly present. However, Chaffin[7] presents empirical support for the fact that coerced treatments for offenders are not less effective. With careful attention to the nature of the offender's involvement in the therapeutic process, treatment can be useful and successful for offenders, even though it is coerced. Clinicians treating offenders work with many clients who do not seek treatment voluntarily, as few offenders voluntarily seek such treatment.

While individual treatment is often conducted with offenders, group treatment is typically considered the treatment of choice. Behavioral treatments conducted on an individual basis can be useful, as an offender's deviant arousal pattern is always unique and behavioral interventions must be targeted in an individualized fashion; but interventions targeted at the meaning of sexual abuse, victim empathy, and cognitive distortions concerning sexuality and sexual relationships are often best conducted in a group format. Offenders are able to learn from and have the experience of teaching and helping each other in these areas of difficulty. Group therapy also provides considerable emotional support for participants when the group is functioning well.[34] Isolation and stigmatization—key problems for offenders, given the secretive and shameful nature of offenses against children—are greatly eased for offenders being treated in group therapy. Mutual confrontation of minimization and emotional denial is another important aspect of the treatment process, and this is also facilitated in group therapy. Offenders who have abused within their family benefit, as does the family, from family therapy sessions late in the treatment process. It is essential when family members sit together to discuss the abuse that the offender not minimize the significance of the abuse or attempt to externalize responsibility for the offending behavior onto other family members or circumstances external to the offender. That is why this vital aspect of the treatment process, for families where reconciliation is planned, must wait until enough treatment has occurred that the offender has a sense of full responsibility for the abuse and awareness of the impact of the abuse on the victim and all other family members.

GOALS OF TREATMENT

Goals and objectives of offender treatment involve the offender's learning nonabusive pathways for expression of needs and impulses and ceasing the offending behavior. Commonly utilized and accepted goals and objectives are

- acknowledgement of the offending behavior,
- developing empathy for the victim,
- locating and clarifying cognitive distortions related to the abusive behavior,
- understanding the cycle of offensive behavior,
- developing social skills to address impulses and needs in a nonabusive fashion, and
- relapse prevention.

Certainly these goals are nearly universal in treatment of child sexual offenders, but they are also widely utilized in other forms of offender treatment.

As noted, acknowledgement of the offending behavior must exist for offender-specific treatment to begin. Typically, however, many details of the abusing are minimized or unrecognized at the initiation of the treatment. One of the early treatment tasks is a thorough review of the specifics of the offenses. This specificity is often facilitated in group treatment, where offenders who have been engaged in treatment for some time are able to confront and encourage newcomers to tell their story more fully. While necessary for the offending pattern to be addressed, such specificity of offense behaviors is also helpful for beginning work on victim empathy, a widely recognized goal of offender treatment. In fact, Lesak and Ivan[19] report research suggesting that deficits in empathy are a central aspect of sexual offenders. Specific discussion of the offending behaviors, with appropriate support and confrontation from the therapist, creates a significant likelihood that the offender's denial of the significance of the abuse for the victim will begin to moderate. The denial or lack of recognition of the negative impact of the sexual abuse on the victim is one of the central factors facilitating abusive behaviors for offenders. This is most clearly true for incestuous offenders.

Identification and clarification of cognitive distortions related to offending behavior have been a central part of offender treatment since the pioneering work of Gene Abel and Judith Becker. Empirical research has been inconsistent in identifying the presence of cognitive distortions in child sexual offenders,[27] but treatment efforts invariably focus on the attitudes and beliefs of the offender with respect to the abusive behaviors and those individuals affected by the abusive behavior. Such distorted beliefs concerning sexuality and relationships, like denial of the behavior's negative impact on the victim, enable and support the offending behavior. Cognitive distortions that are almost stereotypical of child sexual offenders—for example, that sexual contact with children does not harm them if it is not overtly violent—are frequently encountered in offenders and represent an important focus of the treatment process. Also present, in addition to beliefs that enable offending behavior, are cognitive distortions that inhibit appropriate behaviors. For example, an offender's attitudes and beliefs that adults, both male and female, are emotionally threatening and that the offender does not have the skills to address and cope with such emotional threats inhibit and complicate the pursuit of adult relationships for emotional gratification and need satisfaction. Identifying and clarifying such cognitive distortions, in combination with social skill development, opens possibilities for nonabusive relationships to be developed and enhanced.

Another major offender treatment goal is the establishment of the offender's understanding of the cycle of his or her offending behavior, sometimes referred to as the offense chain.[32] A pattern of increased withdrawal and resentment is typical prior to offense incidents, as is a period of shame and remorse after offense incidents, accompanied by decisions never to act on the impulses again. The loneliness and isolation following the period of withdrawal generate depression and resentment that often justify the abusive behavior in the offender's mind. One study[30] found that loneliness and lack of intimacy characterize sexual offenders. A repeated pattern regarding offense behaviors is also common to many forms of impulsive or acting-out behaviors. Extensive therapeutic work on the cycle of offending behavior is most helpful to offenders, who often claim that their abusive behaviors "just happened." This attitude represents a form of denial, but it is clear that these attitudes toward offending behavior reflect a lack of situational and psychological awareness that is essential for self-regulated behavior. Recognizing and understanding offense cycles aids offenders in believing that they have the tools for self-regulation of the behaviors that have caused difficulty in their lives.

Understanding offense cycles also aids the therapist in focusing where social skills training and relapse prevention efforts need to be focused. Offenders withdraw into an emotionally isolated state due to perceived frustration and incompetence in meeting their relationship and life goals. Social skills training for assertion, relationship development, or conflict resolution can help the offender meet needs in a way that will not lead to withdrawal and isolation. Relapse prevention focuses on areas in the individual's offense cycle where circumstances, emotions, and beliefs coincide in a manner that the offender has come to recognize will lead to abusive behavior. Final stages of treatment should include an individualized relapse prevention plan, to provide pro-social alternatives to circumstances that the offender has identified as times when relapse may occur.

CONCLUSIONS

Treatment of offenders is a vast area of clinical endeavor that has increasingly been recognized as productive and useful. Research on recidivism and treatment outcomes has justified the attitude that many offenders can be successfully treated if targeted treatment goals are pursued with individuals who acknowledge their offense and demonstrate motivation for treatment. The relevant question now is not whether offenders can be treated successfully but what type of offender can be treated successfully with which form of therapeutic intervention. The field of offender treatment has followed the path of psychotherapy outcome studies of years ago. Originally, researchers and clinicians struggled with the question of whether psychotherapy worked. Later the question became what form of psychotherapy would be successful with what type of patient. Clinicians engaging in treatment of offenders are challenged, as they address this complexity of outcomes, to find the delicate balance between a focus on society's safety from abuse and the individual offender's needs.

R E F E R E N C E S

1. Adler N, Schutz J. Sibling adolescent offenders. *Child Abuse Negl* 1995;19:811–819.

2. American Psychiatric Association. *Diagnostic and statistical manual of mental disorders,* 4th ed. Washington, DC: American Psychiatric Press. 1994.

3. Becker J, Quinsey V. Assessing suspected child molesters. *Child Abuse Negl* 1993;17:169–174.

4. Becker J, Kaplan M, Cunningham-Rathner B, Kavoussi R. Characteristics of adolescent incest sexual perpetrators. *J Fam Viol* 1986;1:85–97.

5. Briere J. *Child abuse trauma: Theory and treatment of the lasting effects.* Newbury Park, CA: Sage Publications. 1992.

6. Campbell J (ed.). *Assessing dangerousness: Violence by sexual offenders, batterers, and child abusers.* Thousand Oaks, CA: Sage Publications. 1995.

7. Chaffin M. Research in action: Assessment and treatment of child sexual abusers. *J Interpers Viol* 1994;9:224–237.

8. Fehrenbach P, Monastersky C. Characteristics of female adolescent sexual offenders. *Am J Orthopsychiatry* 1988;58:148–151.

9. Finkelhor D. *A sourcebook on child sexual abuse.* Newbury Park, CA: Sage Publications. 1986.

10. Freud S. Three essays on the theory of sexuality. In Strachey J (ed.), *The complete psychological works of Sigmund Freud,* vol. 7, pp. 125–245. London: Hogarth Press. 1905/1953.

11. Freund K. A laboratory method for diagnosing predominance of homo- or hetero-erotic interest in the male. *Behav Res Ther* 1963;1:85–93.

12. Freund K. Erotic preference in pedophilia. *Behav Res Ther* 1967;5:339–348.

13. Gil E, Johnson T. *Sexualized children: Assessment and treatment of sexualized children and children who molest.* Rockville, MD: Launch Press. 1993.

14. Green A, Kaplan M. Psychiatric impairment and childhood victimization experiences in female child molesters. *J Am Acad Child Adolesc Psychiatry* 1994;33:954–961.

15. Kafka M. Successful antidepressant treatment of nonparaphilic sexual addictions and paraphilias in men. *J Clin Psychiatry* 1991;52:60–65.

16. Kaufman K, Hilliker D, Daleiden E. Subgroup differences in the modus operandi of adolescent sexual offenders. *Child Maltreat* 1996;1:17–24.

17. Kaufman K, Wallace A, Johnson C, Reeder M. Comparing female and male perpetrators' modus operandi: Victims' reports of sexual abuse. *J Interpers Viol* 1995;10:322–333.

18. Kolko D. Individual cognitive behavioral treatment and family treatment for physically abused children and their offending parents: A comparison of clinical outcomes. *Child Maltreat* 1996;4:322–342.

19. Lesak D, Ivan C. Deficits in intimacy and empathy in sexually aggressive men. *J Interpers Viol* 1995;10:296–308.

20. Maletzky B. The cognitive/cognitive treatment of the sexual offender: The decline of behavior therapy. Editorial. *Sexual Abuse: J Res Treat* 1996;8:261–265.

21. Marshall W. The sexual offender: Monster, victim, or everyman? *Sexual Abuse: J Res Treat* 1996;8(4):317–335.

22. Marshall W, Barbaree H, Eccles A. Early onset and deviant sexuality in child molesters. *J Interpers Viol* 1991;6:323–335.

23. Marshall W, Jones R, Ward T, Johnston P, Barbaree H. Treatment outcome with sex offenders. *Clin Psychol Rev* 1991;11:465–485.

24. Murphy C, O'Leary K. Research paradigms, values and spouse abuse. *J Interpers Viol* 1994; 9:207–223.

25. Nagayama Hall G. Sexual offender recidivism revisited: A meta-analysis of recent treatment studies. *J Consult Clin Psychol* 1995;63:802–809.

26. O'Brien M. Taking sibling incest seriously. In Patton M (ed.), *Family sexual abuse: Frontline research and evaluation,* 75–92. Thousand Oaks, CA: Sage Publications. 1991.

27. Quinsey V, Lalumiere M. *Assessment of sexual offenders against children.* Thousand Oaks, CA: American Professional Society on the Abuse of Children, with Sage Publications. 1996.

28. Quinsey V, Harris G, Rice M, Lalumiere M. Assessing treatment efficacy in outcome studies of sex offenders. *J Interpers Viol* 1993;8:512–523.

29. Scalia J. Psychoanalytic insights and the prevention of pseudo success in the cognitive-behavioral treatment of batterers. *J Interpers Viol* 1994;9:548–555.

30. Seidman B, Marshall W, Hudson S, Robertson P. An examination of intimacy and loneliness in sex offenders. *J Interpers Viol* 1994;9:518–534.

31. Smith W, Monastersky C. Assessing juvenile sexual offenders' risk of reoffending. *Crim Just Behav* 1986;13:115–140.

32. Ward T, Louden K, Hudson S, Marshall W. A descriptive model of the offense chain for child molesters. *J Interpers Viol* 1995;10:452–472.

33. Worling J. Adolescent sibling-incest offenders: Differences in family and individual functioning when compared to adolescent non-sibling sex offenders. *Child Abuse Negl* 1995;19:633–643.

34. Yalom I. *The theory and practice of group psychotherapy.* 2nd ed. New York: Basic Books. 1975.

Chapter 22

Treatment-Resistant Families

Richard J. Gelles, Ph.D.

Some families in which child abuse or neglect occurs must be classified as "treatment-resistant." Contributing to this categorization is a constellation of factors—among them, sociological and psychological attributes and deficits, resistance to change or treatment and lack of readiness to change, and the necessary duration of treatment. These families are dangerous to the child, and the longer a child is in an abusive and neglectful environment, the greater the risk of physical and psychological harm. The parent who is young and who has the characteristics of early onset of violent behavior, antisocial personality disorder, substance abuse, social isolation, and poverty may be most dangerous and is least likely to be treated effectively. For treatment-resistant families, the intervention of choice is the termination of parental rights and a permanent placement outside the family for the child or children.

GENERAL CONSIDERATIONS

In the three decades since the modern rediscovery of child abuse and neglect, the study and treatment of child maltreatment has gone through a variety of changes, even paradigm shifts. Kempe and colleagues' benchmark article, "The Battered Child Syndrome,"[19] ushered in a period during which psychopathology was considered the main cause of abuse and neglect, while social factors were viewed as playing no important causal role. The 1970s saw the psychopathology model replaced by a variety of social and sociopsychological models that emphasized factors such as social disadvantage, distressed family functioning, social learning, and social and cultural approval of violence.[9,10,14,24]

When causal models changed, so did treatment and intervention. When child maltreatment was conceptualized as arising out of psychopathology, child welfare agencies tended to remove children from abusive or neglectful parents and provide counseling or psychotherapy for maltreating caretakers. When child maltreatment was envisioned as arising out of poverty, lack of education about child development, social isolation, and stress, children might still be removed from the home, but psychological services were augmented with support services, such as day care, homemakers, parenting classes, and other forms of hard and soft services designed to add resources to families while reducing or ameliorating stressors. By the 1980s there was an increased effort to keep children in the home while providing families and caretakers with social and psychological resources and services.

Throughout the transformation of the causal models, philosophies, and treatments, one philosophy seems to have persisted: that *all* abusive families can be helped. At the core of this philosophy is the cultural ideology that all parents are capable of being caring and loving. No matter how horrific the abuse or how fractured the family, according to this philosophy, the family can be treated and treatment can be successful if the quantity and quality of treatment are sufficient.

Consistent with this ideology, if treatment "fails," that is, the family or caretakers do not engage in or respond to the treatment process or they reabuse, reneglect, reinjure, or even kill their children, the failure is not attributed to the parents but to inadequate treatment. Failure is thought to be the result of insufficient resources, too few caseworkers, overworked caseworkers, undertrained caseworkers, or a failure to properly implement the intervention. Failure is rarely attributed to the family or caretakers' being treatment-resistant.

In the child abuse and neglect literature, the premise is rarely found that some families who come into the child welfare system are "untreatable." What portion of the more than one million substantiated cases of child maltreatment each year[32] are treatment-resistant? My best estimate is that between 10 and 15 percent of parents and caretakers engage in harmful behavior, are not even considering changing their behavior, and have a constellation of social and psychological attributes that would make them treatment-resistant according to the definitions that will be set forth in this chapter.

What are the characteristics of treatment-resistant families? First, the family or caretakers are dangerous. Second, they do not respond to the various types of intervention. The type of intervention, the intensity or "dose" of intervention, and the expertise of the provider do not affect the level of risk or danger in the family and do not decrease the abuse and neglect.

A treatment-resistant family may also be one that simply will not engage in the intervention. Here the issue is not so much that the family or caretaker does not respond to the proffered treatment but that they do not actually accept or become involved in the treatment *process*.

A third type of impediment to treatment is the time factor. A family may engage in and actually respond to treatment but not do so within a time frame that is in the best interests of their children's safety and development. Unlike substance abuse, alcohol abuse, mental illness, or other physiological or psychological problems or conditions, child maltreatment involves someone other than the individual with the condition or problem being treated. There is no real limit on how long it should take to treat alcoholism, drug abuse, or depression (aside from the limits set by managed care). Relapse is a normal and expected part of the change process. Although others may be affected by the relapse or lack of change, it is the individual in treatment who is most directly affected by the course of the treatment. Such is not the case for abuse and neglect treatment. If an abusive parent relapses or does not change, the child is the victim—both in terms of the harm inflicted by abuse and neglect and the harm that results from a lack of permanent caretaking. The unique aspect of treatment for child abuse perpetrators is that the longer the treatment takes, the less likely a child is to have permanent caretaking. I will have more to say about this later in this chapter.

HOW EFFECTIVE IS TREATMENT
FOR CHILD ABUSE?

Before examining the issue of treatment-resistant families, it is useful to consider the effectiveness of the various treatments and combinations of treatments that are offered and provided to caretakers and families who maltreat their children. How effective are they? In fact, if we use the normal standards for scientific evidence in evaluation research to judge the effectiveness of treatments for abuse and neglect, our answer must be either, "we don't know," or "not very effective."

Although there is a great deal of anecdotal evidence about the effectiveness of interventions, and some interventions indeed show promise, from a purely scientific point of view we have little hard evidence for the effectiveness of treatment. The National Academy of Sciences has convened two panels to examine child abuse and neglect. The first panel's report, *Understanding Child Abuse and Neglect* (1993), stated that the fragmentary nature of research in this area inhibited the panel's ability to evaluate the strengths and limitations of the intervention process.[21] A second panel, charged with assessing the effectiveness of family violence interventions in general, reviewed thousands of publications on family violence interventions and found 135 evaluations that met the panel's standards for scientific evaluations.[22] Of these, most were evaluations of social service child maltreatment interventions, but few offered convincing evidence that these interventions were effective.

Among the better evaluations of an intervention is the evaluation research on home health visitors. David Olds and his colleagues looked at the effectiveness of a home-visiting family support program during pregnancy and for the first two years after birth for low-income, unmarried, teenage first-time mothers.[23] Nineteen percent of a sample of poor unmarried teenage girls who received no services during their pregnancy were reported for subsequent child maltreatment. In contrast, among poor, unmarried teenage mothers who were provided with a full complement of home visits by a nurse during pregnancy and for the first two years, 4 percent were the subjects of confirmed cases of child abuse and neglect reported to the state child protection agency.

Another review, of evaluations of 88 child maltreatment programs that were funded by the federal government between 1974 and 1982,[3] found that there was no correlation between a given set of services and the likelihood of further maltreatment of children. In fact, the more services a family received, the worse the family got and the more likely children were to be maltreated. This puzzling finding may result from the fact that the most difficult families received the most services, and these are the families that are least likely to change. Receiving a larger amount of services may actually increase a family's level of stress and problems rather than ameliorating them. It is possible for families to receive more services than they can handle. Having to meet appointments for counseling, welfare benefits, and job training as well as having to adapt to an influx of home visitors and services may increase stress and actually reduce a family's level of functioning.

The evaluation reviewed indicated that lay counseling, group counseling, and parent education classes resulted in more positive treatment outcomes. The optimal treatment period appeared to be between 7 and 18 months. The most successful projects were those that separated children from abusive parents by placing them in foster homes or requiring the maltreating adult to move out of the house. Perhaps the success of these interventions was not in the treatment of the parents and caretakers but in separating the child from the abuser.

For a time, intensive family preservation services were thought to be the most promising interventions for treating child maltreatment. Intensive family preservation services are an alternative to the "business-as-usual" family preservation/family reunification child welfare casework used by child welfare agencies. The intensive family preservation services movement began in Tacoma, Washington, in 1974. Child psychologists David Haapala and Jill Kinney developed a program they called Homebuilders, with a grant from the National Institute of Mental Health. The goal of the program was to work intensively with families *before* a child was removed. There are now many variations of intensive family preservation services in use across the country. The core goal of such programs is to maintain children safely in the home or to facilitate a safe and lasting reunification. Intensive family preservation services were designed for families that have a serious particular crisis threatening the stability of the family and the safety of the family members.

Although there are many variations of intensive family preservation services, the essential feature is that such programs are short-term crisis intervention. Services are meant to be provided in the client's home. The length of the sessions can be variable. Unlike traditional family preservation services, intensive family preservation services are available seven days a week, twenty-four hours a day. Perhaps the most important feature of intensive family preservation services is that caseloads are small—caseworkers may have only two or three cases. In addition, the length of time is brief and fixed at a specific number of weeks. Both hard and soft services are provided. Hard services include food stamps, housing, homemaker services; soft services include parent education classes and individual and/or family counseling.

The initial evaluations of intensive family preservation services were uniformly enthusiastic. The programs were claimed to have reduced the placement of children outside the home, reduced the cost of out-of-home placement, and, at the same time, assured the safety of children. Foundation program officers and program administrators claimed that families involved in intensive family preservation services had low rates of placement and "100 percent safety records."[1,8] There have been at least 46 evaluations of intensive family preservation services of one form or another.[16,20] Of these and of nearly 850 published articles on intensive family preservation, only 10 studies performed meaningful evaluations, included outcome data demonstrating effectiveness, and used a control group of some kind. In California, New Jersey, and Illinois, the evaluations used randomly assigned control groups, included outcome data, and had large enough samples to allow for rigorous evaluation. In all three studies, there were either small or insignificant differences between the group receiving intensive family preservation services and the control group receiving traditional casework services. Even in terms of placement avoidance, there was no difference between the two groups, thus suggesting that earlier claims that intensive family preservation services were successful in reducing placement were because of the low overall rate of placement by child welfare agencies.

Most importantly, the outcome measures of most evaluations have not included data specifically designed to measure child outcome. Thus, it is also impossible to verify the claim of the safety record of intensive family preservation services. In summary, the empirical case for intensive family preservation has yet to be made.

There are numerous reasons why intensive family preservation services, specifically, and the broader range of efforts at family reunification, are not effective treatments. First, it is possible that intensive family preservation services, in and of themselves, are simply not effective. The theory behind the program may be faulty and the programs themselves, therefore, may not be addressing the key mechanisms that cause child abuse. Second, the programs may be effective but not being implemented properly by the agencies and workers that are using them. When the evaluation data for the Illinois Family First program were made public,[30] an initial reaction was that there was considerable variation in how intensive family preservation was being implemented at the different sites in Illinois and that the overall implementation was not true to the Homebuilders model of intensive family preservation. The lack of evidence of effectiveness was blamed on the programs' not being properly implemented. Third, the theory behind the intensive program may be accurate and the program itself may be appropriate, but the "dose" may be too small. It may be that more services are necessary or the length of the intervention should be increased. If this is true, however, it would partially negate the cost-effectiveness claims for intensive family preservation services.

Because even the most promising effort to treat abusive and neglectful caretakers has not demonstrated widespread effectiveness, both practitioners and policy makers need to be cautious in their assumptions about the effectiveness of treatment. Nonetheless, the fact that the case cannot be made for the effectiveness of treatment does not, in and of itself, support an argument that some or many families are untreatable. The following section suggests that one of the reasons why evaluations of treatment programs show either no or minimal effectiveness is that some families and caretakers are indeed resistant to treatment.

TYPES OF MALTREATERS

Most current child welfare programs, including intensive family preservation services, assume that abuse and maltreatment are one end of a continuum of parenting behavior. The continuum model rejects a psychiatric or psychological "kind of person" explanation for maltreatment. Abusers and neglectors are not defective, deviant, or sick individuals; rather, they experience a "tipping point" or a "deficit" of parental skills and resources. In the former, stresses or problems pile up until a "tipping point" pushes parents from caring to maltreating. These stressors can be poverty, unemployment, marital conflict, alcohol or other substance abuse, social isolation, sexual difficulties, physical illness, or child-produced stressors such as colic, developmental delays, and delinquency. When the tipping point is reached, overstressed parents either actively lash out and physically abuse their children or passively neglect their children.

Alternatively, a "deficit" approach assumes that some parents lack the personal, social, or economic resources necessary to be effective parents. Inadequacy of resources is seen as the cause of abuse, so it is concluded that adding resources such as psychological counseling, parent education, treatment for substance abuse, or home visitors will help parents to meet their own needs and the needs of their children. Based on these models, the goal of most child welfare interventions is to add resources or remove stresses or both and to make the home safe again, so that children can be reunified with their parents.

An alternative to the continuum model is the conceptualization that there are different types of abusers.[11,13] Rather than seeing abuse and neglect as arising out of a surplus of risk factors or a deficit of resources, this model supposes that there may be distinct psychological and social attributes of caretakers who inflict serious or fatal injuries compared to caretakers who commit less injurious acts of maltreatment. If there are different types of maltreaters and different underlying causes for different types of abuse, it is reasonable to assume that a "one size fits all" intervention or policy would not be effective. Moreover, there may be types of abusers or neglectors who are not amenable to treatment.

Research on men who abuse women and on youthful violent offenders is more supportive of a typological conceptualization of violence than a continuum model.[6,7,15,17,18]

In the case of child abuse, the factors that correlate with the most abusive behaviors are:

- young age (between 18 and 30),
- low income or poverty,
- stressful life events,
- social isolation and lack of social support,
- experiencing or witnessing violence as a child, and
- alcohol and/or substance abuse.[13,21,22]

Although men are more violent in and outside the family, the relationship between sex and child abuse is more complex. Biological mothers are the most likely abusers and murderers of children under 1 year of age, while men are more likely to injure and abuse older children. Men who are not biologically related to children in their care are more likely to injure and kill the children than are biological fathers.[2,13,32]

Although there is not a consistent profile of parental psychopathology related to serious child maltreatment, researchers do find that perpetrators with antisocial personality disorders have the highest rates of serious abuse and violence.[21] Research on seriously violent offenders finds that offenders whose onset of violent behavior began before the age of 12 are the least likely to desist in their violent acts in their late 20s and early 30s.[7]

While these factors are correlates of abuse, injury, and even fatal child maltreatment, they cannot be considered predictors of serious abuse, fatal abuse, or dangerousness. The low rate of serious and fatal abuse and the modest correlations between these factors and serious or fatal abuse means that we do not have a set of risk factors that can accurately predict dangerous behavior. However, we do know that the early onset of violent behavior, young age, and antisocial personality disorder, combined with substance abuse, social isolation, and poverty may indicate a type of individual who is more dangerous and is less likely to be treated effectively.

READINESS TO CHANGE

Behind the notion that anyone can abuse a child and all families can be treated, if adequate personal and social resources are available, is the assumption that change is a two-step process, that individuals move directly from engaging in inappropriate, deviant, or dangerous behavior to not engaging in the behavior. Interventions, simply stated, instruct the individual "don't do that" or "do this." Social interventions are designed so that the client "does not do that" or acquires the resources to "do this." The assumption is that any reasonable person does not want to "do that" and simply needs help to "do this."

Research on behavioral change clearly demonstrates, however, that change is not simply a two-step process. Rather, changing behavior is a dynamic, ongoing process that progresses through a number of stages. Research also has found that there are cognitive aspects to behavioral change that can be measured.[25-28]

One of the reasons child welfare interventions have such modest success rates may be that they require action of the client but are often provided to individuals and families who are not ready to make active change, maybe not even to consider it. Prochaska and his colleagues call these the "contemplation" and "precontemplation" stages of change. Others have described individuals in these stages as "denying" or "ambivalent" about the need for change.

I have discussed the application of Prochaska's transtheoretical model of change to child maltreatment fully elsewhere.[12,13] The virtues of this instrument for child mal-

Severity of Risk

Stage of Change	High	Low
Precontemplation	No reunification High likelihood of terminating parental rights	Parent education classes
Contemplation		
Preparation		
Action	Family preservation only with close monitoring	Family preservation Reunification recommended
Maintenance		

Figure 22.1   Two Dimensions of Risk Assessment for Child Abuse and Neglect
Source: Adapted from Prochaska et al.[25–28]

treatment assessment are that it can classify caretakers into one of the five stages of change (precontemplation, contemplation, preparation, action, and maintenance) and that the main constructs of the model (decisional balance, self-efficacy, and the processes of change) can be assessed.

With regard to precontemplation and contemplation, Prochaska and his colleagues found that, for a set of 15 different health and mental health problems, 40 to 60 percent of a representative sample of 6,000 people who were still engaging in problem behaviors (i.e., not yet in the action stage of change) were in the precontemplation stage and the rest were in the contemplation stage.[29] It is reasonable to assume that similar percentages of abusive families in the child welfare system are in the precontemplation or contemplation stage for changing their abuse and neglect of their children.

What I believe makes these individuals and families treatment-resistant is the combination of high risk, early stage of readiness to change, and long duration of time before change will occur (see figure 22.1).

Caretakers who do not recognize or admit to the harm they have inflicted on their children, by acts of either omission or commission, are not going to respond to an action-oriented intervention such as intensive family preservation, a parenting class, additional social resources, or even psychotherapy. Precontemplation- or contemplation-stage abusers remain risks to their children. They are also unlikely to respond to conventional interventions or treatments.

The transtheoretical model of change would argue that clinicians should match interventions to an abuser's readiness to change and have a goal of moving a precontemplative caretaker to contemplation. However, such a course of intervention takes time. As noted earlier, while time may not be a critical issue for smoking cessation or drug or alcohol abuse, it is critical for child safety and health. The longer a child is in an abusive and neglectful environment, the greater the risk of physical and psychological harm. Moreover, the older a child gets, the less likely a child is to be adopted. Thus, while child welfare agencies struggle to engage a high-risk, precontemplative caretaker in an intervention, the probability decreases that an adoptive home for the child will be available if treatment fails.

Thus, the last component of a classification of "treatment-resistant" is how long it is likely to take to successfully intervene with a maltreating caregiver. For those caretakers in the upper left cell of figure 22.1, high-risk precontemplators, the likelihood of change within 12 to even 18 months is low (based on research on the process of change for other behaviors). From the eyes of the child, and using a child's sense of time and need for permanence, treatment of these families and caretakers is impractical.

CONCLUSION

A portion of parents and caretakers who maltreat their children are treatment-resistant. They have engaged in behavior that is so harmful and so dangerous that they should be considered at high risk to engage in such behavior again. Psychometrically sound risk assessment and assessments of dangerousness notwithstanding, the best predictor of an individual's future behavior is past behavior.

Some parents and caretakers are resistant to treatment because they have a combination of psychological and social attributes that suggests a low likelihood that interventions will be effective. Individuals who have begun their violent behaviors at young ages, are diagnosed with antisocial personality disorders, have alcohol or other substance abuse problems, and who are young, poor, and disengaged from social networks tend to continue their violent careers for longer periods of time than other perpetrators of violent and abusive behavior.

Also, some parents and caretakers are at such an early stage of readiness to change their behavior that treatment, if it could be effective, would have to be provided over a long period of time. Most importantly, precontemplators, who do not believe that they have a problem that requires change, are unresponsive to action-based treatment programs.

Finally, decisions to treat perpetrators of abuse must take into account the permanence interests of the children involved. Decisions about treatment or intervention should be made with a child's sense of time and a child's need for permanence as the main criteria for choice of intervention. For treatment-resistant families, the intervention of choice would be to terminate parental rights and seek a permanent placement for the child or children.

Finally, a caveat: it is not possible to predict who will be treatment-resistant without knowing the parents' or caretakers' actual behavior toward their children. There is no way of assessing who is or is not going to respond to treatment without a complete knowledge of their caretaking behavior.

R E F E R E N C E S

1. Barthel J. *For children's sake: The promise of family preservation.* New York: Edna McConnell Clark Foundation. 1991.

2. Daly M, Wilson M. *Homicide.* New York: Aldine de Gruyter. 1988.

3. Daro D, Cohn AH. Child maltreatment evaluations efforts: What have we learned? In Hotaling GT, Finkelhor D, Kirkpatrick JT, Straus MA (eds.), *Coping with family violence: Research and policy perspectives,* 275–287. Newbury Park, CA: Sage Publications. 1988.

4. Daro D, Gelles R. Public attitudes and behaviors with respect to child abuse prevention. *J Interper Viol* 1992;7:517–531.

5. DiClemente CC, Prochaska JO, Gibertini M. Self-efficacy and the stages of self-change of smoking. *Cogn Ther Res* 1985;9:181–200.

6. Dutton DG, Golant SK. *The batterer: A psychological profile.* New York: Basic Books. 1995.

7. Elliott DS. Serious violent offenders: Onset, developmental course, and termination (American Society of Criminology Presidential Address.) *Criminology* 1994;32:1–21.

8. Forsythe P. Homebuilders and family preservation. *Child Youth Serv Rev* 1992;14:37–47.

9. Garbarino J. The human ecology of child maltreatment. *J Marr Fam* 1977;39:721–735.

10. Gelles RJ. Child abuse as psychopathology: A sociological critique and reformulation. *Am J Orthopsychiatry* 1973;43:611–621.

11. Gelles RJ. Physical violence, child abuse, and child homicide: A continuum of violence or distinct behaviors? *Hum Nature* 1991;2:59–72.

12. Gelles RJ. "Using the transtheoretical model of change to improve risk assessment in cases of child abuse and neglect." Roundtable presented at the 4th International Family Violence Research Conference, Durham, NH, 1995.

13. Gelles RJ. *The book of David: How preserving families can cost children's lives.* New York: Basic Books. 1996.

14. Gil D. *Violence against children: Physical child abuse in the United States.* Cambridge: Harvard University. 1970.

15. Gondolf EW, Fisher ER. *Battered women as survivors: An alternative treating learned helplessness.* Lexington, MA: Lexington Books. 1988.

16. Heneghan AM, Horwitz SM, Leventhal JM. Evaluating intensive family preservation programs: A methodological review. *Pediatrics* 1996;97:535–542.

17. Holtzworth-Munroe A, Stuart GL. Typologies of batterers: Three subtypes and the differences among them. *Psychol Bull* 1994;116:476–497.

18. Jacobson NS, Gottman JM, Waltz J, Rushe R, Babcock J, Holtzworth-Munroe A. Affect, verbal content, and psychophysiology in the arguments of couples with a violent husband. *J Consult Clin Psychol* 1994;62:982–988.

19. Kempe CH, Silverman FN, Steele BF, Droegemueller W, Silver HK. The battered child syndrome. *JAMA* 1962;181:107–112.

20. Lindsey D. *The welfare of children.* New York: Oxford University Press. 1994.

21. National Research Council. *Understanding child abuse and neglect.* Washington, DC: National Academy Press. 1993.

22. National Research Council. *Assessing family violence interventions.* Washington, DC: National Academy Press. 1997.

23. Olds DL, Henderson CR Jr, Tatelbaum R, Chamberlin R. Preventing child abuse and neglect: A randomized trial of nurse home visitation. *Pediatrics* 1986;77:65–78.

24. Parke RD, Collmer CW. Child abuse: An interdisciplinary analysis. In Hetherington M (ed.), *Review of child development research,* vol. 5, p. 102. 1975. Chicago: University of Chicago Press. 1975.

25. Prochaska JO, DiClemente CC. Toward a more integrative model of change. *Psychotherapy: Theory, Research and Practice* 1982;19:276–288.

26. Prochaska JO, DiClemente CC. Stages and processes of self-change in smoking: Toward an integrative model of change. *J Consult Clin Psychol* 1983;5:390–395.

27. Prochaska JO, DiClemente CC. *The transtheoretical approach: Crossing traditional boundaries of change.* Homewood, IL: Dow Jones/Irwin. 1984.

28. Prochaska JO, Norcross JC, DiClemente CC. *Changing for good.* New York: Morrow. 1994.

29. Rossi JS. *Stages of change for 15 health risk behaviors in an HMO population.* Paper presented at the meeting of the Society of Behavioral Medicine, New York, 1992.

30. Schuerman J, Rzepnicki TL, Littell JH. *Putting families first: An experiment in family preservation.* New York: Aldine de Gruyter. 1994.

31. U.S. Advisory Board on Child Abuse and Neglect. *A nation's shame: Fatal child abuse and neglect in the United States.* Washington, DC: U.S. Department of Health and Human Services. 1995.

32. U.S. Department of Health and Human Services, National Center on Child Abuse and Neglect. *Child maltreatment 1995: Reports from the states to the National Center on Child Abuse and Neglect.* Washington, DC: U.S. Government Printing Office. 1997.

Chapter 23

Medicolegal Aspects of Child Abuse

John E. B. Myers, J.D.

Children's statements during examinations and interviews have forensic as well as medical significance. Under certain circumstances, the child's statements are inadmissible as evidence, due to the hearsay rules of evidence. There are, however, important exceptions. They include the "excited utterance" exception, disclosure under the doctrine of "fresh complaint," statements made during diagnostic or treatment services, and the "residual" and "child hearsay" exceptions. Interviewing techniques must include the avoidance of suggestive or leading questions. Confidentiality and privileged communication have well-defined boundaries, and child abuse reporting laws override confidentiality and privilege. A professional called upon to appear in court as an expert witness should review only those portions of the record needed for the testimony and should document the parts of the record reviewed. Privileged and nonprivileged materials should be separated in the record. If one takes the record to court, limit what is taken to the intended testimony. If possible, do not take the record to the witness stand, and if it is taken, refer to it only if necessary. Expert testimony usually takes one of three forms: an opinion, an answer to a hypothetical question, or a lecture providing information to the judge or jury. Be prepared for cross-examination, understanding that the defense attorney will try to raise doubts about the expert testimony. This is done by trying to limit the expert's ability to explain, by undermining the expert's assumptions, by impeaching the expert with a "learned treatise," or by raising the issue of the expert's bias toward the prosecution.

FORENSIC IMPLICATIONS OF CHILDREN'S DISCLOSURE STATEMENTS DURING PHYSICAL EXAMINATIONS AND INTERVIEWS

Many children disclose abuse to medical professionals. The diagnostic importance of children's disclosure statements is described elsewhere in this text. Children's statements during examinations and interviews have forensic as well as medical significance. This section provides a description of the critical forensic importance of documenting children's disclosure statements and addresses the use of suggestive and leading questions with children.

Children's Statements Describing Abuse Are Hearsay

Medical professionals are aware of the forensic importance of medical and laboratory evidence of abuse. They may, however, be less cognizant of the important legal implications of children's words during examinations and interviews. If children's statements are properly documented, they may be admissible in subsequent legal proceedings, that is, become legal evidence of abuse or neglect. Indeed, in some cases, the child's statements to professionals are the most compelling evidence of maltreatment. Suppose, for example, that while 4-year-old Beth is being examined by a physician, the child points to her genital area and says, "Daddy put his pee-pee in me down there. Then he took it out and shook it up and down until white stuff came out." Beth's words are compelling evidence of abuse. In subsequent criminal proceedings against Beth's father, the prosecutor calls the examining physician as a witness and asks the physician to repeat Beth's words and to describe her pointing gesture for the jury. Before the doctor can speak, however, the father's defense attorney objects that Beth's words and gesture are hearsay. The rule in all states is that hearsay is inadmissible in criminal and civil litigation unless the particular hearsay statement meets the requirements of an exception to the rule against hearsay.

To determine whether Beth's description of abuse is hearsay, analyze Beth's words in terms of the following definition. A child's words are hearsay if three requirements are fulfilled: (1) the child's words were intended by the child to describe something that happened; *and* (2) the child's words were spoken before the court proceeding at which the words are repeated by someone who heard the child speak; *and* (3) the child's words are offered in court to prove that what the child said actually happened.[20,21,22]

Analysis of Beth's words describing abuse reveal that they are hearsay. First, Beth intended to describe something that happened. Second, Beth spoke prior to the proceeding where the prosecutor asks the physician to repeat her words. Finally, the prosecutor offers Beth's words to prove that what the child said actually happened.

Beth's words are not the only hearsay, however. Her gesture pointing to her genital area is also hearsay. The gesture was nonverbal communication intended by Beth to describe the abuse.

The judge will sustain the defense attorney's hearsay objection unless the prosecutor persuades the judge that Beth's words and gesture meet the requirements of an exception to the rule against hearsay. In this, as in many other child abuse cases, the prosecutor's ability to convince the judge that the child's hearsay statement meets the requirements of an exception depends as much on the conduct of the physician as on the legal acumen of the prosecutor. If the doctor knew what to watch for and document when Beth disclosed the abuse, the prosecutor has a better chance of persuading the judge to allow the doctor to repeat Beth's powerful hearsay statement.

Although the rule against hearsay has many exceptions, only a few play a day-to-day role in child abuse and neglect litigation. Five hearsay exceptions are briefly discussed below.

The Excited Utterance Exception

An excited utterance is a hearsay statement that relates to a startling event. The statement must be made while the child is under the acute emotional stress caused by the startling event. Excited utterances can be used in court even though they are hearsay. Judges consider all relevant circumstances to determine whether a hearsay statement is an excited utterance. Professionals can document the following important factors:

Nature of the event.   Some events are more startling than others, and judges consider the likely impact a particular event would have on a child of the alleged victim's age and experience.

Amount of time elapsed between the startling event and the child's statement relating to the event.   The more time that has passed between a startling event and a child's statement describing it, the less likely a judge is to conclude that the statement is an excited utterance. Although passage of time is important, time alone is not dispositive. Judges have approved delays ranging from a few minutes to several hours.

First safe opportunity.   In many cases, abused children remain under the control of the abuser for minutes or hours after the abusive incident. When the child is finally released to a trusted adult, the child has the first safe opportunity to disclose what happened. A child's statement at the first safe opportunity may qualify as an excited utterance even though considerable time has elapsed since the abuse occurred.

Indications the child was emotionally upset when the child spoke.   Judges consider whether the child was crying, frightened, or otherwise upset when the statement was made. If the child was injured or in pain, a judge is more likely to find the words an excited utterance.

Child's speech pattern.   In some cases, the way the child speaks (e.g., pressured or hurried speech) indicates emotional excitement.

Extent to which the child's statement was spontaneous.   Spontaneity is a critical factor in the excited utterance exception. The more spontaneous the statement, the more likely it meets the requirements of this exception.

Number and type of questions used to elicit the child's statement.   Asking questions does not necessarily destroy the spontaneity required for the excited utterance exception. As questions becomes leading, however, spontaneity may dissipate, undermining applicability of this exception.

Fresh Complaint of Sexual Assault

A child's initial disclosure of sexual abuse may be admissible in court under an ancient legal doctrine called fresh complaint of rape or sexual assault. In most states, a child's fresh complaint is not, technically speaking, hearsay.

Statements to Professionals Providing Diagnostic or Treatment Services

Most states have an exception to the hearsay rule for certain statements to professionals providing diagnostic or treatment services. The professional may be a physician, nurse, or technician. This exception is commonly called the diagnosis or treatment exception. The exception includes the child's statement describing medical history. Also included are statements describing present symptoms, pain, and other sensations. The exception does include the child's description of the cause of illness or injury.

In many cases, the child is the one who provides the information that is admissible under the diagnosis or treatment exception. On occasion, however, an adult describes the child's history and symptoms to the professional. As long as the adult's motive is to obtain treatment for the child, the adult's statements are admissible under this exception.

The primary rationale for the diagnosis or treatment exception is that hearsay statements to professionals providing diagnostic or treatment services are reliable. Reliability is presumed because the patient has a strong incentive to be truthful with the professional. This rationale is also applicable for many older children and adolescents. Some young children, however, may not understand the need for accuracy and candor with health care providers. When a child does not understand that personal well-being may be affected by the accuracy of what is said, the primary rationale for the diagnosis or treatment exception evaporates, and the judge may rule that the child's hearsay statement does not satisfy the exception.

The diagnosis or treatment exception has its clearest application with children receiving traditional medical care in a hospital, clinic, or physician's office. Most children have at least some understanding of doctors and nurses and of the importance of telling the clinician "what really happened." Judges are less certain about the applicability of the diagnosis or treatment exception with psychotherapy. In psychotherapy, the child may not understand the importance of accuracy, thus undermining the rationale of the exception. If, however, the child understands the need for accuracy with the mental health professional, most judges conclude that the exception applies.

To increase the probability that a child's statements satisfy the diagnosis or treatment exception to the rule against hearsay, the professional can take the following steps.

Discuss with the child the importance of providing accurate information and of being completely forthcoming. For example, the physician might say, "Hello, I'm Doctor Jones, and I'm going to give you a checkup to make sure everything is okay. While you are here today, I'll ask you some questions so I can help you. It's important for you to listen carefully to my questions. When you answer my questions, be sure to tell me everything you know. Okay? Tell me only things that really happened. Don't pretend or make things up. Will you do that for me?" Document the discussion in the child's chart.

Document how the information disclosed by the child is pertinent to diagnosis or treatment. The diagnosis or treatment exception requires that the information supplied to the professional and being considered for exception be pertinent to diagnosis or treatment.

If the child identifies the perpetrator, document why knowing the identity of the perpetrator is pertinent to diagnosis or treatment. For example, knowing the identity of the perpetrator may be important to determining whether it is safe to send the child home. The physician also needs to know the perpetrator's identity if sexually transmitted disease is a possibility.

The Residual Exception and the Child Hearsay Exception

Many states have a hearsay exception known as a residual or catch-all exception, which allows use in court of reliable hearsay statements that do not meet the requirements of one of the traditional exceptions, such as the excited utterance exception. A majority of states also have a special hearsay exception for statements by children in child abuse cases. These child hearsay and residual exceptions allow use in court of children's reliable hearsay statements that do not fit into another exception.

When a child's hearsay statement is offered under a residual or child hearsay exception, the most important question is whether the statement is reliable. Professionals who interview, examine, and treat children play an indispensable role in documenting the information judges consider when determining whether children's statements are sufficiently reliable to be admitted under a residual or child hearsay exception.

Spontaneity of statement. The more spontaneous the child's statement, the more likely a judge will find it reliable.

Statements elicited by questioning. The reliability of a child's statement may be influenced by the type of questions asked. When questions are suggestive or leading, the possibility increases that the questioner influenced the child's statement. It should be noted, however, that suggestive questions are sometimes necessary to elicit information from children, particularly when the information is embarrassing.[10,12,16,22,24,27,30]

Consistency of statements. Reliability may be increased if the child's description of abuse is consistent over time. Consistency regarding core details is most important. Inconsistency regarding peripheral details is marginally relevant.

Child's affect and emotion when making statement. When a child's emotions are consistent with the child's statement, the reliability of the statement may be enhanced.

Play or gestures that corroborate the statement. The play or gestures of a young child may strengthen confidence in the child's statement. For example, the child's use of anatomic dolls may support the reliability of the child's statement.[22]

Developmentally unusual sexual knowledge. A young child's developmentally unusual knowledge of sexual acts or anatomy supports the reliability of the child's statement.[7,8,21,22]

Idiosyncratic detail. Presence in a child's statement of idiosyncratic details of sexual acts points toward reliability. Jones and McQuiston write that "[i]diosyncracy in the sexual abuse account is exemplified by children who describe smells and tastes associated with rectal, vaginal, or oral sex."[13]

Child's belief that disclosure might lead to punishment of the child. Children hesitate to make statements they believe may get them in trouble. If a child believed disclosing abuse could result in punishment, confidence in the child's statement may increase.

Child's or adult's motive to fabricate.   Evidence that the child or an adult had a motive to fabricate allegations of abuse impacts reliability.

Medical evidence of abuse.   The child's statement may be corroborated by medical evidence (see chapters 1 and 6).

Changes in child's behavior.   When a child's behavior alters in a way that corroborates the child's description of abuse, it may be appropriate to place increased confidence in the child's statement.[22]

Importance of Documentation

None of the foregoing factors is a litmus test for reliability. In evaluating reliability, judges consider the totality of the circumstances, and professionals can assist the legal system by documenting anything that indicates that the child was or was not telling the truth when describing abuse.

Medical professionals are in an excellent position to document children's hearsay statements. Without careful documentation of *exactly* what questions are asked and *exactly* what children say, the professional will not be likely to remember months or years later, when the professional is called as a witness and asked to repeat what the child said. Documentation is needed not only to preserve the child's words but also to preserve a record of the factors indicating that the child's hearsay statements meet the requirements of an exception to the hearsay rule.

USE OF SUGGESTIVE OR LEADING QUESTIONS DURING INTERVIEWS OF CHILDREN

There is no single "correct" way to interview children who may be abused or neglected.[12,27,22] Increasingly, however, defense attorneys challenge the way professionals talk to children.[21,22,24] Defense attorneys are particularly fond of criticizing leading questions. A leading question is a question that contains a suggestion of what the answer should be. Thus, a leading question is a suggestive question—a question that tempts a child to give a particular answer.

When talking to a child who may be a victim of abuse, the professional should create an atmosphere in which the child feels comfortable. Initial questioning should be as nonsuggestive and nonleading as possible.[12,22,27] The professional might begin with open-ended questions such as, "Can you tell me why you are here today?" If the child does not respond to open-ended questions—and many children do not—the professional then focuses the child's attention on a particular topic. When focused questions are used, the professional proceeds along a continuum, usually beginning with questions that simply focus the child's attention on a particular subject, and then, when necessary, moving to more specific questions. Highly specific questions sometimes cross the line into leading questions.

Experienced professionals are skeptical of advice to begin interviews of young children with open-ended questions like, "Why are we here today?" Few young children understand, let alone disclose abuse in response to, such questions. Nevertheless, just as physicians are aware of the need for "defensive medicine" in other areas of practice, use of nonsuggestive, open-ended questions with children helps immunize professionals from legal challenge. A defense attorney has difficulty attacking a professional who begins an interview with open-ended questions and who moves to more focused and, finally, mildly leading questions only when open-ended questions prove unproductive. Thus, the professional has little to lose and much to gain, forensically, by starting interviews with open-ended questions.

Although suggestive and leading questions should be avoided when possible, many occasions arise when suggestive and even mildly leading questions are necessary. The dynamics of abuse often work against disclosure.[30,32] Many abused children are threatened into silence. Others are ambivalent about disclosure. In Lawson and Chaffin's study of children with documented sexually transmitted disease,[15] 57 percent of the children initially denied that they had been abused.

The psychological dynamics of abuse are not the only barriers to disclosure. The developmental immaturity of young children further complicates the interview process. Young children are not as adept as older children and adolescents at responding to open-ended questions.[10,22,24,27] It is not that young children have poor memories.[6,28,29] Rather, young children often need cues to trigger their memories. In some cases, the necessary memory cue is a mildly leading question. When mildly leading questions are postponed until less-suggestive methods have proved unsuccessful, the professional is warranted in asking mildly leading questions.[22,23]

PROTECTION OF CONFIDENTIAL RECORDS AND PRIVILEGED COMMUNICATIONS

Abused and neglected children interact with many professionals. Each professional who comes in contact with the child documents the interaction. Needless to say, much of this information is confidential, and it must be protected from inappropriate disclosure.

Confidentiality arises from three sources: the broad ethical duty to protect confidential information, laws that make certain records confidential, and privileges that apply in legal proceedings.

Ethical and Legal Duty to Safeguard Confidential Information

The ethical principles of medicine, nursing, and other professions require professionals to safeguard confidential information revealed by patients. The principles of medical ethics of the American Medical Association require physicians to "safeguard patient confidences within the constraints of the law."[1] The Hippocratic oath states that "whatsoever I shall see or hear in the course of my profession . . . if it be what should not be published abroad, I will never divulge, holding such things to be holy secrets." The Code of Nurses of the American Nurses Association states that nurses safeguard the patient's right to privacy by carefully protecting information of a confidential nature.[2]

Every state has laws that make certain records confidential. Some of the laws pertain to records compiled by government agencies, such as child protective services, public hospitals, and the juvenile court. Other laws govern records created by professionals and institutions in the private sector, such as physicians, psychotherapists, and private hospitals.

Privileged Communications

The ethical duty to protect confidential information applies in *all* settings. In legal proceedings, however, certain professionals have an additional duty to protect confidential information. The law prohibits disclosure during legal proceedings of confidential communications between certain professionals and their patients. These laws are called privileges.[20]

Unlike the across-the-board ethical obligation to protect confidential patient information, privileges apply only in legal proceedings. Privileges clearly apply when professionals testify in court and are asked to reveal privileged information. Privileges also apply during legal proceedings outside the courtroom. For example, in most civil cases, and in some criminal cases as well, attorneys take pretrial depositions of potential witnesses. If questions are asked during a deposition that call for privileged information, the professional or one of the attorneys should raise the issue of privilege.

Communication between a patient and a professional is privileged when three requirements are fulfilled. First, the communication must be between a patient and a professional with whom privileged communication is possible. All states have some form of physician-patient privilege. Not all professions are covered by privilege statutes, however. For example, most states have a privilege for confidential communication between certain psychotherapists and their patients. If the patient communicates with a psychotherapist who is not covered by privilege law, however, no privilege applies. (A privilege may apply if the therapist not covered by a privilege is working under the supervision of a therapist who is covered by a privilege.) Of course, the fact that a privilege does not apply does nothing to undermine the therapist's ethical duty to protect confidential information.

In legal proceedings, the presence or absence of a privilege is important. In court, a professional may have to answer questions that require disclosure of information the professional is ethically bound to protect. By contrast, the professional generally does not have to answer questions that require disclosure of privileged information. Thus, in legal proceedings, a privilege gives added protection to confidentiality, protection that is not available under the ethical duty to protect confidential information.

The second requirement for a privilege to apply is that the patient must seek professional services. The patient must consult the professional to obtain advice or therapy. If the patient enters therapy, the privilege applies to confidential communications leading up to and during therapy. If the patient does not formally enter therapy, the privilege may nevertheless apply to confidential communications between the patient and the professional. For example, a patient may consult a physician who refers the patient to a second professional. In most states, communication between the patient and the referring physician is privileged even though the patient does not receive treatment from the referring doctor.

The third requirement of privilege law is that only communications that the patient intends to be confidential are privileged. The privilege generally does not attach to communications that the patient intends to be released to other people.

The fact that a third person is present when a patient discloses information may or may not eliminate the confidentiality required for a privilege. The deciding factor usually is whether the third person is needed to assist the professional. For example, suppose a physician is conducting a physical examination and interview of a child. The presence of a nurse during the examination does not undermine the confidentiality of information revealed to the doctor. Furthermore, presence of the child's parents need not defeat confidentiality. Again, the important factor is whether the third person is needed to assist the professional. A privilege is not destroyed when colleagues consult about cases.

Privileged communications remain privileged when the relationship with the patient ends. In most situations, the patient's death does not end the privilege.

The privilege belongs to the patient, not the professional. In legal parlance, the patient is the "holder" of the privilege. As the privilege holder, the patient can prevent the professional from disclosing privileged information in legal proceedings. For example, suppose a treating physician is subpoenaed to testify about a patient. While the physician is on the witness stand, an attorney may ask a question that calls for privileged information. At that point, the patient's attorney should object. The patient's attorney asserts the privilege on behalf of the privilege holder—the patient. The judge then decides whether a privilege applies.

If the patient's attorney fails to object to a question calling for privileged information, or if the patient is not represented by an attorney, the professional may assert the privilege on behalf of the patient. Indeed, the professional may have an ethical duty to assert the privilege if no one else does. The professional might turn to the judge and say, "Your honor, I would rather not answer that question, because answering would require disclosure of information I believe is privileged." When the judge learns that a privilege may exist, the judge decides whether the question should be answered.

DISCLOSURE OF CONFIDENTIAL AND PRIVILEGED INFORMATION

Patient Consent

Patient consent plays the central role in release of confidential or privileged information. As Gutheil and Appelbaum[11] observe, "with rare exceptions, identifiable data [about patients] can be transmitted to third parties only with the patient's explicit consent" (p. 5). A competent adult may consent to release of information to attorneys, courts, or anyone else. The patient's consent should be fully informed and voluntary. The professional should explain any disadvantages of disclosing confidential information. For example, the patient may be told that release to most third persons may waive privileges that would otherwise apply.

A professional who discloses confidential information without patient consent can be sued. With an eye toward such lawsuits, Gutheil and Appelbaum write: "[I]t is probably wise for therapists always to require the written consent of their patients before releasing information to third parties. Written consent is advisable for at least two reasons: (1) it makes clear to both parties involved that consent has, in fact, been given; (2) if the fact, nature or timing of the consent should ever be challenged, a documentary record exists. The consent should be made a part of the patient's permanent chart."[11]

When the patient is a child, parents normally have authority to make decisions about confidential and privileged information. When a parent is accused of abusing or neglecting a child, however, it may be inappropriate for the parent to make decisions regarding the child's confidential information. In the event of a conflict between the interests of the child and the authority of the parents, the judge may appoint someone else, such as a guardian ad litem, to make decisions about confidential and privileged information.

Limitations on Privilege

Every privilege has limitations established by law. In most states, for example, the physician-patient privilege has numerous limitations. Mueller and Kirkpatrick[20] write that "[m]ost states recognize numerous exceptions to the physician-patient privilege that significantly limit its scope. For example, the privilege is often made inapplicable in criminal cases" (p. 466).

Subpoenas

A subpoena is issued by a court at the request of an attorney. A subpoena is a court order, and it cannot be ignored. Disobedience of a subpoena can be punished as contempt of court.

The two types of subpoenas are: (1) a subpoena requiring an individual to appear at a designated time and place to provide testimony, sometimes called a subpoena *ad testificandum,* and (2) a subpoena requiring a person to appear at a designated time and place and to bring records or documents designated in the subpoena. A subpoena for records is sometimes called a subpoena *duces tecum.*

A subpoena does not override privileges such as the physician-patient and psychotherapist-patient privileges. The subpoena requires the professional to appear, but it does not mean the professional has to disclose privileged information. The judge decides whether a privilege applies and whether the professional has to answer questions or release records.

Before responding to a subpoena, the professional should contact the patient or, in the case of a child, a responsible adult. The patient may desire to release confidential or privileged information.

It is often useful, with the patient's permission, to communicate with the attorney issuing the subpoena. In some cases, the conversation lets the attorney know the professional has nothing that can assist the attorney, and the attorney withdraws the subpoena. Even if the attorney insists on compliance with the subpoena, the telephone conversation may clarify the limits of relevant information in the professional's possession. Naturally, care is taken during such conversations to avoid discussing confidential or privileged information.

If doubts exist concerning how to respond to a subpoena, consult an attorney. Needless to say, legal advice should not be obtained from the attorney who issued the subpoena.

REVIEWING CLIENT RECORDS BEFORE OR DURING TESTIMONY

When a professional is asked to testify, portions of the child's medical record may be reviewed to refresh the professional's memory. In some cases, the professional leaves the record at the office; sometimes the record is taken to court. In most cases, it is appropriate to review pertinent records prior to testifying. Indeed, such review is often essential for accurate and detailed testimony. Professionals should be aware, however, that reviewing records before or during testimony may compromise the confidentiality of the records.

While the professional is on the witness stand, the attorney for the alleged perpetrator may ask whether the professional reviewed the child's record and, if so, may request the judge to order the record produced for the attorney's inspection. In most states, the judge has authority to order the record produced. In favor of disclosure, the judge considers the attorney's right to cross-examine the professional and the extent to which the record will assist cross-examination. Against disclosure, the judge evaluates the impact on the child of disclosing confidential information. The outcome turns on which of these factors predominates. When records are reviewed *before* testifying, the judge is unlikely to order the record disclosed to the attorney for the alleged perpetrator. If the professional takes the record to court and refers to it *while* testifying, however, the judge is likely to order the record disclosed.

Protecting Records from Disclosure

Whether a professional reviews a child's record before or during testimony, a judge is more likely to require disclosure of nonprivileged records than records that are protected by physician-patient or psychotherapist-patient privileges. Unfortunately, in most states, the law is unsettled regarding the impact of record review on privileged communications. With the law unsettled, simple steps can be taken to reduce the likelihood that reviewing records will jeopardize confidentiality. Before implementing any of these recommendations, however, consult an attorney.

First, when reviewing a child's record before going to court, limit the review to those portions of the record that are needed to prepare for testifying. Document which parts of the record were reviewed and which not reviewed. In this way, if the judge orders the record disclosed to the attorney for the alleged perpetrator, an argument can be made that disclosure should be limited to portions of the record actually used to prepare for testifying.

Second, professionals may wish to organize records so that privileged information is maintained separately from nonprivileged information. When a record organized in this manner is reviewed before testifying, it is sometimes possible to avoid review of privileged communications. This done, if a judge orders the record disclosed, the judge may be willing to limit disclosure to nonprivileged portions of the record. Although this approach entails the burden of separating records into privileged and nonprivileged sections, and may not persuade all judges, the technique is worth considering, especially for professionals who testify regularly.

Third, if it is necessary to take the record to court, consider taking only the portions of the record that will be useful during testimony and leaving the remainder at the office.

Fourth, if the record is taken to court, perhaps the record can remain in the briefcase rather than be taken to the witness stand. Make no mention of the record unless it becomes necessary to refer to it while testifying. Once the record is used during testimony, the attorney for the alleged perpetrator may have a right to inspect it.

Again, legal advice should be obtained before implementing any of the foregoing suggestions. Some of the recommendations may not be permitted in some states.

CHILD ABUSE REPORTING LAWS OVERRIDE CONFIDENTIALITY AND PRIVILEGE

Child abuse reporting laws require professionals to report suspected child abuse and neglect to designated authorities.[14] The reporting laws override the ethical duty to protect confidential client information. Moreover, the reporting requirement overrides privileges for confidential communications between professionals and their patients.

Although reporting laws abrogate privileges, abrogation usually is not complete. In many states, professionals may limit the information they report to that which is specifically required by law. Information that is not required to be reported remains privileged.

Psychotherapist's Duty to Warn Potential Victims about Dangerous Clients

In 1974, the California Supreme Court ruled in *Tarasoff v. Regents of the University of California*[33] that a psychotherapist has a legal duty to warn the potential victim of a psychiatric patient who threatens the victim. The duty to warn overcomes both the ethical duty to protect confidential information and the psychotherapist-patient privilege. If the therapist fails to take reasonable steps to warn the victim, and the patient carries out the threat, the therapist can be sued.[22]

Since the *Tarasoff* case was decided, judges have grappled with the difficult question of when professionals have a legal duty to warn potential victims. Unfortunately, in most states, the law remains unsettled. Most judges agree that there is a legal duty to warn potential victims, but judges have not achieved consensus on when the duty applies. In 1985, California enacted a statute[4] that limits the duty to warn to situations in which "the patient has communicated to the psychotherapist a serious threat of physical violence against a reasonably identifiable victim or victims" (*California Civil Code* § 43.92).

Emergencies

In emergencies, a professional may have little choice but to release confidential information without prior authorization from the patient. The law allows release of confidential information in genuine emergencies.[11]

Court-Ordered Examinations

A judge may order an individual to submit to a medical examination or a psychological evaluation to help the judge decide the case. Because everyone knows from the outset that the professional's report will be shared with the judge and the attorneys, the obligation to protect confidential information is limited.

OBLIGATION TO REPORT SUSPECTED ABUSE AND NEGLECT

Professionals who work with children are required to report suspected abuse and neglect to designated authorities.[14] The list of mandated reporters includes physicians, nurses, mental health professionals, social workers, and day care providers. In most states, mandated reporters have no discretion whether to report. Reporting is mandatory, not optional.

The reporting requirement is triggered when a professional possesses a prescribed level of suspicion that a child is abused or neglected. The terms used to describe the triggering level of suspicion vary slightly from state to state, and include "cause to believe," "reasonable cause to believe," "known or suspected abuse," and "observation or examination which discloses evidence of abuse." Despite shades of difference, the basic meaning of the reporting laws is the same across the country. Reporting is required when a professional has evidence that would lead a reasonable professional to believe abuse or neglect is likely to have occurred.

The duty to report does not require the professional to "know" that abuse or neglect occurred. All that is required is information that raises a reasonable suspicion of maltreatment. A mandated reporter who postpones reporting until all doubt is eliminated probably violates the reporting law.

A substantial number of reporting laws authorize designated professionals to photograph or radiograph children without parental consent.

GIVING EXPERT TESTIMONY IN CHILD ABUSE LITIGATION

Expert testimony plays a critical role in child abuse litigation.[23] Such testimony is provided by physicians, nurses, psychologists, social workers, and other professionals. Before a professional may testify as an expert witness, the judge must be convinced that the professional possesses sufficient knowledge, skill, experience, training, or education to qualify as an expert. Normally, the proposed expert takes the witness stand and answers questions about educational accomplishments, specialized training, and relevant experience.

Preparation for Expert Testimony

When preparing to testify, an expert witness should meet with the attorney who has requested the testimony. Nothing about pretrial conferences is ethically or legally improper. Chadwick[5] observes that "[f]ace-to-face conferences between. . . attorneys and [expert witnesses] are always desirable, and rarely impossible" (p. 936).

Form of Testimony

Expert testimony usually takes one of three forms: an opinion, an answer to a hypothetical question, or a lecture providing background information for the judge or jury. The most common form of expert testimony is an opinion, although in child sexual abuse cases, expert testimony often takes the form of a lecture designed to help jurors understand the psychological dynamics of sexual abuse.

Opinion Testimony

Expert witnesses are permitted to offer professional opinions. For example, in a physical abuse case, a physician could testify that, in the doctor's opinion, the child has battered child syndrome, and the child's injuries are not accidental. In a neglect case, an expert could offer an opinion that a child's failure to thrive is caused by parental behavior.

The expert must be reasonably confident of the opinion. Lawyers use the term "reasonable certainty" to describe the necessary degree of confidence. Unfortunately, "reasonable certainty" is not easily defined. How certain must the expert be to be reasonably certain? It is clear that expert witnesses may not speculate or guess. It is equally clear that experts do not have to be completely certain before offering opinions. Thus, the degree of certainty lies somewhere between guesswork and absolute certainty.

In the final analysis, the reasonable certainty standard provides little guidance. A more useful way to assess the strength of expert testimony looks beyond reasonable certainty and asks questions that shed light on the factual and logical strength of the expert's opinion: In formulating the opinion, did the expert consider all relevant facts? Did the expert have adequate understanding of pertinent clinical and scientific principles? Did the expert use methods of assessment that are appropriate, reliable, and valid? Are the expert's assumptions and conclusions reasonable? Is the expert reasonably objective? In the end, the issue is whether the expert's reasoning is logical, consistent, and reasonably objective.

The Hypothetical Question

In some cases, expert testimony is elicited in response to a hypothetical question asked by the attorney who requested the expert's testimony. A hypothetical question contains facts that closely parallel the facts of the actual case on trial. In a physical abuse case, for example, the attorney might say, "Now doctor, let me ask you to assume that all of the following facts are true." The attorney then describes injuries suffered by a *hypothetical* child. After describing the hypothetical child, the attorney asks, "Doctor, based on these hypothetical facts, do you have an opinion, based on a reasonable degree of medical certainty, whether the hypothetical child's injuries were accidental or nonaccidental?" The doctor gives an opinion about the *hypothetical* child's injuries. The jury then applies the information supplied by the doctor regarding the hypothetical child to the injuries suffered by the actual child in the case on trial.

In bygone days, expert witnesses nearly always testified in response to a hypothetical question; but the hypothetical question is a cumbersome device, and it gradually fell into disfavor. Today, expert witnesses usually take the more direct approach of offering an opinion about the child in the case on trial, rather than an opinion about a hypothetical child. In modern trials, it is usually the cross-examining attorney who resorts to hypothetical questions. The cross-examiner seeks to undermine the expert's opinion by presenting a hypothetical set of facts that differs from the facts described by the expert. The cross-examiner then asks, "Now Doctor, if the hypothetical facts I have suggested to you turn out to be true, would that change your opinion?" Chadwick[5] observes that it is "common to encounter hypothetical questions based on hypotheses that are extremely unlikely, and the [expert] witness may need to point out the unlikelihood" (p. 967).

A Background Lecture to Educate the Jury

An expert may testify in the form of a lecture that provides the jury with background information on technical, clinical, or scientific issues. This form of expert testimony plays an important role in child sexual abuse litigation when the defense asserts that a child's delayed reporting or recantation means the child cannot be believed. When the defense attacks the child's credibility in this way, judges allow an expert witness to inform the jury that it is not uncommon for sexually abused children to delay reporting and to recant. Equipped with this background information, the jury is in a better position to evaluate the child's credibility.[21]

Physical Abuse Cases

When physical abuse is alleged, the most common defense is that the child's injuries were accidental. Expert testimony plays a key role in proving nonaccidental injury. Judges routinely allow physicians to testify that a child has battered child syndrome. A physician may testify that a child's injuries are probably not accidental. In addition, judges allow physicians to describe the means used to inflict injury. For example, a physician may testify that a skull fracture was probably caused by a blow from a blunt instrument, such as a fist. Experts are permitted to estimate the amount of force required to inflict injury. Judges generally allow physicians to state whether a caretaker's explanation for injuries is reasonable. Judges allow expert witnesses to describe shaken baby syndrome, Munchausen syndrome by proxy, and other evidence of nonaccidental injury.

When physical abuse is suspected, the following information, if present, should be documented in the child's chart: (1) unexplained injury, (2) implausible explanation offered by caretaker, (3) caretakers with inconsistent explanations, (4) caretakers' claims that injuries were inflicted by a sibling, and (5) delay in seeking medical care for serious or life-threatening conditions.

Sexual Abuse Cases

Expert testimony regarding child sexual abuse can be divided into two categories: expert testimony describing medical evidence of sexual abuse and expert testimony regarding the psychological effects of sexual abuse. Although these categories overlap, the distinction is important.

Medical and Laboratory Evidence

Uncertainty continues regarding some aspects of medical and laboratory evidence of sexual abuse (see chapter 1). Nevertheless, when medical or laboratory evidence is available, judges permit medical professionals to describe such evidence. Moreover, judges allow physicians to describe the results of examinations aided by colposcopy. Judges permit physicians to use photographs and other visual aids to illustrate their testimony.

Psychological Effects

Expert testimony regarding the psychological effects of sexual abuse is usefully divided into two categories. In the first category, the expert offers an opinion that a particular child was sexually abused or that a child has a diagnosis of sexual abuse or symptoms consistent with sexual abuse. Expert testimony in this category focuses directly on the ultimate issue before the court—Was this child abused? Expert psychological testimony of this type is controversial.[19,21,22]

The second category of expert testimony regarding the psychological effects of sexual abuse is less controversial than the first. In the second category, the expert does not offer an opinion that a particular child was sexually abused. Rather, the expert's testimony has the more limited purpose of explaining to the jury that certain behavior, such as delayed reporting and recantation, is relatively common in sexually abused children. As explained earlier, such expert testimony is permitted when the attorney for the alleged perpetrator attacks the child's credibility by attempting to persuade the jury to disbelieve the child because the child delayed reporting or recanted.

Testimony by Mental Health Experts

When it comes to expert testimony from mental health professionals, commentators and judges disagree over whether such professionals should testify that particular children were sexually abused.[19,21,22,23] Melton and Limber[18] write that "under no circumstances should a court admit the opinion of an expert about whether a particular child has been abused" (p. 1230). Contrary to this position, many professionals believe that, in some cases, properly qualified and experienced professionals can reach diagnostic decisions that help the court decide whether children were sexually abused.[21,22]

Testimony to Rehabilitate Children's Credibility

One of the basic rules of the American legal system is that the credibility of a witness cannot be supported or bolstered until the witness's credibility has been attacked. The process that attorneys use to attack witnesses is called impeachment. In child sexual abuse litigation, two forms of impeachment are particularly common. First, the defense attorney may assert that a child's behavior is inconsistent with allegations of abuse. For example, defense counsel may argue that a child should not be believed because the child did not report abuse for a substantial period of time or because the child recanted. Such impeachment is legitimate. When the defense concentrates on delay, recantation, and certain other behaviors, however, the prosecutor is generally allowed to respond with expert testimony to inform jurors that such behavior is relatively common in sexually abused children.

In the second form of impeachment, the defense attorney seeks to undermine the child's credibility by arguing that developmental differences between adults and children render children as a group less credible than adults. Defense counsel may assert that children are highly suggestible and have poor memories. In response to such impeachment, the prosecutor may offer expert testimony to inform jurors that children have adequate memories and are not as suggestible as many adults believe.[12,16,21,22,23,24,28,29]

The following guidelines are suggested for professionals providing expert testimony to rehabilitate children's impeached credibility.

1. The prosecutor should tell the judge and the defense attorney which behavior(s) the expert will discuss. For example, if the defense attorney limits the attack on the child's credibility to delay in reporting, the prosecutor informs the judge and defense counsel that the expert's testimony will be limited to helping the jury understand delay. The expert who serves the limited function of rehabilitating a child's credibility should limit testimony to the behavior emphasized by the defense attorney and should not offer a broad ranging lecture on children's reactions to sexual abuse.

2. In many cases, expert rehabilitation testimony is limited to a description of behaviors seen in sexually abused children as a group, and the expert avoids mentioning the child in the present case.

3. If it is appropriate to refer to the child in the present case, avoid referring to the child as a "victim."

4. In most sexual abuse cases, avoid reference to syndromes such as child sexual abuse accommodation syndrome.[32] One does not need to use the word *syndrome* to help the jury understand that delay in reporting, recantation, and inconsistency are relatively common in sexually abused children.

Although experts are allowed to rehabilitate children's credibility by explaining behaviors such as delayed reporting and recantation, experts are *not* permitted to testify that particular children told the truth or that sexually abused children as a group generally tell the truth about abuse.

Expert Testimony Regarding Syndromes

The legal system is comfortable with medical syndromes that are offered in court to prove physical abuse. Thus, judges routinely allow expert testimony on battered child syndrome, shaken baby syndrome, and Munchausen syndrome by proxy. When it comes to sexual abuse however, there is no syndrome—medical or psychological—that detects or diagnoses sexual abuse. Although no psychological syndrome is pathognomonic of sexual abuse, several psychological syndromes play subsidiary roles in child sexual abuse litigation. Five psychological syndromes are briefly discussed below.

Child Sexual Abuse Accommodation Syndrome

Summit[32] described child sexual abuse accommodation syndrome (CSAAS). CSAAS includes five characteristics commonly observed in sexually abused children:

- secrecy
- helplessness
- entrapment and accommodation
- delayed, conflicted, and unconvincing disclosure
- retraction

Summit's purpose in describing CSAAS was to provide a common language for professionals working to protect sexually abused children, not to create a diagnostic device. Summit observes that "[t]he accommodation syndrome is neither an illness nor a diagnosis, and it can't be used to measure whether or not a child has been sexually abused."[17]

The accommodation syndrome does *not* detect sexual abuse. Rather, CSAAS assumes that abuse occurred and explains the child's reaction to it.

The accommodation syndrome has a place in the courtroom, not as proof that a child was abused, but to help explain why many sexually abused children delay reporting their abuse and why some children recant allegations of abuse. When the syndrome is confined to this explanatory purpose, it serves a useful forensic function.

Rape Trauma Syndrome

Rape trauma syndrome (RTS) was described by Burgess and Holmstrom in 1974 as "the acute phase and long-term reorganization process that occurs as a result of forcible rape or attempted forcible rape. This syndrome of behavioral, somatic, and psychological reactions is an acute stress reaction to a life-threatening situation."[3]

Although expert testimony on RTS is used most frequently in litigation involving adult victims, RTS is sometimes useful in child sexual abuse litigation. Expert testimony on RTS has been offered by prosecutors for two purposes: to prove lack of consent to sexual relations, and to explain certain behaviors, such as delay in reporting rape, which jurors might misconstrue as evidence that rape did not occur.

Proving lack of consent.   In rape cases involving adult victims, the evidence often focuses on whether the victim consented. Courts are divided on the admissibility of RTS to prove lack of consent. Some courts reject RTS as a means of proving lack of consent. In *People v. Taylor,*[26] for example, the New York Court of Appeals wrote that "evidence of rape trauma syndrome does not by itself prove that the complainant was raped" (p. 135). The court concluded that "evidence of rape trauma syndrome is inadmissible when it inescapably bears solely on proving that a rape occurred" (p. 138). The California Supreme Court reached a similar result in *People v. Bledsoe,*[25] in which the court ruled that "expert testimony that a complaining witness suffers from rape trauma syndrome is not admissible to prove that the witness was raped" (p. 301). In contrast to the New York and California courts, several other courts state that RTS is admissible when the defendant asserts that the woman consented.[21] In *State v. Marks,*[31] for example, the Kansas Supreme Court wrote that "[w]hen consent is the defense in a prosecution for rape qualified expert psychiatric testimony regarding the existence of 'rape trauma syndrome' is relevant and admissible" (p. 1294). It should be remembered that when the victim is a child, consent is not generally an issue because children are legally incapable of consenting to sexual relations.

Rape trauma syndrome to explain the victim's behavior following the attack.   Most courts allow expert testimony on RTS to rehabilitate a child or adult victim's credibility after the defense attorney attacks the victim's credibility by emphasizing delayed reporting and other behaviors that jurors might construe as evidence that the rape did not occur. In *People v. Bledsoe,*[25] for example, the California Supreme Court wrote that "expert testimony on rape trauma syndrome may play a particularly useful role by disabusing the jury of some widely held misconceptions about rape and rape victims, so that it may evaluate the evidence free of the constraints of popular myths" (p. 457). In *People v. Taylor,*[26] the New York Court of Appeals approved expert testimony explaining why a rape victim might not appear upset following the assault. Courts that allow RTS to explain behaviors observed in rape victims place limits on such evidence. Thus, several court decisions state that the expert should describe behaviors observed in rape victims as a group and should not refer to the victim in the case at hand.[21]

Posttraumatic Stress Disorder

Judges generally permit qualified experts to testify that a patient has a diagnosis of posttraumatic stress disorder.[21]

Parental Alienation Syndrome

Gardner[9] describes parental alienation syndrome (PAS) as a psychiatric disorder that is observed in some parents fighting over custody of children in divorce court. One parent—the alienating parent—programs the child to revile the other parent. When one divorcing parent accuses the other of abusing their child, PAS is used to support an argument that the accusation is a lie. Of course, false accusations do arise in bitter custody disputes. On the other hand, many accusations appear to be true. In still other cases, the accusation is unfounded but the accusing parent makes the accusation in the good-faith belief that abuse happened. The important point here is that PAS does not help distinguish true from false accusations. PAS is not diagnostic. The syndrome does not detect false accusations or, for that matter, true accusations. Unfortunately, PAS is often used unfairly to attack the credibility of parents—usually mothers—who allege abuse. In the final analysis, everyone would be better off to discontinue use of the term *parental alienation syndrome* and to evaluate accusations of abuse on their individual merits.

CROSS-EXAMINATION AND IMPEACHMENT OF EXPERT WITNESSES

Testifying begins with direct examination. During direct examination, the expert witness answers questions from the attorney who asked the expert to testify. After direct examination, the opposing attorney has the right to cross-examine. Cross-examination is sometimes followed by redirect examination. Redirect examination affords the attorney who asked the expert to testify an opportunity to clarify issues that were discussed during cross-examination.

Cross-examination causes anxiety. The following discussion is intended to demystify cross-examination by explaining six techniques commonly used by cross-examining attorneys.

Raise Doubts about the Expert's Testimony

At the end of the case, the attorneys will present closing arguments. One goal of the closing argument is to persuade the jury to disbelieve certain witnesses. With the closing argument in mind, the opposing attorney uses cross-examination to raise doubts about the expert's testimony. During closing argument, the attorney reminds the jury of those doubts.

Leading Questions

The attorney conducting *direct* examination is generally not allowed to ask leading questions. By contrast, the cross-examiner is permitted to do so, and some attorneys ask *only* leading questions during cross-examination. The cross-examiner attempts to control the expert by using leading questions that require short, specific answers; answers the attorney wants the jury to hear. The cross-examiner keeps the witness hemmed in with leading questions and seldom asks why or how something happened. How and why questions permit the witness to explain, and explanation is precisely what the cross-examiner does not want.

Limit the Expert's Ability to Explain

When an expert attempts to explain an answer, the cross-examining attorney may interrupt and say, "Please just answer yes or no." If the expert persists, the cross-examiner may ask the judge to admonish the expert to limit answers to the questions asked. Experts are understandably frustrated when an attorney thwarts efforts at clarification. It is sometimes proper to say, "Counsel, it is not possible for me to answer with a simple yes or no. May I explain myself?" Chadwick[5] advises that "[w]hen a question is posed in a strictly 'yes or no' fashion, but the correct answer is 'maybe,' the witness should find a way to express the true answer. A direct appeal to the judge may be helpful in some cases" (p. 967). Many judges permit witnesses to explain themselves during cross-examination if the jury needs more information to make sense of the witness's testimony.

Remember that after cross-examination comes redirect examination, during which the attorney who asked the expert to testify is allowed to ask further questions. During redirect examination, the expert has an opportunity to clarify matters that were left unclear during cross-examination.

Undermine the Expert's Assumptions

One of the most effective cross-examination techniques is to commit the expert witness to the facts and assumptions that support the expert's opinion and then to dispute one or more of those facts or assumptions. Consider, for example, a case in which a physician testifies on direct examination that a child experienced vaginal penetration. The cross-examiner begins by committing the doctor to the facts and assumptions underlying the opinion. The attorney might say, "So Doctor, your opinion is based exclusively on the history, the physical examination, and on what the child told you. Is that correct?" "And there is nothing else you relied on to form your opinion. Is that correct?" The cross-examiner commits the doctor to a specific set of facts and assumptions so that when the attorney disputes those facts or assumptions, the doctor's opinion cannot be justified on some other basis.

Once the cross-examiner pins down the basis of the doctor's opinion, the examiner attacks the opinion by disputing one or more of the facts or assumptions that support it. The attorney might ask whether the doctor's opinion would change if certain facts were different. The attorney might press the doctor to acknowledge alternative explanations for the doctor's conclusion. The attorney might ask the doctor whether experts could come to different conclusions based on the same facts. Finally, the cross-examiner might confront the doctor with a hypothetical question that favors the examiner's client.

Rather than attack the doctor's assumptions and conclusions during cross-examination, the attorney may limit cross-examination to pinning the doctor down to a limited set of facts and assumptions and then, when the doctor has left the witness stand, offer another expert to contradict those facts and assumptions.

Impeach the Expert with a Learned Treatise

The judge may allow a cross-examining attorney to undermine an expert's testimony by confronting the expert with books or articles (called "learned treatises") that contradict the expert. The rules on impeachment with learned treatises vary from state to state. There is agreement on one thing, however. When an expert is confronted with a sentence or a paragraph selected by an attorney from an article or chapter, the expert has the right to put the selected passage in context by reading surrounding material. The expert might say to the cross-examining attorney, "Counsel, I cannot comment on the sentence you have selected unless I first read the entire article. If you will permit me to read the article, I'll be happy to comment on the sentence that interests you."

Raise the Possibility of Bias

The cross-examiner may raise the possibility that the expert is biased in favor of one side of the litigation. For example, if the expert is part of a multidisciplinary child abuse team, the cross-examiner might proceed as follows:

Q: Now, Doctor, you are employed by Children's Hospital, isn't that correct?

A: Right.

Q: At the hospital, are you a member of the multidisciplinary team that investigates allegations of child abuse?

A: The team performs medical examinations and interviews. We do not investigate as the police investigate. But yes, I am a member of the hospital's multidisciplinary child abuse team.

Q: Your team regularly performs investigative examinations and interviews at the request of the prosecuting attorney's office, isn't that correct?

A: Yes.

Q: When you complete your investigation for the prosecutor, you prepare a report for the prosecutor, don't you?

A: A report and recommendation are prepared and placed in the child's medical record. Upon request, the team provides a copy of the report to the prosecutor and, I might add, to the defense.

Q: After your team prepares its report and provides a copy to the prosecutor, you often come to court to testify as an expert witness for the prosecution in child abuse cases, isn't that right, Doctor?

A: Yes.

Q: Do you usually testify for the prosecution rather than the defense?

A: Correct.

Q: In fact, would I be correct in saying that you always testify for the prosecution and never for the defense?

A: I am willing to testify for the defense, but so far I have always testified for the prosecution.

Q: Thank you, Doctor. I have no further questions.

Clearly, the cross-examiner is seeking to portray the doctor as biased in favor of the prosecution. Notice, however, that the cross-examiner is too cunning to ask, "Well then, Doctor, isn't it a fact that because of your close working relationship with the prosecution, you are biased in favor of the prosecution?" The cross-examiner knows that the answer to that question is a truthful and indignant "No." So the cross-examiner refrains from asking directly about bias, and simply plants seeds of doubt in the jurors' minds. When it is time for the defense to give its closing argument, the defense attorney will remind the jury of the doctor's close working relationship with the prosecution, "a relationship, ladies and gentlemen of the jury, that is just a little too cozy." What is the antidote to this tactic? First, the doctor may find an opportunity to indicate lack of bias during cross-examination itself. Second, remember that cross-examination is followed by redirect examination. During redirect, the prosecutor may ask, "Doctor, in light of the defense attorney's questions about your job on the multidisciplinary team, are you biased in favor of the prosecution?" Now the doctor can set the record straight.

CONCLUSION

The professions of medicine and law sometimes seem like ships passing in the night. Yet, if children are to be protected, physicians and attorneys must put aside their differences and work together. Only genuine interdisciplinary cooperation holds realistic hope of reducing the tragic number of abused and neglected children.

REFERENCES

1. American Medical Association. *Principles of medical ethics.* Chicago: American Medical Association. 1989.

2. American Nurses Association. *Code for nurses.* Washington, DC: American Nurses Association. 1985.

3. Burgess A, Holmstrom L. Rape trauma syndrome. *Am J Psychiatry* 1974;131:981–986.

4. *California civil code.* St. Paul, MN: West Publishing. 1999.

5. Chadwick DL. Preparation for court testimony in child abuse cases. *Pediatr Clin North Am* 1990;37:955–970.

6. Fivush R. Developmental perspectives on autobiographical recall. In Goodman GS, Bottoms BL (eds.), *Child victims, child witnesses: Understanding and improving children's testimony.* New York: Guilford Press. 1992.

7. Friedrich WN, Brambsch P, Broughton K, Beilke RL. Normative sexual behavior in children. *Pediatrics* 1991;88:456–464.

8. Friedrich WN, Brambsch P, Damon L, et al. Child sexual behavior inventory: Normative and clinical comparisons. *Psychol Assess* 1992;4:303–311.

9. Gardner RA. *The parental alienation syndrome: A guide for mental health and legal professionals.* Cresskil, NJ. Creative Therapeutics. 1992.

10. Goodman GS, Bottoms BL. *Child victims, child witnesses: Understanding and improving testimony.* New York: Guilford. 1993.

11. Gutheil TG, Appelbaum PS. *Clinical handbook of psychiatry and the law.* New York: McGraw-Hill. 1982.

12. Hewitt SK. *Assessing allegations of sexual abuse in preschool children: Understanding small voices.* Thousand Oaks, CA: Sage. 1998.

13. Jones DPH, McQuiston M. *Interviewing the sexually abused child.* Denver, CO: C. Henry Kempe National Center for the Prevention and Treatment of Child Abuse and Neglect. 1985.

14. Kalichman SC. *Mandated reporting of suspected child abuse: Ethics, law, and policy.* Washington, DC: American Psychological Association. 1993.

15. Lawson L, Chaffin M. False negatives in sexual abuse disclosure interviews: Incidence and influence of caretaker's belief in abuse cases of accidental abuse disclosure by diagnosis of STD. *J Interpers Viol* 1992;7:532–542.

16. Lyon TD. The new wave in children's suggestibility research: A critique. *Cornell Law J* 1999;84;1004–1086.

17. Meinig MB. Profile of Roland Summit. *Violence Update* 1991;1:6–7.

18. Melton GB, Limber S. Psychologists' involvement in cases of child maltreatment. *Am Psychol* 1989;44:1225–1233.

19. Melton GB, Petrila J, Poythress N, Slobogin C. *Psychological evaluations for the courts.* 2nd ed. New York: Guilford. 1997.

20. Mueller CB, Kirkpatrick LC. *Federal evidence.* 2nd ed. Rochester, NY: Lawyers Cooperative Publishing. 1994.

21. Myers JEB. *Evidence in child abuse and neglect cases.* 2nd ed. New York: Aspen Law and Business. 1997.

22. Myers JEB. *Legal issues in child abuse and neglect practice.* Thousand Oaks, CA: Sage. 1998.

23. Myers JEB, Bays J, Becker JV, Berliner L, Corwin DL, Saywitz KJ. Expert testimony in child sexual abuse litigation. *Nebraska Law Rev* 1989; 68:1–145.

24. Myers JEB, Saywitz KJ, Goodman GS. Psychological research on children as witnesses: Practical implications for forensic interviews and courtroom testimony. *Pacific Law J* 1996;28:3–92.

25. *People v. Bledsoe,* 681 P.2d 291, California 1984.

26. *People v. Taylor,* 552 N.E.2d 131, New York 1990.

27. Poole DA, Lamb ME. *Investigative interviews of children.* Washington, DC: American Psychological Association. 1998.

28. Quas JA, Goodman GS, Bidrose S, Pipe ME, Craw S, Ablin DS. Emotion and memory: Children's long-term remembering, forgetting, and suggestibility. *J Exper Child Psychol* 1999;72:235–270.

29. Ricci CM, Beal CR. Child witnesses: Effect of event knowledge on memory and suggestibility. *J Appl Dev Psychol* 1998;19:305–317.

30. Saywitz KJ, Goodman GS, Nicholas E, Moan SF. Children's memories of a physical examination involving genital touch: Implications for reports of child sexual abuse. *J Consult Clin Psychol* 1991;59:682–691.

31. *State v. Marks,* 647 P.2d 1292 Kansas 1982.

32. Summit RC. The child sexual abuse accommodation syndrome. *Child Abuse Negl* 1983; 7:177–193.

33. *Tarasoff v. Regents of the University of California,* 551 P.2d 334, California 1976.

PART VII

Child Maltreatment and Society

Chapter 24

Understanding the Consequences of Childhood Victimization

Cathy Spatz Widom, Ph.D.

The consequences of childhood victimization are complex, with multiple determinants that require multidimensional models for explanation. Attempts at understanding must consider the child, the parents and family, the community, and the various interactions of these entities. Children who are victimized are likely to be affected in a number of ways—neurologically, cognitively, behaviorally and socially, and psychologically and emotionally—which may also be interactive, setting off a cascade of dysfunction. In addition, the consequences of any child's victimization may be influenced by the age, gender, and ethnicity of the child, and dysfunction that occurs as a result of victimization at one stage of development will go on to lay the groundwork for subsequent dysfunctional behaviors. Much remains to be learned about the mechanisms by which maltreatment influences later dysfunction, but a number of forces may be at work, including maladaptive means of coping, modeling of abusive and violent behaviors, attachment disorders, and the physical and personality changes that are a result of abuse.

GENERAL CONSIDERATIONS

The model for much of contemporary thinking about child maltreatment is based on an ecological view of child development.[16,24,71] It emphasizes the importance of social context and the need to consider the child in the framework of the broader environment in which he or she develops. A series of concentric circles or embedded boxes has typically been used to illustrate this model (see figure 24.1A)[134] The child is depicted as embedded or existing within the context of a family and families as embedded in a larger social system that includes neighborhoods, communities, and broader cultures.

Figure 24.1B presents a somewhat different model. Like the traditional model this one acknowledges that abused and neglected children live within families and, in turn, these families exist within larger social units. This modified ecological model assumes that behavior is complex and multiply determined, explicitly recognizing the importance of individual child, parent and family, and neighborhood and/or community characteristics. This model recognizes that behavior does not occur in a vacuum and that early patterns of adaptation or maladaptation influence later adaptation, but not necessarily in a simple,

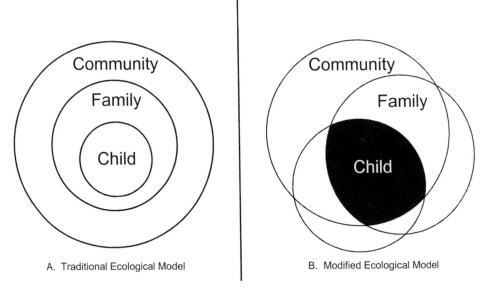

A. Traditional Ecological Model   B. Modified Ecological Model

Figure 24.1   Models of Child Developmental Environment

linear manner. This perspective reflects the influence of interactionist theorists such as Magnusson and Torestad[119] who emphasize that individuals develop in reciprocal interactions with their environments. Furthermore, the model assumes that risk factors may overlap and interact synergistically with each other, creating a "pile up" effect.[125,181] Genetic and neurobiological factors are also likely to play a role in determining consequences of childhood victimization.[108]

Attempts to understand the consequences of childhood victimization must first take into account characteristics of the child. For example, a number of studies have found that personality characteristics play an important role in the etiology of later behaviors. A child who is irritable, has temper tantrums, fights with other children and siblings, sets fires, is destructive, uncontrollable, or shows extreme defiance of authority is more at risk for certain types of deviant behavior outcomes than children with less difficult temperaments and personality characteristics, regardless of whether or not he or she has experienced childhood abuse or neglect.

Parental and familial characteristics are important, as well, to understanding outcomes associated with childhood victimization. For example, Gibbin et al.[77] found that the provision of appropriate play materials and maternal involvement were more discriminating in predicting outcome than abuse/control status alone. Thus, the presence or absence of abuse may interact with other aspects of the child's environment to determine outcome. Terr[171] found that preexisting family pathology contributed to individual differences in the long-term adjustment of children kidnapped and held for 48 hours in an underground hideout. Four years after the kidnapping, the children from troubled families were more maladjusted than children from healthier families.

Child abuse and neglect are often committed by biological parents, and these parents may have certain characteristics (e.g., alcohol or drug problems or criminal behavior) which influence psychological and behavioral outcomes for their offspring, directly or indirectly. A number of studies suggest that abusive parents [29,82,93,126,176,177] and neglectful parents[13] have drug problems. Furthermore, characteristics of parents and families have been found to influence out-of-home placement decisions for abused and neglected children.[155,189] Thus, it is critical to disentangle the contribution of family factors from outcomes associated with childhood victimization.

There is also emerging evidence that the long-term impact of childhood trauma may depend on characteristics of the community (which can refer to small block groups, local neighborhoods, census tracts, or larger contexts such as cities, states, or counties) or practices of the community and the justice and social service systems in which the child lived at the time of the abuse or neglect. Some ways of handling or responding to incidents of abuse or neglect may act to buffer the child and, in turn, lead to better outcomes for that child, whereas other responses may act to exacerbate the problems of these already vulnerable children. Indeed, some have suggested that the relationship between childhood victimization and problem behaviors in later life may be in part a function of juvenile justice system practices which disproportionately label and adjudicate maltreatment victims as juvenile offenders.[168] It has been suggested[73] that delinquency may be one eventual consequence of maltreatment, because some of the behavioral responses to maltreatment are officially defined as delinquent. An example is a child who becomes estranged from her parents or prosocial peers and then develops friendships with antisocial peers. In turn, this association with delinquent friends leads to the adoption of a delinquent lifestyle, including substance abuse and violence.

Figure 24.1B depicts the child's environment with circles that in some areas overlap and in some do not. Although the child lives largely within the context of a family, this model emphasizes that the child also spends time outside (and independent of) the family unit and in the larger community. The areas of nonoverlap of child and family will change with the age of the child; as the child gets older, he or she is likely to spend more time outside the family and in the community and with peers. Some children, particularly neglected children, may experience increasing amounts of unsupervised time, spent in ways of which parents are unaware. For example, if a child begins to use drugs as an escape from an abusive home environment, he or she is likely to associate with drug-using peers. This exposure to drug-using peers, in turn, may increase the likelihood that he or she will continue to use drugs and that the use may escalate. Brook et al.[25] described such a feedback loop, and particularly its effect on youngsters who are "detached" from their parents.

Figure 24.1B also calls attention to aspects of the developing child that may occur and exist outside both family and community. That is, there may be experiences unique to the child, independent of family and/or community context. These areas of nonshared experience (areas of nonoverlap in the figure) may be particularly important to the subsequent development of severely abused or neglected children. Childhood victims, especially incest victims, may learn to "tune out" or dissociate during abuse experiences and may extend this approach to other domains of functioning.[85]

This modified ecological model emphasizes that experiences of families may also lie in part outside the neighborhood and community and yet may also be influenced in major ways by the surrounding environment or context. Families may be isolated or insulated from the larger social contact. Indeed, the lack of social support systems and associated social isolation are important characteristics associated with families at high risk for physical and sexual abuse of children.[72,136]

The modified ecological model also stresses the need to consider the interactions of child, family, and community factors. Some community characteristics (e.g. high social disorganization) may interact with characteristics of the child (abused or neglected) or the family (unemployment) to magnify risk for certain outcomes. Characteristics of the child and family or characteristics of the child and community may have effects that are conditional on one another.

BASIC ASSUMPTIONS OF THE MODEL

This modified ecological model incorporates some basic assumptions about the consequences of child maltreatment, which are discussed in detail below:

- Childhood victimization has the potential to affect multiple domains of functioning.
- Consequences of childhood victimization may differ depending on the age of the child at time of occurrence.
- Deficits or dysfunctional behaviors at one developmental period lay the groundwork for subsequent dysfunctional behaviors.
- Consequences of childhood victimization are likely to differ by gender and ethnicity.
- Neighborhood and community level factors affect consequences.
- Positive effects of protective factors or interventions are theoretically possible at all ages.

Victimization Can Affect Multiple Domains of Functioning

Figure 24.2 illustrates potential negative outcomes across different domains of functioning, beginning in early childhood and extending into adulthood (working down the columns). *Neurological and medical* consequences may range from minor injuries to severe brain damage and even death. Early studies of abused and neglected children documented significant intellectual and neuromotor handicap, noting higher incidences of growth retardation, central nervous system damage, physical defects, mental retardation, and serious speech problems.[57,122,133,160] *Cognitive and intellectual* effects may be manifested in attentional problems, learning disorders, or poor school performance.[123,142,193] *Behaviorally and socially,* not only are abused and neglected children destructive to themselves, but their behavior is also potentially destructive to others. The consequences can range from poor peer relations and physical aggression[55,102] to antisocial and violent behaviors[110,112,116,148,186,187] to alcohol and substance abuse problems,[104,129,130,131,152,192] promiscuity,[29,105] prostitution,[8,191] and teenage pregnancy.[28] *Psychological and emotional* consequences can include low self-esteem, anxiety, and depression,[4,27,96,98,114,144] posttraumatic stress disorder,[22,23,60,127,141,153,154,159] dissociation,[5,20,31,52,146,151,161] multiple personality disorder,[38,101,147] somatization and somatoform disorders,[51] and suicide attempts.[45,79,180,190]

These and other studies illustrate the wide variety of negative outcomes for which abused and neglected children are potentially at increased risk. Unfortunately, empirical support for some of these consequences remains sparse and it is possible that at least some of these outcomes may not be uniquely associated with early childhood victimization. While methodological problems will not be reviewed here,[21,33,132,188,194] some caveats are important. Few prospective studies have traced outcomes for abused and neglected children beyond adolescence and into adulthood, and much of our existing knowledge is based on retrospective reports. Many studies have sampled from in- and outpatient samples, a characteristic which may restrict the generalizability of the findings, since many

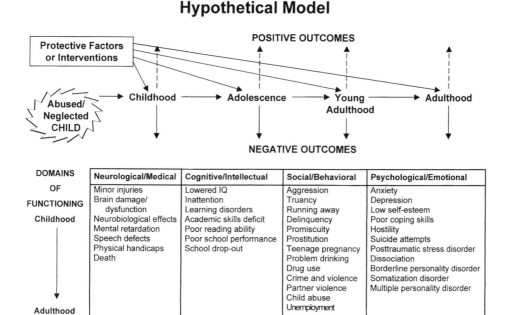

Figure 24.2   Potential Effects of Abuse and Neglect on Domains of Functioning over the Life Span

childhood victims do not seek later treatment or professional services. Also, those who use such services may have higher rates of problem behaviors than those who do not seek treatment, leading to an overestimation of subsequent problems among childhood victims.

Certain outcomes may represent a direct pathway from abuse and/or neglect in childhood through adolescence, to young adulthood, and adulthood. For example, an abused child who externalizes his problems might show aggressive behavior in early childhood (working down the column labeled "Social/Behavioral") and might continue to be delinquent in adolescence and to engage in crime and violent behavior in adulthood. Given the stability of aggressive behavior,[62,139,149,192] such a sequence of behaviors would not be hard to imagine. One might also expect a further direct link to adult abusive behavior in the home (as in partner violence or child abuse).

On the other hand, for some children the consequences of childhood victimization may not lead to aggression, delinquency, or violent behavior but may be manifested by other forms of dysfunctional or deviant behavior, particularly for those children who have adopted an internalizing style of responding.

Consequences Depend on Child's Age at Occurrence

Little is known about the age-relatedness of the effects of abuse and neglect. The model presented here is based on a dynamic view of development that assumes that childhood victimization that occurs at one age is likely to have different consequences from victimization that occurs at other ages. Is there a critical time period before which or after which the effects of these early experiences are magnified or minimized? Maccoby has argued that "we cannot be upset by events whose power to harm we do not understand; we cannot be humiliated by failure to handle problems where solutions are someone else's responsibility; we cannot be distressed by anticipating other's contemptuous or critical reactions to our weaknesses if we are not aware of other's probable reactions and if our egos are not yet invested in appearing strong and competent. So younger children are buffered against many phenomena that would produce distress in older people."[118,p219]

In considering the effects of abuse and neglect on children at different ages, it is useful to consider the developmental literature on children's responses to other forms of stressful life events. For example, one study[200] found that a child moved from a foster home to a permanent adoptive home before the age of 6 months tended to show only transitory distress. By contrast, in children between the ages of 7 and 12 months, such a change involved more pervasive disturbances. Similarly, the age period of greatest risk for the stress of hospital admission has been found to be between 6 months and 4 years of age;[157] children below the age of 6 or 7 months being relatively immune because they have not yet developed selective attachments and are therefore not able to experience separation anxiety. The lower vulnerability of children above the age of 4 years or so probably results from their having the cognitive skills to understand the situation. Children's responses to parental divorce also have been found to vary by age and level of development.[178]

There has been some speculation in the literature that the older the child at the time of the abuse incident, the greater the subsequent disturbances.[175] Some studies of children and adolescents have reported greater disturbances associated with abuse during the preteen and teenage years compared to abuse at younger ages.[1,143,163,167] On the other hand, studies have reported that abuse at younger ages was associated with greater trauma.[40,64,100,128,156,197] Nevertheless, after reviewing the literature on the effects of sexual abuse, Berliner[17] concluded that age of onset of abuse had not been consistently associated with the severity of impact. Similarly, Beitchman et al.[14] concluded that "findings regarding the relation between age of onset and severity of outcome are inconclusive."

Two possible explanations[14] have been suggested for the inconsistencies in findings. First, if victims are assessed as children, the full extent of the consequences may not be manifest. As children grow and develop, new symptoms associated with their abuse may emerge. Prospective longitudinal studies would permit the examination of this hypothesis. Second, it is possible that age of onset is related to the duration and type of abuse experience, and this might confound outcomes. Young children may not have suffered the abuse for a long period of time and may not have experienced the use of force and threats, which may be more common aspects of sexual abuse with older children and adolescents.[78,143]

Earlier Dysfunctional Behaviors Promote Later Ones

The modified ecological model assumes that deficits or dysfunctional behaviors that appear at one age will continue to exert an influence at the next age, unless an intervention occurs or a protective factor is introduced. For example, in the neurological/medical domain, malnutrition in infancy may lead to impaired cognitive and intellectual functioning in toddlers, and this in turn may affect IQ and, in turn, affect school performance in a negative way. Deficits in IQ or cognitive ability laid down in early childhood may lead to impaired performance in elementary or secondary school and then to impaired functioning as a young adult. At the same time, with decreased cognitive functioning, lowered self-esteem may result, either from the childhood victimization directly (feelings of low self-worth, that the child was somehow responsible for the abuse or neglect) or as a by-product of lowered cognitive functioning and poor social and interpersonal skills. Dysfunctional behaviors, such as running away or substance use, may serve as an escape mechanism for abused and neglected children and, in turn, may lead to a lowering of self-esteem; actions that to the children may seem like solutions to their problems may lead to further problems at later stages.

Consequences May Differ by Gender and Ethnicity

Gender

At least with prepubertal children, gender differences in response to most kinds of stressful events seem to operate in the same direction. Boys appear to be more vulnerable than girls.[58,88,157,178,179] Do boys and girls respond in similar ways to the experiences of early abuse and neglect? If gender differences exist, do they parallel gender differences in socialization experiences?

Surprisingly little research has compared the consequences of child abuse and neglect for males and females separately. While some studies have reported gender differences in response to abuse[46,68,83,115,173,187,190] others have not.[43,44] Using two different alcohol use-related outcomes, researchers[94,192] found that abused and neglected females were at increased risk for alcohol abuse (measured by arrests related to alcohol and/or drug use and alcohol abuse/dependence diagnoses), whereas males were not. In contrast, another study[116] reported that abused and neglected males were at increased risk for diagnosis of antisocial personality disorder in young adulthood, while females were not.

Early clinical reports on the connections of childhood abuse and neglect to violence primarily described violent male adolescents. Studies of sexual promiscuity and teenage pregnancy among child abuse victims have utilized samples of females, and primarily females who were sexually abused. For each of these sex-linked outcomes (violence in males, sexuality in females), studying the nonstereotypic sex may yield important insights. Finkelhor[65] called attention to the need to study males who have been sexually abused in childhood, at the same time that we continue to attend to the research and treatment needs of female childhood sexual abuse victims. It may also be instructive to examine the extent to which sexually abused males are sexually promiscuous and involved in paternity as teenagers (even if they are not responsible for the care of the child).

Although gender differences in the consequences of child abuse and neglect have not received much attention, some writers have discussed differences in the manifestations of distress, suggesting some conformity to gender roles.[47,48,91,185] Downey et al.[48] have suggested that gender differences in the consequences of abuse may parallel the gender differences in expressions of psychopathology and that aggression and depression may be different expressions of the same underlying distress, perhaps reflecting different strategies for maintaining self-esteem in the face of perceived rejection. For example, one might expect males to direct their suffering in an outward (externalizing) direction, as in aggression, and females to direct their pain inwardly (internalizing), with self-destructive behaviors and depression.

However, some additional factors complicate the study of gender differences in consequences of childhood victimization. First, some of the lack of attention to gender differences in consequences may result from the small number of male victims of sexual abuse in most studies and lower rates of reporting of childhood sexual abuse in males.[65] Second, males and females are not necessarily subject to the same forms of maltreatment.[1,80] Since males and females may experience different types of abuse or neglect, any differences in their responses to maltreatment may be a function of the type of maltreatment, rather than gender differences. It may be that the type of childhood abuse or neglect, rather than gender, is the critical variable in determining a person's risk for subsequent problem behaviors. Third, there are differences in the prevalence of certain forms of psychopathology and psychiatric diagnoses by gender,[150,185] which at least suggests interactions in outcome patterns by gender.

Ethnicity

Korbin[103] has called attention to the importance of culture in defining and understanding child abuse. At least one report comparing the profiles of Chinese American, Native Indian, and Anglo-Canadian children and abusers has suggested that there may be important cultural differences in the role of substance abuse.[107] Earlier work on the cycle of violence[187] found that African American abused and neglected children (as compared to African American children who were not abused or neglected) were at increased risk of arrest for a violent crime, a pattern of arrest not found for whites in the sample.

Racial and ethnic minority children may encounter discrimination against their race, color, language, life style, and family styles that affects their self-esteem and exacerbates the initial and lasting effects of earlier childhood victimization.[198] In a paper on the epidemiology of trauma, Norris[138] reported complex findings regarding race, which she felt "highlighted the importance of specifying the cultural context in which traumatic events occur." These findings suggest the need to examine more fully racial and ethnic differences in consequences, as well as the role of family and community factors, especially since poor and ethnic minority children are more likely to be identified as maltreated than children from more affluent white families.[137]

If differences in ethnic or racial backgrounds result in differences in the community's or legal system's response to abused and neglected children, it seems important to identify these differences, particularly if they relate to subsequent levels of violence in these children. A comparison of two samples of adolescents—one sent to a correctional facility and the other admitted to a state psychiatric hospital—in one urban area during a one-year time period found that the most powerful distinguishing factor between the two groups was race.[111] Seventy-one percent of the hospitalized adolescents were white, and 67 percent of the incarcerated adolescents were black. The study, published in 1980, noted that "clinical and epidemiological findings indicate clearly that many seriously psychiatrically disturbed, aggressive black adolescents are being channeled to correctional facilities while their equally aggressive white counterparts are directed toward psychiatric treatment facilities."[111,p1216] Not only would this practice "reinforce the stereotypes instead of demolishing them"[35] but it would also perpetuate the segregation of white and black violently disturbed adolescents.

A more recent study, this one examining the role of clinical and institutional interventions in children's recovery from sexual abuse,[135] found that children of color received later and less outpatient therapy than did white children and were more likely to be placed outside the home and to be hospitalized for psychiatric diagnoses than be left at home and treated as outpatients. If the abuse or neglect experiences of some children are being identified at a later point in the process, then there is less opportunity to intervene positively in these children's lives and more time for dysfunctional behaviors to become firmly entrenched. If earlier identification of abuse and neglect leads to *positive* interventions, then this should minimize negative outcomes. The longer society waits to intervene, the more difficult the change process becomes and the less time positive influences have to affect the developing child. Furthermore, abused and neglected children may become angry and hostile in response to the abuse or may adopt what has been called a "hostile world view."[41] In turn, these angry and hostile feelings may give way to antisocial and violent behavior patterns.

Community Factors Affect Consequences

Factors at the neighborhood and community level are contextual variables that also need to be considered in understanding the impact of childhood abuse and neglect. Early work of Garbarino and his colleagues found that childhood maltreatment rates by neighborhood were highly correlated with socioeconomic measures, family structure, and residential satisfaction.[72,74] More recently, using census and administrative agency data, Coulton et al.[39] found that child maltreatment rates were related to indicators of community breakdown and disorganization. Children who lived in neighborhoods characterized by poverty, high population turnover, and high rates of female-headed households were at higher risk of maltreatment than other children.

Maltreating families have frequently been characterized as having limited contact with relatives, neighbors, and friends. For example, family studies suggest that abusive families may perceive their social relationships differently than nonabusive families do.[145] Some research[145] has also suggested that neglectful families are less likely than their similarly low-income neighbors to interact socially with their neighbors or to perceive their neighbors as helpful and are more likely to be seen as marginal and avoided. However, this association between social isolation and child maltreatment has been challenged.[162]

Contextual variables also include the family's or community's reaction to the abuse or neglect experience.[22,81,171] For example, some ways of handling or responding to incidents of abuse or neglect may act to buffer the child and, in turn, lead to better outcomes for that child. Other responses may act to exacerbate susceptibility of these already vulnerable children. For example, although premature babies generally do relatively poorly in school, the long-term disadvantage for the premature infants was especially marked if the child was raised in an unstable, disturbed family setting.[50]

Positive Effects of Protective Factors Possible at All Ages

Studies of the impact of childhood abuse and neglect find substantial groups of individuals who appear to have little or no symptomatology.[36,97,121,124,167,172,187,190] A number of explanations for these findings can be offered, including inadequate measurement techniques by researchers and denial on the part of the victims. It is also possible that some characteristics of the child (good coping skills) or the child's environment (a relationship with a significant and supportive person) may have acted to buffer the individual from long-term negative consequences. Figure 24.2 calls attention to the role of what Garmezy[75] has called protective factors—those dispositional attributes, environmental conditions, biological predispositions, and positive events that can act to mitigate early negative experiences.

What are some of the possible mediating variables, the attributes and experiences that may act to buffer abused and neglected children from negative outcomes? It is conceivable that high (or above average) intelligence and good scholastic attainment exert a protective effect. Intelligence may play a direct role or it may operate as a protective influence by enhancing such other factors as school performance, problem-solving skills, or levels of self-esteem. Frodi and Smetana[69] found that, if one controls for IQ, differences between the abilities of maltreated and nonmaltreated children to discriminate emotions disappeared. High-IQ children maintained good achievement test performance at both low and high levels of stress, whereas low-IQ children showed a drop in performance under high stress.[76]

Although Werner and Smith[183] were not studying abused children, their findings are also relevant. In their longitudinal study of nearly 700 children in Hawaii, followed from birth to age 18, they found that the most resilient children were those with high infant intelligence, high verbal skills, and high self-esteem in adolescence and who were from families characterized by smaller size, low discord, and fewer absent fathers or working mothers.[182]

Empirical findings suggest that a person's cognitive appraisal of life events strongly influences his or her response.[106] The same event may be perceived by different individuals as irrelevant, benign, positive, or threatening and harmful. In thinking about the effects of abuse and neglect, it is likely that the child's cognitive appraisal of these events will determine at least in part whether they are experienced as neutral, negative, or harmful. In part, this might reflect the system's response to the abusive or neglectful experience or the individual child's perception of the experience. Cognitive appraisal may be particularly important in abuse involving older children who have the cognitive skills necessary to process the event.[118]

In a 14-year longitudinal study of 2,000 families,[201] 35 families with abused children were identified. Abused children (n=9) who survived the trauma of their childhood seemingly unscathed and grew up to be well-adjusted individuals (n=9) were compared with the rest of the abused children, who showed a high degree of psychosocial pathology. A number of variables distinguished the two groups of children, including level of fatalism, self-esteem, cognitive abilities, self-destructiveness, hope and fantasy, behavior patterns, and external support. The interpretation was that the perception of the well-adjusted group of their good personal resources—intellectual potential, good self-image, and hope—coupled with relatively sound external resources, tipped the scale in their favor.

Despite problems with the concept and measurement of temperament,[11] there is evidence that infants and young children with different temperaments may elicit different parental behaviors.[12] In some cases, temperament may protect the child; in others, temperament may place the child at risk by negatively affecting parent-child interactions.[140] There is some support for the notion that children with difficult temperaments are singled out for abuse.[66] For example, one study[189] found that victims of physical abuse tended to be described by their mothers as "difficult" children. However, other researchers have not found this to be the case.[46,165]

Temperament most likely interacts with early childhood experiences to exacerbate or minimize a child's level of risk for the development of subsequent problem behaviors.[140] In an analysis of characteristics associated with the avoidance of delinquency in abused and neglected children, Widom[189] found that a small group of children (n=51, 6.6%) who had indications of early behavior problems in their records were more likely to have extensive criminal histories as adolescents than other abused and/or neglected children. In contrast to the abused and neglected children with no mention of behavior problems in childhood, children with a history of behavior problems were over eight times as likely to be arrested.

Clinicians and child protection service workers have stressed the importance of a significant person in the lives of abused and neglected children, yet little systematic evidence of their role as buffers for victimized children exists. One study[75] identified the presence of a supportive family member as one of the important themes in the lives of children who overcame adversity. In a follow-up study,[117] children who had recovered from their childhood maltreatment had had the support of an adult. Another investigation[61] found few competent survivors among physically or emotionally neglected children, but the children who were more likely to be competent were those whose mothers showed some interest in them and were able to respond to them emotionally. For sexually abused children, one positive mediating variable appears to be the presence of a supportive, positive relationship with a nonabusive parent or sibling.[37]

Although out-of-home placements and foster care are interventions designed to positively affect the development of abused and neglected children, the role of these experiences remains controversial and ethically complex.[155] While critics have argued against foster care and out-of-home placement experiences, some evidence suggests that out-of-home placement for some abused and neglected children may not be detrimental to their long-term development and that early stable placements may be associated with better outcomes.[189] Having a relationship with a significant person, such as a foster parent, may serve as a protective factor for abused and/or neglected children.

Research is needed to examine the role of placements as buffers in the lives of abused and neglected children. For example, it is unknown whether there are critical time periods after which interventions become substantially less effective. The limited data on behavioral change suggests that interventions may be more effective in the early stages of development than at later stages.[164,174] However, once problem behaviors have occurred, later interventions are more labor intensive and face more entrenched behavior patterns than when efforts are targeted at younger children. Furthermore, interventions at later ages must deal simultaneously with the existence of problem behaviors and the prevention of new ones.

Early interventions should focus on eliminating factors that decrease a child's capacity for normal cognitive and/or neurological maturation. Once behavior problems have been identified, intervention efforts can be aimed at reducing the likelihood of further problem behaviors. Children who develop problem behaviors and who are inattentive or hyperactive are, in turn, likely to be at increased risk for delays or deficits in social skills. Interventions may then be aimed at the development of good social skills in an age appropriate manner, to decrease the chance for disruption in the child's peer relationships and his or her relationships with adults.

The modified ecological model also recognizes that what may be risk factors or protective factors for abused and neglected children may not be risk or protective factors for nonabused and non-neglected children and that outcomes will depend on the social context and other factors. For example, divorce may be associated with increased risk for children from advantaged backgrounds, but it may, in fact, be protective for children living in highly disorganized or dysfunctional households.

POTENTIAL CAUSAL LINKS BETWEEN CHILDHOOD VICTIMIZATION AND LATER DYSFUNCTION

The processes linking childhood victimization with later negative consequences may have an immediate impact or a delayed outcome, apparent only some time after the abuse. It is likely that there are many ways in which the experience of early childhood victimization influences later behaviors and increases the risk for certain problem behaviors. It is also likely that the mechanisms vary depending on characteristics of the child (such as age at the time of the abuse or neglect, gender, ethnicity, and temperament), family, and community. It is possible that problem behaviors occur only in conjunction with certain other characteristics associated with abusive and/or neglectful families (i.e., poverty, unemployment, stress, or alcohol and drug problems). Although most of the mechanisms described below represent developments within the child, other mechanisms suggest consequences that may result from external influences. That is, child abuse and/or neglect may not directly cause problem behaviors, but these outcomes may be an indirect by-product of these early experiences.

Immediate Sequelae

Childhood victimization may lead to immediate sequelae that then have an irremediable effect on the subsequent development of the child. Dykes[53] has described infants who were shaken so vigorously that they sustained intracranial and intraocular bleeding with no signs of external trauma. Being abused or neglected as a child may result in brain dysfunction as a result of direct brain injury or as a result of malnutrition. Forms of physical abuse like battering or of severe neglect (e.g., that induces dehydration, diarrhea, or failure to thrive) may lead to developmental retardation, which, in turn, may affect school performance and behavior (e.g., causing truancy). Some empirical support is provided by a study of Barbadian children[70] which found that malnourished children ages 5–11 years old had significantly lower IQ scores than a matched control group. The malnourished children also exhibited more attention deficits, poorer social skills, and less emotional stability, in comparison to the controls. (For a more detailed discussion of these immediate sequelae, see chapters 1 [sexual abuse], 7 [physical abuse], and 12 [neglect].)

Modeling (Social Learning)

From a social learning perspective, physical aggression between family members provides a likely model for aggressive behavior as well as for the appropriateness of such behavior within the family.[9,63] Children learn behavior, at least in part, by imitating someone else's behavior, and this effect is particularly potent when the model observed is someone of high status (such as a parent) or a successful person. Children learn to be aggressive by observing aggression in their families and in the surrounding community.[63] White and Straus[184] suggested that physical punishment "lays the groundwork for the normative legitimacy of all types of violence." According to this view, "each generation learns to be violent by being a participant in a violent family."[170] Numerous studies have documented that observing violence leads to increased risk for further aggression and violence[92,95,196] and that aggressive parents tend to produce aggressive children.[10,54,59,120]

However, modeling does not fully explain the consequences of childhood victimization. The hypothesis that children model their parents' behavior and thus learn violent behavior in itself is not adequate as an explanation of adult violence. Alone, this explanation would have a difficult time explaining the fact that although girls are more likely to be sexually abused than boys, females rarely commit sexual abuse as adults. On the other hand, modeling may explain a predisposition to behave in aggressive or violent ways, whose specific manifestation may be a function of characteristics outlined as important in the earlier discussion of assumptions.

Failure in Attachment

Bowlby's[18,19] attachment theory has also influenced explanations of developmental outcomes of abused and neglected children. The assumption is that infants develop an "internal working model" of the world which functions as a framework for further interaction with the physical and interpersonal environment and involves expectations about the way the world functions.[3] Attachment provides a secure base from which to explore, develop, and solve problems. Inconsistent, haphazard care or rejection of the infant may lead to the development of an insecure-avoidant child, likely to interpret neutral or even friendly behavior as hostile and to show inappropriate aggressive behavior.

Dodge et al. have suggested that the experience of physical abuse leads to chronic aggressive behavior by promoting development of an internal working model of the world that includes hostile social-information-processing patterns. They suggest that the experience of severe physical harm is associated with later violent behavior through the "acquisition of a set of biased and deficient patterns of processing social provocative information."[46,p1679] They found that physically harmed 4-year-old children showed deviant patterns of processing social information at age 5 and that these patterns were related to aggressive behavior.

As Cicchetti, Toth, and Lynch noted, "attachment theory provides a framework within which to conceptualize an expanding relational network that is organized around explicit styles of interaction and that ultimately reflects, in relational style, the original family members (i.e., the parents) that set the emotional tone for subsequent family development."[34] In a family system that accepts violence and intimidation as a viable strategy, the parent may be the victimizer (of the child) and also the victim.

Bodily Changes

The experiences of early abuse and neglect may lead to bodily changes that, in turn, relate to the development of antisocial behavior and aggression. As a result of being beaten continually, a child might become desensitized to future painful or anxiety-provoking experiences. This desensitization might influence the child's later behavior, making him or her less emotionally and physiologically responsive to the needs of others, callous and lacking in empathy, and lacking remorse or guilt. On the other hand, this desensitization might also work to protect the individual in later life, by providing certain "steeling" effects with which to overcome stress and adverse life events. Whether desensitization occurs and whether it serves a positive or negative function remains unanswered empirically.

If the stress of abuse or neglect occurs during critical periods of development, it may give rise to abnormal brain chemistry, which may in turn lead to aggressive behavior at later points in life.[56] It is also possible that childhood victimization and later behaviors are related in part through brain neurotransmitters.[108] Studies of nonhuman primates have suggested that rearing experiences may be associated with changes in central nervous system neurotransmitter activity in both norepinephrine and serotonin monamine systems.[90] Research findings indicate that rearing conditions affect reactivity, which influences levels of both norepinephrine and serotonin.[89] Peer-reared monkeys (a laboratory analogue to being neglected or reared without parental figures) showed aggressive behavior and low levels of 5-HIAA (a crude indicator of serotonin turnover) and consumed significantly more alcohol than mother-reared controls.[89] While the extent to which findings from this work on nonhuman primates can be generalized to humans is not known, this research holds promise for understanding individual differences in reactivity and behavior. It may be particularly useful in examining mechanisms by which childhood victimization leads to later dysfunctional behavior, given the ethical constraints of comparable research with humans.

Maladaptive Styles of Coping

Abuse or neglect may lead to the development of certain styles of coping that might be less than adaptive. For example, early abuse or neglect might encourage the development of impulsive behavioral styles that are related to deficiencies in problem-solving skills, inadequate school performance, or less than adequate functioning in occupational spheres.

Substance abuse is another maladaptive—and prevalent—style of coping. Researchers have speculated that substance abuse may serve a number of coping functions for abused and neglected children:

- to escape emotionally and/or psychologically from an abusive environment or from depression[49,78,83,98,199]
- to reduce feelings of isolation and loneliness[166]
- to self-medicate[2,30,42,49,83,84,113,166]
- to increase self-esteem[44]

Some forms of coping that appear less than adaptive may be adaptive under certain circumstances. For example, running away from home may be an effective means of coping with an abusive home situation, although it may ultimately place the child at higher risk of exposure to subsequent victimization and negative relationships. Dysfunctional behaviors such as substance use and abuse or running away may provide escape for abused and neglected children; however, these surface solutions to problems at one stage may lead ultimately to more deeply entrenched problems at later ages. That is, adaptations that may appear functional at one point in a child's development (avoiding an abusive parent, desensitizing oneself against feelings, or running away) may later compromise the person's ability to draw upon the environment in a more adaptive and flexible way.

It is unclear whether abused and/or neglected children actually have inadequate coping skills due to maltreatment or whether inadequate coping skills are simply a function of behaviors or cognitive dysfunctions established at an earlier point in time. Early childhood victimization experiences may lead directly to altered patterns of behavior that are in place in rudimentary form during childhood but become manifest only some years later. Disordered patterns of adaptation may lie dormant, only to surface during times of increased stress or in conjunction with particular circumstances.[169]

Changes in Self-concept or Attributional Styles

Childhood victimization may alter the child's self-concept, attitudes, or attributional styles; this change may then influence the person's response to later situations. For example, the clinical literature has identified low self-esteem as one of the major characteristics of childhood victims.[8,40,85] Lowered self-esteem may result from childhood victimization directly, caused by the child's feelings of low self-worth, derived from the idea that he or she was somehow responsible for the abuse or neglect. Low self-esteem may also be indirectly related to abuse and neglect as a by-product of lowered cognitive functioning and poor social and interpersonal skills.

Changed Environments or Chain of Events

Finally, problem behaviors may result from the chain of events that occur subsequent to the victimization, rather than from the victimization experience itself. For example, child abuse and/or neglect may lead to changes in environment or family conditions and render the child at increased risk for running away, delinquency, or other problem behaviors.

CONCLUSIONS

The study of childhood victimization has been developing rapidly, with heightened recognition of the need for more sophisticated and controlled research designs. At the same time, findings from an increasing number of studies suggest the need for multidimensional models to explain the consequences of childhood victimization. A modified ecological model is presented here, incorporating a combination of internal and external factors and explicitly recognizing that behavior (functional and dysfunctional) occurs in a social context. Research is needed to disentangle and test some of these complex relationships. Analytic strategies need to be developed to deal with these embedded models and multiple possible outcomes, which may differ by gender, ethnicity, or age at the time of childhood victimization. We need to examine the role of protective factors and to determine whether they function for abused and neglected children as they do with nonvictimized children. Finally, we need further research that systematically examines mechanisms whereby childhood victimization is linked to subsequent outcomes.

REFERENCES

1. Adams-Tucker C. Proximate effects of sexual abuse in childhood: A report on 28 children. *Am J Psychiatry* 1982;139:1252–1256.
2. Agnew R. Toward a general strain theory. *Crim* 1992;30:47–87.
3. Ainsworth MDS, Blehar MC, Waters E, et al. *Patterns of attachment.* Hillsdale, NJ: Lawrence Erlbaum Associates. 1978.
4. Allen DM, Tarnowski KJ. Depressive characteristics of physically abused children. *J Abnorm Child Psychol* 1989;17:1–11.

5. Anderson G, Yasenik L, Ross CA. Dissociative experiences and disorders among women who identify themselves as sexual abuse survivors. *Child Abuse Negl* 1993;17:677–686.

6. Augoustinos M. Developmental effects of child abuse: Recent findings. *Child Abuse Negl* 1987;11:15–27.

7. Bagley C, Ramsay R. Sexual abuse in childhood: Psychosocial outcomes and implications for social work practice. *J Soc Work Hum Sexuality* 1986;4:1–2,33–47.

8. Bagley C, Young L. Juvenile prostitution and child sexual abuse: A controlled study. *Can J Comm Ment Health* 1987;6:5–26.

9. Bandura A. *Aggression: A social learning analysis.* Englewood Cliffs, NJ: Prentice-Hall. 1973.

10. Bandura A, Walters RH. *Adolescent aggression.* New York: Ronald. 1959.

11. Bates JE. The concept of difficult temperament. *Merrill-Palmer Quarterly* 1980;26:299–319.

12. Bates JE. In Kohnstamm GA, Bates JE, Rothbart MK (eds.), *Temperament in childhood,* 321. Chichester, England: Wiley. 1989.

13. Bath HI, Haapala DA. Intensive family preservation services with abused and neglected children: An examination of group differences. *Child Abuse Negl* 1993;17:213–225.

14. Beitchman JH, Zucker KJ, Hood JE, et al. A review of the short-term effects of childhood sexual abuse. *Child Abuse Negl* 1991;15:537–556.

15. Beitchman JH, Zucker KJ, Hood JE, et al. A review of the long-term effects of child sexual abuse. *Child Abuse Negl* 1992;16:101–118.

16. Belsky J. Child maltreatment: An ecological integration. *Am Psychol* 1981;35:320–335.

17. Berliner L. Effects of sexual abuse on children. *Violence Update* 1991;1:1,8,10–11.

18. Bowlby J. Forty-four juvenile thieves. *Int J Psychoanal* 1944;25:107–128.

19. Bowlby J. *Maternal care and mental health.* Geneva: World Health Organization. 1951.

20. Braver M, Bumberry J, Green K, et al. Childhood abuse and current psychological functioning in a university counseling center population. *J Coun Psychol* 1992;39:252–257.

21. Briere J. Methodological issues in the study of sexual abuse effects. *J Consult Clin Psychol* 1992;60:196–203.

22. Briere J, Runtz M. Symptomatology associated with childhood sexual victimization in a nonclinical adult sample. *Child Abuse Negl* 1988;12:51–59.

23. Briere J, Runtz M. Childhood sexual abuse: Long-term sequelae and implications for psychological assessment. Special issue: Research on treatment of adults sexually abused in childhood. *J Interpers Viol* 1993;8:312–330.

24. Bronfenbrenner U. *The ecology of human development.* Cambridge: Harvard University Press. 1977.

25. Brook JS, Whiteman M, Finch S. Role of mutual attachment in drug use: A longitudinal study. *J Am Acad Child Adolesc Psychiatry* 1993;32:982–989.

26. Browne A, Finkelhor D. Impact of child sexual abuse: A review of the research. *Psychol Bull* 1986;99:66–77.

27. Burnam MA, Stein JA, Golding JM, et al. Sexual assault and mental disorders in a community population. *J Consult Clin Psychol* 1988;56:843–850.

28. Butler JR, Burton LM. Rethinking teenage childbearing: Is sexual abuse a missing link? *Fam Rel* 1990;39:73–80.

29. Cavaiola A, Schiff M. Behavioral sequelae of physical and/or sexual abuse in adolescents. *Child Abuse Negl* 1988;12:181–188.

30. Cavaiola A, Schiff M. Self-esteem in abused chemically dependent children. *Child Abuse Negl* 1989;13:327–334.

31. Chu JA, Dill DL. Dissociative symptoms in relation to childhood physical and sexual abuse. *Am J Psychiatry* 1990;147:887–892.

32. Cicchetti D, Carlson V (eds.). *Child maltreatment: Theory and research on the causes and consequences of child abuse and neglect.* New York: Cambridge University Press. 1989.

33. Cicchetti D, Rizley R. Developmental perspectives on the etiology, intergenerational transmission, and sequelae of child maltreatment. *New Dir Child Dev* 1981;11:31–55.

34. Cicchetti D, Toth SL, Lynch M. The developmental sequelae of child maltreatment: Implica-

tions for war-related trauma. In Leavitt LA, Fox NA (eds.), *The psychological effects of war and violence on children.* Hillsdale, NJ: Lawrence Erlbaum Associates. 1993.

35. Comer J. *Beyond black and white.* New York: Quadrangle. 1972.

36. Conte JR, Schuerman JR. Factors associated with an increased impact of child sexual abuse. *Child Abuse Negl* 1987;11:201–211.

37. Conte JR, Schuerman JR. The effects of sexual abuse on children: A multidimensional view. *J Interpers Viol* 1988;2:380–390.

38. Coons PM, Milstein V. Psychosexual disturbances in multiple personality: Characteristics, etiology, and treatment. *J Clin Psychiatry* 1986;47:106–110.

39. Coulton CJ, Korbin J, Su M, et al. Community level factors and child maltreatment rates. Unpublished paper, Center for Urban Poverty and Social Change, Mandel School of Applied Social Sciences, Case Western Reserve, Cleveland, OH. 1995.

40. Courtois CA. The incest experience and its aftermath. *Victimology* 1979;4:337–347.

41. Crittendon PM, Ainsworth MDS. Child maltreatment and attachment theory. In Cicchetti D, Carlson V (eds.), 432. *Child maltreatment.* New York: Cambridge University Press. 1989.

42. Dembo R, Dertke M, Borders S, et al. The relationship between physical and sexual abuse and tobacco, alcohol and illicit drug use among youths in a juvenile detention center. *Int J Addict* 1988;23:351–378.

43. Dembo R, Williams L, La Voie L, et al. Physical abuse, sexual victimization, and illicit drug use: Replication of a structural analysis among a new sample of high-risk youths. *Violence Vict* 1989;4:121–137.

44. Dembo R, Williams L, La Voie L, et al. A longitudinal study of the relationship among alcohol use, marijuana/hashish use, cocaine use, and emotional/psychological functioning problems in a cohort of high risk youths. *Int J Addict* 1990;25:1341–1382.

45. DeWilde EJ, Kienhorst IC, Diekstra RF, et al. The relationship between adolescent suicidal behavior and life events in childhood and adolescence. *Am J Psychiatry* 1992;149:45–51.

46. Dodge KA, Bates JE, Pettit GS. Mechanisms in the cycle of violence. *Science* 1990;250(21 December):1678–1683.

47. Dohrenwend BP, Dohrenwend BS. Sex differences in psychiatric disorders. *Am J Sociology* 1976;81:1447–1459.

48. Downey G, Feldman S, Khuri J, et al. Maltreatment and childhood depression. In Reynolds WM, Johnson HF (eds.), *Handbook of depression in children and adolescents.* New York: Plenum Press. 1994.

49. Downs WR, Miller BA, Testa M. The impact of childhood victimization experiences on women's drug use. Paper presented at the annual meeting of the American Society of Criminology, San Francisco, CA, November 20–23, 1991.

50. Drillen CM. *The growth and development of the prematurely born infant.* Baltimore: Williams and Wilkins. 1964.

51. Dubowitz H, Black M, Harrington D, et al. A follow-up study of behavior problems associated with child sexual abuse. *Child Abuse Negl* 1993;17:743–754.

52. Dubowitz H, Black M, Starr RH, et al. A conceptual definition of child neglect. *Crim Just Behav* 1993;20(1):8–26.

53. Dykes L. The whiplash shaken infant syndrome: What has been learned? *Child Abuse Negl* 1986;10:211–221.

54. Egeland BE, Sroufe LA. Attachment and early maltreatment. *Child Dev* 1981;52:44–52.

55. Egeland BE, Sroufe LA, Erickson M. The developmental consequences of different patterns of maltreatment. *Child Abuse Negl* 1983;7:459–469.

56. Eichelman B. Neurochemical and psychopharmacologic aspects of aggressive behavior. *Annu Rev Med* 1990;41:149–158.

57. Elmer E. *Children in jeopardy: A study of abused minors and their families.* Pittsburgh: University of Pittsburgh Press. 1967.

58. Eme RF. Sex-related differences in the epidemiology of child psychopathology. In Widom CS (ed.), *Sex roles and psychopathology,* 279. New York: Plenum. 1984.

59. Eron L, Walder LO, Lefkowitz MM. *Learning aggression in children.* Boston: Little Brown. 1971.

60. Famularo R, Fenton T, Kinscherff R, et al. Maternal and child posttraumatic stress disorder in cases of child maltreatment. *Child Abuse Negl* 1994;18:27–36.

61. Farber EA, Egeland B. Invulnerability among abused and neglected children. In Anthony EJ, Cohler B (eds.) *The invulnerable child,* 253. New York: Guilford. 1987.

62. Farrington DP. Childhood aggression and adult violence: Early precursors and later life outcomes. In Pepler DJ, Rubin KH (eds.), *The development and treatment of childhood aggression.* Hillsdale, NJ: Lawrence Erlbaum Associates. 1991.

63. Feshbach S. Child abuse and the dynamics of human aggression and violence. In Gerbner J, Ross CJ, Zigler E (eds.), *Child abuse: An agenda for action.* New York: Oxford University Press. 1980.

64. Finkelhor D. *Sexually victimized children.* New York: Free Press. 1979.

65. Finkelhor D. Early and long-term effects of child sexual abuse: An update. *Prof Psychol: Res Pract* 1990;21:325–330.

66. Friedrich W, Boriskin JA. The role of the child in abuse: A review of the literature. *Am J Orthopsychiatry* 1976;46:580–590.

67. Friedrich WH, Einbender AJ, Luecke WJ. Cognitive and behavioral characteristics of physically abused children. *J Consult Clin Psychol* 1983;51:313–314.

68. Friedrich WH, Urquiza AJ, Beilke RL. Behavior problems in sexually abused young children. *J Pediatr Psychol* 1986;11:47–57.

69. Frodi A, Smetana J. Abused, neglected, and nonmaltreated preschoolers' ability to discriminate emotions in others: The effects of IQ. *Child Abuse Negl* 1984;8:459–465.

70. Galler JR, Ramsey F, Solimano G, et al. The influence of malnutrition on subsequent behavioral development. II. Classroom behavior. *J Am Acad Child Psychiatry* 1983;24:16–22.

71. Garbarino J. The human ecology of child maltreatment: A conceptual model for research. *J Marr Fam* 1977;39:721–735.

72. Garbarino J, Crouter A. Defining the community context for parent-child relations: The correlates of child maltreatment. *Child Dev* 1978;49(3):604–616.

73. Garbarino J, Plantz M. Part I: Review of the literature. In Gray E, Garbarino J, Planz M (eds.), *Child abuse: Prelude to delinquency?,* 5. Washington, DC: U.S. Department of Justice, Office of Juvenile Justice and Delinquency Prevention. 1986. (Findings of a research conference conducted by the National Committee for Prevention of Child Abuse, 7–10 April 1984.)

74. Garbarino J, Sherman D. High-risk neighborhoods and high-risk families: The human ecology of child maltreatment. *Child Dev* 1980;51(1):188–198.

75. Garmezy N. Children under stress: Perspectives on antecedents and correlates of vulnerability and resistance to psychopathology. In Rabin AI, Arnoff J, Barclay AM, et al (eds.), *Further explorations in personality.* New York: Wiley. 1981.

76. Garmezy N, Masten A, Tellegen A. The study of stress and competence in children: A building block for developmental psychopathology. *Child Dev* 1984;55:97–111.

77. Gibbin PT, Starr RH, Agronow SW. Affective behavior of abused and control children: Comparison of parent-child interactions and the influence of home environment variables. *J Genet Psychol* 1984;144:69–82.

78. Gomes-Schwartz B, Horowitz JM, Sauzier M. Severity of emotional distress among sexually abused preschool, school-age, and adolescent children. *Hosp Comm Psychiatry* 1985;36:503–508.

79. Green AH. Self-destructive behavior in battered children. *Am J Psychiatry* 1978;135:579–582.

80. Gutierres S, Reich JA. A developmental perspective on runaway behavior: Its relationship to child abuse. *Child Welfare* 1981;60:89–94.

81. Harris T, Brown GW, Bifulco A. Loss of parent in childhood and adult psychiatric disorder: A tentative overall model. *Dev Psychopathol* 1990;2:311–328.

82. Harrison PA, Edwall GE, Hoffmann NG, et al. Correlates of sexual abuse among boys in treatment for chemical dependency. *J Adolesc Chem Depend* 1990;1:53–67.

83. Harrison PA, Hoffmann NG, Edwall GE. Sexual abuse correlates: Similarities between male and female adolescents in chemical dependency treatment. *J Adolesc Res* 1989;4:385–399.

84. Harrison PA, Hoffmann NG, Edwall GE. Differential drug use patterns among sexually abused adolescent girls in treatment for chemical dependency. *Int J Addict* 1989;24:499–514.

85. Herman J. *Father-daughter incest.* Cambridge: Harvard University Press. 1981.

86. Herman J, Hirschman L. Father-daughter incest. *Signs* 1977;2:735–756.

87. Herrenkohl RC, Herrenkohl EC. Some antecedents and developmental consequences of child maltreatment. In Rizley R, Cicchetti D (eds.), *New directions for child development, developmental perspectives on child maltreatment,* 11:57. San Francisco: Jossey-Bass. 1981.

88. Hetherington EM. Divorce, a child's perspective. *Ann Prog Child Psychiatry Child Dev* 1980;1980:277–291.

89. Higley JD, Hasert MF, Suomi SF, et al. A nonhuman primate model of alcohol abuse: Effects of early experience, personality and stress on alcohol consumption. *Proc Natl Acad Sci USA* 1991;88(16):7261–7265.

90. Higley JD, Suomi SJ. Temperamental reactivity in non-human primates. In Kohnstamm GA, Bates JE, Rothbart MK (eds.), *Temperament in childhood,* 153. New York: John Wiley. 1989.

91. Horwitz AV, White HR. Gender role orientations and styles of pathology among adolescents. *J Health Soc Behav* 1987;28:158–170.

92. Huesmann LR, Eron LD, Lefkowitz MM, et al. Stability of aggression over time and generation. *J Abnorm Psychol* 1984;20:1120–1134.

93. Hussey DL, Singer M. Psychological distress, problem behaviors, and family functioning of sexually abused adolescent inpatients. *J Am Acad Child Adolesc Psychiatry* 1993;32:954–961.

94. Ireland T, Widom CS. Childhood victimization and risk for alcohol and drug arrests. *Int J Addict* 1994;29:235–274.

95. Kalmuss D. The intergenerational transmission of marital aggression. *J Marr Fam* 1984;46:11–19.

96. Kaufman J. Depressive disorders in maltreated children. *J Am Acad Child Adolesc Psychiatry* 1991;30:257–265.

97. Kaufman J, Zigler E. Do abused children become abusive parents? *Am J Orthopsychiatry* 1987;57:186–192.

98. Kazdin A, Moser J, Colbus D, et al. Depressive symptoms among physically abused and psychiatrically disturbed children. *J Abnorm Psychol* 1985;94:298–307.

99. Kendall-Tackett KA, Williams LM, Finkelhor DJ. The impact of sexual abuse on children: A review and synthesis of recent empirical studies. *Psychol Bull* 1993;113:164–180.

100. Kinard EM. Emotional development in physically abused children. *Am J Orthopsychiatry* 1980;50:686–696.

101. Kluft RP (ed.). *Childhood antecedents of multiple personality.* Washington, DC: American Psychiatric Press. 1985.

102. Kolko DJ, Moser JT, Weldy SR. Medical/health histories and physical evaluation of physically and sexually abused child psychiatric patients: A controlled study. *J Fam Viol* 1990;5(4):249–267.

103. Korbin JE. The cross-cultural context of child abuse and neglect. In Kempe CH, Helfer RE (eds.), *The battered child,* 3rd ed., 21. Chicago: University of Chicago Press. 1980.

104. Ladwig GB, Anderson MD. Substance abuse in women: Relationship between chemical dependency of women and past reports of physical abuse and/or sexual abuse. *Int J Addict* 1989;24:739–754.

105. Laumann EO, Gagnon JH, Michael RT, et al. *The social organization of sexuality: Sexual practices in the United States.* Chicago: University of Chicago Press. 1994.

106. Lazarus RS, Launier R. Stress-related transactions between person and environment. In Pervin LA, Lewis M (eds.), *Perspectives in interactional psychology.* New York: Plenum. 1978.

107. Leung SMR, Carter JE. Cross-cultural study of child abuse among Chinese, Native Indians, and Anglo-Canadian children. *J Psychiatr Treat Eval* 1983;5:37–44.

108&109. Lewis DO. From abuse to violence: Psychophysiological consequences of maltreatment. *J Am Acad Child Adolesc Psychiatry* 1992;31:383–391.

110. Lewis DO, Pincus J, Shanok S, et al. Psychomotor epilepsy and violence in a group of incarcerated adolescent boys. *Am J Psychiatry* 1982;139:882–887.

111. Lewis DO, Shanok SS, Cohen RJ, et al. Race bias in the diagnosis and disposition of violent adolescents. *Am J Psychiatry* 1980;137:1211–1216.

112. Lewis DO, Shanok SS, Pincus JH, et al. Violent juvenile delinquents: Psychiatric, neurological, psychological, and abuse factors. *J Am Acad Child Adolesc Psychiatry* 1979;18:1161–1167.

113. Lindberg FH, Distad LJ. Survival responses to incest: Adolescents in crisis. *Child Abuse Negl* 1985;9:521–526.

114. Lipovsky JA, Saunders BE, Murphy SM. Depression, anxiety, and behavior problems among victims of father-child sexual assault and nonabused siblings. *J Interpers Viol* 1989;4:452–468.

115. Livingston R. Sexually and physically abused children. *J Am Acad Child Adolesc Psychiatry* 1987;26:413–415.

116. Luntz BK, Widom CS. Antisocial personality disorder in abused and neglected children grown up. *Am J Psychiatry* 1994;151:670–674.

117. Lynch MA, Roberts J. *Consequences of child abuse.* New York: Academic Press. 1982.

118. Maccoby EE. Social-emotional development and response to stressors. In Rutter M, Garmezy N (eds.), *Stress, coping, and development in children.* New York: McGraw-Hill. 1983.

119. Magnusson D, Torestad B. A holistic view of personality: A model revisited. *Annu Rev Psychol* 1993;44:427–452.

120. Main M, Goldwyn R. Predicting rejection of her infant from mother's representation of her own experience: Implications for the abused-abusing intergenerational cycle. *Child Abuse Negl* 1984;8(2):203–217.

121. Mannarino AP, Cohen JA. A clinical-demographic study of sexually abused children. *Child Abuse Negl* 1987;10:17–23.

122. Martin HA, Beezley P, Conway EF, et al. The development of abused children. *Adv Pediatr* 1974;21:25–73.

123. Martin JA, Elmer EE. Battered children grown up: A follow-up study of individuals severely maltreated as children. *Child Abuse Negl* 1992;16:75–88.

124. McCord J. A forty-year perspective on effects of child abuse and neglect. *Child Abuse Negl* 1983;7:265–270.

125. McCubbin HI, Patterson JM. The family stress process: The double ABCX Model of adjustment and adaptation. *Marr Fam Rev* 1983;6:7–37.

126. McGaha JE. Alcoholism and the chemically dependent family: A study of adult felons on probation. *J Offend Rehabil* 1993;19(3/4):57–69.

127. McLeer SV, Callaghan M, Henry D, et al. Psychiatric disorders in sexually abused children. *J Am Acad Child Adolesc Psychiatry* 1994;33:313–319.

128. Meiselman K. *Incest.* San Francisco: Jossey-Bass. 1978.

129. Miller B. Investigating links between childhood victimization and alcohol problems. In Martin SE (ed.), *Alcohol and interpersonal violence: Fostering multidisciplinary perspectives.* Rockville, MD: U.S. Government Printing Office; NIH Publication No. 93–3496 (NIAAA Research Monograph No. 24). 1993.

130. Miller B, Downs W, Gondoli D. Delinquency, childhood violence, and the development of alcoholism in women. *Crime and Delinquency* 1989;35:94–108.

131. Miller B, Downs W, Gondoli D, et al. The role of childhood sexual abuse in the development of alcoholism in women. *Violence Vict* 1987;2:157–172.

132. Milner JS. Physical child abuse perpetrator screening and evaluation. Special Issue: Physical child abuse. *Crim Just Behav* 1991;18:47–63.

133. Morse CW, Sahler OJ, Friedman SB. A 3-year follow-up study of abused and neglected children. *Am J Dis Child* 1970;120:439–446.

134. National Research Council, Committee on Behavioral and Social Sciences. *Losing generations: Adolescents in high-risk settings.* Washington, DC: National Academy Press. 1993.

135. Newberger CM, Gremy IM. The role of clinical and institutional interventions in children's recovery from sexual abuse. Paper presented at the Fourth International Family Violence Research Conference, 21–24 July 1995, Durham, NH.

136. Newberger EH, Newberger CM, Hampton RL. Child abuse: The current theory base and future research needs. *J Am Acad Child Psychiatry* 1983;22:262–268.

137. Newberger EH, Reed RB, Daniel JH, et al. Pediatric social illness: Toward an etiological classification. *Pediatrics* 1977;50:178–185.

138. Norris FH. Epidemiology of trauma: Frequency and impact of different potentially traumatic events on different demographic groups. *J Consult Clin Psychol* 1992;60:409–418.

139. Olweus D. Stability of aggressive reaction patterns in males: A review. *Psychol Bull* 1979; 86:852–875.

140. Patterson GR, Debaryshe BD, Ramsey E. A developmental perspective on antisocial behavior. *Am Psychol* 1989;44:329–335.

141. Pelcovitz D, Kaplan S, Goldenberg B, et al. Post-traumatic stress disorder in physically abused adolescents. *J Am Acad Child Adolesc Psychiatry* 1994;33:305–312.

142. Perez C, Widom CS. Childhood victimization and long-term intellectual and academic outcomes. *Child Abuse Negl* 1994;18:617–633.

143. Peters JJ. Children who are victims of sexual assault and the psychology of offenders. *Am J Psychother* 1976;30:398–421.

144. Peters SD. *The relationship between childhood sexual victimization and adult depression among Afro-American and white women.* Ph.D. diss., University of California, Los Angeles, 1984.

145. Polansky NA, Gaudin JM, Ammons PW, et al: The psychological ecology of the neglectful mother. *Child Abuse Negl* 1985;9(2):265–275.

146. Putnam FW. Dissociation as a response to extreme trauma. In Kluft RP (ed.), *The childhood antecedents of multiple personality.* Washington, DC: American Psychiatric Press. 1985.

147. Putnam FW, Guroff JJ, Silberman EK, et al. The clinical phenomenology of multiple personality disorder: A review of 100 recent cases. *J Clin Psychiatry* 1986;47:285–293.

148. Rivera B, Widom CS. Childhood victimization and violent offending. *Violence Vict* 1990;5:19–34.

149. Robins LN. Sturdy childhood predictors of adult antisocial behavior: Replications from longitudinal studies. *Psychol Med* 1978;8:611–622.

150. Robins LN, Regier DA (eds.). *Psychiatric disorders in America: The epidemiologic catchment area study.* New York: Free Press. 1991.

151. Roessler TA, McKenzie N. Effects of childhood trauma on psychological functioning in adults sexually abused as children. *J Nerv Ment Dis* 1994;182:145–150.

152. Root MP. Treatment failures: The role of sexual victimization in women's addictive behavior. *Am J Orthopsychiatry* 1989;59:542–549.

153. Rowan AB, Foy DW. Post-traumatic stress disorder in child sexual abuse survivors: A literature review. *J Trauma Stress* 1993;6:3–20.

154. Rowan AB, Foy DW, Rodriguez N, et al. Posttraumatic stress disorder in a clinical sample of adults sexually abused as children. *Child Abuse Negl* 1994;18:51–61.

155. Runyan DK, Gould CL, Trost DC, et al. Determinants of foster care placement for the maltreated child. *Child Abuse Negl* 1982;6:343–350.

156. Russell DEH. *The secret trauma: Incest in the lives of girls and women.* New York: Basic Books. 1986.

157. Rutter M. Epidemiological-longitudinal approaches to the study of development. In Collins WA (ed.). *The concept of development: Minnesota symposia on child psychology,* vol. 15. Hillsdale, NJ: Lawrence Erlbaum. 1982.

158. Rutter M. Stress, coping, and development: Some issues and some questions. In Garmezy N, Rutter M (eds.), 1. *Stress, coping, and development in children.* New York: McGraw-Hill. 1983.

159. Sadeh A, Hayden RM, McGuire JP, et al. Somatic, cognitive and emotional characteristics of abused children in a psychiatric hospital. *Child Psychiatry Hum Dev* 1994;24:191–200.

160. Sandgrund A, Gaines RW, Green AH. Child abuse and mental retardation: A problem of cause and effect. *J Ment Def* 1974;79:327–330.

161. Saunders EA. Rorschach indicators of chronic childhood sexual abuse in female borderline inpatients. *Bull Menninger Clin* 1991;55:48–71.

162. Seagull EAW. Social support and child maltreatment: A review of the evidence. *Child Abuse Negl* 1987;11:41–52.

163. Sedney MA, Brooks B. Factors associated with a history of childhood sexual experience in a nonclinical female population. *J Am Acad Child Adolesc Psychiatry* 1984;23:215–218.

164. Shure MB, Spivack G. Interpersonal problem-solving in young children: A cognitive approach to prevention. *Am J Community Psychol* 1982;10:341.

165. Silver LR, Dublin CC, Lourie RS. Does violence breed violence? Contributions from a study of the child abuse syndrome. *Am J Psychiatry* 1969;126:152–155.

166. Singer M, Petchers M, Hussey D. The relationship between sexual abuse and substance abuse among psychiatrically hospitalized adolescents. *Child Abuse Negl* 1989;13:319–325.

167. Sirles EA, Smith JA, Kusama H. Psychiatric status of intrafamilial child sexual abuse victims. *J Am Acad Child Adolesc Psychiatry* 1989;28:225–229.

168. Smith CP, Berkman DJ, Fraser WM. *A preliminary national assessment of child abuse and neglect and the juvenile justice system: The shadows of distress.* Washington, DC: Office of Juvenile Justice and Delinquency Prevention. 1980.

169. Sroufe LA, Rutter M. The domain of developmental psychopathology. *Child Dev* 1984; 55:17–29.

170. Straus MA, Gelles RJ, Steinmetz SK. *Behind closed doors: Violence in the American family.* Garden City, NY: Anchor Press. 1980.

171. Terr LA. Chowchilla revisited: The effects of psychiatric trauma four years after a school bus kidnapping. *Am J Psychiatry* 1983;140:1543–1550.

172. Tong L, Oates K, McDowell M. Personality development following sexual abuse. *Child Abuse Negl* 1987;11:371–383.

173. Toray T, Coughlin C, Vuchinich S, et al. Gender differences associated with adolescent substance abuse: Comparisons and implications for treatment. *Fam Rel* 1991;40:338–344.

174. Tremblay RE, McCord J, Pulkkinen L, et al. Treating antisocial child behavior. Paper presented at the Third Symposium of Violence and Aggression, Saskatoon, Saskatchewan, 24–27 June 1990.

175. Tsai M, Feldman-Summers S, Edgar M: Childhood molestation: Variables related to differential impact of psychosexual functioning in adult women. *J Abnorm Psychol* 1979;88:407–417.

176. Van Hasselt VB, Ammerman RT, Glancy LJ, et al. Maltreatment in psychiatrically hospitalized dually diagnosed adolescent substance abusers. *J Am Acad Child Adolesc Psychiatry* 1992; 31:868–874.

177. Wallen J, Berman K. Possible indicators of childhood sexual abuse for individuals in substance abuse treatment. *J Child Sexual Abuse* 1992;1:63–74.

178. Wallerstein JS. Children of divorce: Stress and developmental tasks. In Garmezy N, Rutter M (eds.), *Stress, coping and development in children.* New York: McGraw-Hill. 1983.

179. Wallerstein JS, Kelly JB. Effects of divorce on the visiting father-child relationship. *Am J Psychiatry* 1980;137:1534–1539.

180. Walsh BW, Rosen P. *Self-mutilation: Theory, research, and treatment.* New York: Guilford. 1988.

181. Webster-Stratton C. Stress: A potential disruptor of parent perceptions and family interactions. *J Consult Clin Psychol* 1990;19(4):302–312.

182. Werner EE. Vulnerability and resiliency among children at risk for delinquency. Paper presented at the annual meeting of the American Society of Criminology, Denver, CO, 1983.

183. Werner EE, Smith RS. *Vulnerable but invincible: A longitudinal study of resilient children and youth.* New York: McGraw-Hill. 1982.

184. White SO, Straus MA. The implications of family violence for rehabilitation strategies. In Martin SE, Sechrest LB, Redner R (eds.), *New directions in the rehabilitation of criminal offenders.* Washington, DC: National Academy Press. 1981.

185. Widom CS. Sex roles, criminality, and psychopathology. In Widom CS (ed.), *Sex roles and psychopathology.* New York: Plenum Press. 1984.

186. Widom CS. Child abuse, neglect, and violent criminal behavior. *Crim* 1989;27:251–271.

187. Widom CS. The cycle of violence. *Science* 1989;244:160–166.

188. Widom CS. Does violence beget violence? A critical examination of the literature. *Psychol Bull* 1989;106(1):3–28.

189. Widom CS. The role of placement experiences in mediating the criminal consequences of early childhood victimization. *Am J Orthopsychiatry* 1991;6:195–209.

190. Widom CS. Childhood victimization and risk for adolescent problem behaviors. In Lamb ME, Ketterlinus R (eds.), *Adolescent problem behaviors.* New York: Erlbaum. 1994.

191. Widom CS, Ames MA. Criminal consequences of childhood sexual victimization. *Child Abuse Negl* 1994;18:303–318.

192. Widom CS, Ireland T, Glynn PJ. Alcohol abuse in abused and neglected children followed up: Are they at increased risk? *J Stud Alcohol* 1995;56:207–217.

193. Wodarski JS, Kurtz PD, Gaudin JM, et al. Maltreatment and the school-age child: Major academic, socioemotional and adaptive outcomes. *Soc Work Res Abstr* 1990;35:506–513.

194. Wolfe DA. *Child abuse: Implications for child development and psychopathology.* Newbury Park, CA: Sage. 1987.

195. Wolfe DA. *Preventing physical and emotional abuse of children.* New York: Guilford. 1991.

196. Wolfe DA, Jaffe P, Wilson SK, et al. Children of battered women: The relation of child behavior to family violence and maternal stress. *J Consult Clin Psychol* 1985;53:657–665.

197. Wolfe VV, Gentile C, Wolfe DA. The impact of sexual abuse on children: A PTSD formulation. *Behav Ther* 1989;20:215–228.

198. Wyatt GE. Sexual abuse of ethnic minority children: Identifying dimensions of victimization. *Prof Psychol: Res Pract* 1990;21:338–343.

199. Yamaguchi K, Kandel DB. Patterns of drug use from adolescence to early adulthood—III. Predictors of progression. *Am J Public Health* 1984;74:673–681.

200. Yarrow MR, Campbell JD, Burton RV. Recollections of childhood: A study of the retrospective method. *Monogr Soc Res Child Dev* 1970;135.

201. Zimrin H. A profile of survival. *Child Abuse Negl* 1986;10:339–349.

Chapter 25

Child Abuse Treatment Research: Current Concerns and Challenges

Cris Ratiner, Ph.D.

While research literature about child abuse has grown tremendously in recent years, little attention has been given specifically to treatment issues. Research in the field, which is disproportionately weighted toward the area of sexual abuse, must deal with the heterogenous nature of child maltreatment, which presents obstacles to meaningful research. Other barriers to research are methodological, economic, and logistical. Although there have been calls for narrowing the focus of research in order to yield quantifiable results, an equal case can be made for widening the scope of treatment research so that diverse and far-ranging effects of abuse can be taken into account. Also needed is a bridge between the empirical literature and the working world of practitioners, as well as a discussion of the viability of abuse-specific treatment. One of the greatest impediments to good treatment research today is the increasing control of managed care in medicine, which makes long-term treatment unaffordable for many patients, encourages erroneous diagnostic classification for the purpose of reimbursement, and compromises research efforts with ongoing patients.

GENERAL CONSIDERATIONS

Research efforts into the incidence, prevalence, and consequences of child abuse have multiplied by staggering proportions over the last decade. Researchers and practitioners alike have made significant advances in the epidemiological characterization of child abuse and its associated effects. Inevitably, there has been a concommitant increase in the number of studies devoted to the treatment of child abuse. Yet, this number still represents only a small percentage of the body of child abuse research.[23]

The previous chapters in this text have described current thinking about the treatment of child abuse, with unqualified appeals for further research. The field of childhood trauma is rife with complexities and unanswered questions. Professionals who treat traumatized children are plagued by unavoidable doubt and uncertainty. It is not surprising that the impediments to meaningful research in the treatment of child abuse and neglect are no less imposing.

An inescapable feature of the treatment literature, and of all child abuse literature, which consistently confounds health professionals and researchers is the habit of tackling child abuse as if it were a homogenous phenomenon. It is not. The three traditional categories, physical abuse, neglect, and sexual abuse, have separate histories in the literature, with surprisingly little overlap. Within each of these major categories the call has gone out for multivariate research studies that differentiate particular treatments for different manifestations of each problem.

Another of the great inherent difficulties of conducting research in the treatment of child abuse is the temporal component. In addition to infinite variety in the type of traumatic injury, the limitless variations in course and development pose an extraordinary challenge to even the most obsessive researcher. Different patterns of abuse have elicited widely divergent recommendations. In this regard, the often heard cry for prospective, long-term, and delayed outcome studies assumes even more urgency. Recent studies that attempt to describe abused children's recall of traumatic events and subsequent treatment in adulthood are welcome breakthroughs.[27] Nevertheless, even the most tightly designed treatment studies to date have not been able to study the course of long-term treatment or to conduct outcome studies much after the conclusion of the treatment.[19]

DISPROPORTIONATE EMPHASIS ON SEXUAL ABUSE

The most striking feature of the treatment literature to date is its disproportionate emphasis on child sexual abuse versus other forms of maltreatment. There is no rationale for this imbalance, although speculation might suggest several contributing factors. First, the great attention paid to child sexual abuse in the culture at large, including the sensational media reports of particularly heinous or controversial cases, has undoubtedly played a role.[13] Second, unlike the acts of omission that constitute neglect, acts of commission such as sexually abusive behaviors may present the illusion of a discrete injury that can be studied and addressed. Third, the cultural ingrained difficulty dealing with anything of a sexual nature may play a role. Caring and dedicated child advocates may aggressively pursue its scientific investigation over the study of physical abuse or neglect in an attempt to allay additional anxiety regarding the sexual nature of the maltreatment.

This difference in degree of attention does not, however, reflect the incidence or severity of consequences among forms of child maltreatment. Physical abuse is reported to cause the death of thousands of children each year.[2] Neglect is reported to result in similarly appalling statistics. Multiple studies have shown life-long, severe dysfunction associated with both. One hopes that upcoming years will bring to the other, no less serious, areas of child maltreatment the same degree of scrutiny that has characterized the work on sexual abuse.

Within the category of child sexual abuse, a promising trend in the literature is the development of new theoretical models, such as the posttraumatic stress disorder model[15] and Finkelhor's traumagenic model,[18] as well as the expansion of older models, such as attachment theory,[1] developmental theory,[9] and social learning theory,[4] to include child abuse. The refinement of a theoretical perspective is the necessary first step to conducting meaningful quasi-experimental or experimental research.

Much of the criticism of published child sexual abuse treatment studies centers on methodological flaws that limit the validity and generalizability of the findings. Critics point out that the extant studies are primarily of small sample size, addressed to a highly specific program or treatment modality, and include no comparison group.[20] Further, there is a dearth of information regarding long-term outcome. These criticisms cannot be gainsaid; virtually all researchers would concur. Nevertheless, the risk in enumerating each and every methodological concern at the present time is that researchers will more narrowly restrict the foci of their studies to eliminate statistical problems, when overarching constructs and the multiple phenomena should be fully explicated. At present, there is a gap between the theoretical framing of sexual abuse treatment and the quasi-experimental single project studies being conducted. It is hoped that during the next decade, this tension will be eased.

At present, treatment for physical abuse has not been extensively researched, although physical abuse itself has been a focus of some attention for several decades. As physically abused children often present first and most emergently in hospitals or doctors' offices, reports of their presentation occur often in the medical arena, rather than the psychological one. From a psychological perspective, some of the most important contributions to the future of research have been made in the careful theoretical models presented and discussed by such authors as Bronfenbrenner,[7] Belsky,[3] and Cicchetti.[11]

An ecological focus has led to increased research into intergenerational transmission of abusive or violent behavior,[22] recidivism among families who have received intervention for child battering,[12] and parental attitudes toward physical punishment.[8] These investigations have prompted practitioners to attempt earlier intervention, to establish community-based treatments, and to tend towards familial intervention, including increased case management.

Attention has also been paid to the relationship between economic and societal stress and rates of physical abuse or intrafamilial violence. This has led to an increase in the proportion of studies that examine community-based treatment as well as parental education and treatment.[12] Family-based treatment, parent education programs, and therapeutic day care settings have also been instituted and assessed.[14]

These are all rich and potentially very rewarding avenues of investigation which we hope will continue to be examined in the future. As with other areas of the child maltreatment literature, the research does not address treatment within individual therapy settings. There is a huge array of treatment modalities being offered to physically abused children. One review documented seven different types of treatment: group psychotherapy, parent training, case management, psychodynamic treatment, problem-solving training, relaxation therapy, and stress reduction techniques.[25] Because many, many physically abused children find themselves referred to individual psychotherapists, who might practice any of these treatment approaches, it is vitally important to determine what the different types of treatment address and with what efficacy. In particular, it will be crucial to compare community interventions with individual or group therapies, since they are offered by different segments of the health care community and have not been examined with respect to each other.

The treatment of child neglect may be the least studied form of child abuse. The literature that does exist has often been presented in the context of social support analyses.[14] The social support interventions are based on the belief, derived in part from an ecological model of child maltreatment, that families lacking in support will be more likely in their isolation to violate social norms in their behavior, to express more frustration and anger toward their own members, and to have a higher risk of future child maltreatment. While many of the studies of social support or social networks show improved functioning when they are present, much of the research is equivocal. Clearly, the depth, breadth, and even quantity of research into the treatment of child neglect needs to be dramatically increased.

The small proportion of the literature that covers treatment in relation to the overall explosion in the child abuse literature as a whole is a troubling state of affairs, given that children are being referred for abuse treatment in record numbers.[16] An increasing number of the referrals for assessment and treatment appear at clinicians' doors and on answering machines, with requests for "child abuse expertise" or a "trauma evaluation." Partly in response to the growing sophistication of the field, but probably also in part to the demand, more and more clinicians of all disciplines are offering "child abuse treatment" or "trauma evaluations," but there is so little consensus about the scope of these services that even clinicians may not know what their colleagues are including under the rubric of abuse treatment. This leaves the public at an even greater loss. There is no single abuse treatment or even clinical consensus on what the varieties of abuse treatment might be, so it is often impossible for referring parties to know what to ask for or how to evaluate what is received.

OBSTACLES TO TREATMENT RESEARCH

Why are treatment studies so scarce? There are more potential impediments than could even be enumerated, let alone discussed, in a single book chapter. The legion of obstacles to treatment research includes methodological, economic, and logistical barriers to even the most rudimentary assimilation of information. Rather than cataloguing these impediments it might be worthwhile to highlight some of the thornier problems existing at the present time.

Much of the empirical research does not originate in a clinical perspective. It tries to identify and track symptom patterns that accompany the presence of documented abuse or neglect. While this is important, it does not speak to the clinician's plight in the trenches. So, while most clinicians use the empirical literature to inform their ability to recognize child abuse, they do not find that it presents the benefits, weaknesses, prognostic expectations, or discussions of treatment course that they would find so helpful. The textbooks currently available advocating one particular type of treatment approach or another do so without empirical findings, and often with the author's candid acknowledgment of such.[21]

Perhaps, however, the authors who write these nonempirical texts are on the right track to establishing a viable research dialogue in the treatment of child abuse. The empirical literature stems from an epistemological point of view that seeks to isolate and describe individual symptom clusters and patterns with ever-increasing specificity. Clinical practice, however, with the possible exception of purely behavioral treatments (and even these include such nonsymptom-focused elements as patient-therapist rapport building), is not predicated on the clear-cut, sequential, or even always identifiable presentation of specific symptoms. Most psychotherapy practice is based on theories of personality and development that orchestrate the larger picture of the treatment goals and the nature of the treatment process as a whole.

There is at present no real bridge between the empirical literature and the working world of practitioners. While there are many cries for more quantifiable and less anecdotal material on treatment, it may be that at the present time we actually need more naturalistic studies documenting ongoing treatment. Some relevant questions might be:

- Who is getting referred, by whom, and for what?
- How are the children and their parents addressing treatment?
- Are children and their parents being seen separately?

- What is the course of treatment at each developmental stage, or for different traumatic conditions?
- What does the treatment process sound like?
- What does the patient look like after 10, 20, or 100 sessions?

Some of these questions might initially be better addressed by comprehensive field studies of current treatment, rather than by highly operationalized, narrowly defined studies, which often rest on as yet unproven assumptions.

Pursuing this line of inquiry raises the question of the validity of symptom-driven treatment methods. Few, if any, published articles raise and discuss the essential viability of abuse-specific treatment, although many, many writers take it as axiomatic that the emotional effects of child abuse and/or neglect should be addressed in an explicitly focused treatment.[21] Do clinicians actually need a new "abuse treatment," or would they be better served in their work by enriching their understanding of the epidemiology, risk factors, and putative sequelae of child abuse and using their knowledge and experience to conduct treatment? In the rush to provide child abuse treatment, this question has not been thoroughly discussed or answered.

Again, more anecdotal and qualitative research might be a timely contribution to the dialogue. The clinician sitting with individual patients and their families necessarily looks through different lenses and uses a different set of operating assumptions than does the empirical data-gatherer. One helpful study that begins to close this divide is that of Beutler and Hill,[5] who investigated psychotherapy with adults who were abused as children. It describes "process" and "outcome" variables, which go into the assessment of treatment. This distinction begins to create a language with which to join treatment and descriptive studies.

EXAMINING ASSUMPTIONS

A necessary fact of psychological research is that most of the results of research studies rely on correlational measures for their validity. While the correlational studies are essential to the isolation and characterization of any phenomenon affecting individuals, they do not address causation. Thus, while there is little doubt that abuse of any kind is bad for children and is associated with both deficits in personality and ego functioning and dysfunctional behavior, there is no proof that such symptoms are not in fact caused by other phenomena or by other phenomena in concert with the acts of abuse. Briere[6] referred to this when he reflected that the long-term sequelae of child abuse could possibly be accounted for by another variable. The rush to abuse-specific treatment, while based on the overwhelming evidence that child abuse and neglect are associated with terrible psychological symptoms, is not necessarily, or logically, an improved approach to emotional recovery.

Some of the recent thinking in the field demonstrates these conceptual points. For instance, an interesting line of inquiry examines child sexual abuse within the context of attachment theory. Attachment theory grew out the work of Bowlby, Ainsworth, and others and regards the child's presentation in light of his or her relationship with the primary caretaker(s). It is a body of thought integral to developmental as well as child psychoanalytic theory and practice. The object relations school of psychoanalysis, which has much in common with the attachment group, has long tackled disruptions in functioning and in the ability to relate to others with individual child psychotherapy in conjunction with parent treatment. A consideration of abuse-related symptoms through the lens of this approach raises many previously unasked questions, such as "Would traditional psychotherapy's experience in addressing patterns of attachment have bearing on the treatment of abused children?" Currently this particular theoretical bridge does not exist, but the possibility that this approach could improve treatment does bolster the argument that treatment research should widen its scope even though many of the appeals in the existing literature call for more narrowly circumscribed variables.

It is sometimes assumed that child abuse was inadequately addressed in decades prior to the explosion of public debate on the topic. In fact, there are accounts in the literature as well as anecdotal reports that speak of chillingly casual denials of child abuse by therapists in previous decades. In spite of the great politicization of the topic in recent years, which threatens to discourage thoughtful investigation, therapists and patients alike have a hugely improved and informed standpoint from which to explore the topic, based in part on empirical research that details the warning signs, symptoms, and sequelae of child abuse.[17]

With greater awareness and a fair amount of professional shame, the field has rushed to find new treatments. There is, however, no body of research demonstrating that "old-fashioned" forms of treatment cannot help ameliorate the psychological damage of child abuse, even though there have been assertions to this effect. This may represent a case of the baby being thrown out with the bathwater. It may not. The question, however, appears to have been prematurely closed off in the scientific dialogue.

Another assumption implicit in the current treatment literature is that a child patient's talking about a trauma, or being reminded in sessions of a trauma, is proof of the efficacy of treatment. There is a historical tradition going back at least a century that considers catharsis as the curative factor in all treatment. However, the definition of catharsis may differ from practitioner to practitioner, and it is often reported that interventions which direct or encourage children to talk specifically about traumatic events are curative because the child does so.[6] This assumption has not been addressed in the scientific discussion, but needs to be carefully examined. There are two traditions at work which are diametrically opposed and which have neither been spelled out nor investigated as such. Newer approaches, which advocate frequent therapist-directed verbalizations specifically directed at abuse related statements or behavior, contrast with earlier, psychoanalytic assumptions that premature interpretations will harden the repression and hinder the child's ability to integrate the trauma. Both approaches attempt to help the child overcome traumatic experiences and to reintegrate at a higher level of functioning, but they use fundamentally different methods. Although many therapists report that the actual exchanges in sessions may not differ that much between the two styles, they are in fact based on different assumptions and need to be examined with that in mind.

THE THREAT OF MANAGED CARE

Many of the obstacles to full inquiry into child abuse, as with all research, are political or societal, although such influences are often seen only through the influence of monies spent on grants. Of all the current impediments to good treatment research, the most insidious and menacing of the current decade is the threat posed by the increasing power of managed care providers. The wresting of treatment decisions from clinicians by fiscal agents has already virtually eradicated the possibility of hospital-based inpatient treatment and has interrupted, discontinued, or eliminated outpatient care for countless children. It cannot help but have profound effects on the ability of investigators to examine all theoretically derived treatments for children. Its potential undermining of research may take numerous forms, which merit elaboration.

Most obviously, managed care has made long-term treatment (i.e., more than 20 sessions) unaffordable for the bulk of patients. This makes it all the more difficult to fully examine varying treatment approaches. It may have the effect of removing long-term treatment from the microscope of the researcher before its efficacy with abused children can be assessed. And, while clinical team discussions everywhere are ringing with complaint and frustration at the treatment that is not getting approved for child patients, there have not been even preliminary studies that systematically catalogue or begin to assess the impact of managed care on treatment.

The restrictions that managed care has placed on the type of treatment offered to abused children seriously compromise research efforts with ongoing patients. Because child abuse is not a reimbursable psychiatric diagnosis, clinicians are often endorsing the diagnosis of posttraumatic stress disorder (PTSD) in order to get extra sessions approved for their patients, even though it is not clear that the PTSD model fully applies to child abuse.[7] Alternatively, they are forced to consider other diagnoses, which describe mood or personality disturbances but do not capture the traumatic features of the patient's presentation. Thus, models of treatment are being subtly imposed on patients and their therapists without the benefit of thorough investigation.

As an example of this, consider group psychotherapy as a treatment for child abuse. Group therapy has been tried with physically and sexually abused children and is often advocated, in the belief that it best addresses the sense of stigmatization and social isolation experienced by abused youngsters.[24] As mentioned previously, however, there is simply not enough research to determine that this is unequivocally the case or that group psychotherapy is preferable to individual psychotherapy. Nonetheless, there is enormous pressure on outpatient settings to run groups and place children in them. This author has worked at four different hospitals in the last three years at which administrators pleaded for more group therapy assignments in order to enhance financial viability. In fact, there have been statements made to the effect that certain third-party contracts depend on maintaining a certain percentage of clinic caseload through group treatment. When a certain percentage of incoming patients is mandated to particular treatment modalities, that percentage will inevitably include traumatized children. A clinical direction is thus being dictated by economic forces, rather than by clinical expertise and empirical direction.

These prescriptions are occurring across all areas of treatment and are placing increasing pressure on professionals to provide "fast cures" for problems which are notoriously complicated and often seemingly intractable. There is an unfortunate and unintended synchrony between research, which seeks to isolate specific symptom patterns, and economic arbiters, whose inarguable goal is reducing cost. Both favor the quantifiable and the tangible—the researchers to meet the demands of scientific and statistical methodology, the third-party billers to reduce their costs. While social scientists understand that statistical methods are an approximate and necessarily inexact method of describing an exceptionally complicated reality, the health maintenance organizations and insurance companies may not. Child maltreatment is particularly vulnerable to reductionism, largely because of its complexity.

Disagreements about approaches and modes of therapy within the mental health professions have intensified as the many varieties of mental health practitioners compete for increasingly scarce resources. This poses the hazard of polarization and stifles scholarly discourse at the same time that it heightens the need for careful reflection. When treatments for child abuse were just beginning, greater support existed for experimental social programs and for multimodal simultaneous treatments. In the pioneering Tufts study of sexually exploited children,[26] patients had both a social worker and a therapist. At the present time virtually no one has the luxury of individual therapy, family casework, group psychotherapy, and parent support. The pressure of finding a single "right" treatment for child abuse can be horribly destructive to the necessarily nonlinear process of investigating treatment modalities and their relationships to improvement in the child and family.

CONCLUSION

There may be more agreement about the need for treatment research regarding child abuse and neglect than about any other single issue regarding abuse. It is a dramatic need, in some ways more urgent right now than additional epidemiological studies. The recent sensationalizing of the false memory controversy hints at the backlash that is always present when we speak aloud of something as emotionally distressing as child abuse. Without a firm commitment to scientific dialogue and a growing body of meaningful investigation, we as child advocates run the risk of losing credibility within the scientific and lay communities while increasing numbers of children are referred. The challenges and potential obstacles to valuable, critically sound inquiry are immense, but they must be faced, for the sake of knowledge and for the sake of the children we would help.

REFERENCES

1. Alexander PC.: Application of attachment theory to the study of sexual abuse. *J Consult Clin Psychol* 1992;60:185–195.
2. American Association for Protecting Children. *Highlights of official child neglect abuse reporting.* Denver, CO: American Humane Association. 1984.
3. Belsky J. Child maltreatment, an ecological integration. *Am Psychol* 1980;35:320–335.
4. Berliner L, Wheeler JR. Treating the effects of sexual abuse on children. *J Interpers Viol* 1988;2:415–434.
5. Beutler LE, Hill CE. Process and outcome research in the treatment of adult victims of child sexual abuse: Methodological issues. *J Consult Clin Psychol* 1992;60:204–212.
6. Briere J. Methodological issues in the study of sexual abuse effects. *J Consult Clin Psychol* 1992;60:196–203.
7. Bronfenbrenner U. *The ecology of human development.* Cambridge: Harvard University Press. 1979.
8. Buntain-Ricklefs J, Kemper K, Bell M, Babonis T. Punishments: What predicts adult approval. *Child Abuse Negl* 1994;18:945–955.
9. Celano MP. A developmental model of victims' internal attributions of responsibility for sexual abuse. *J Interpers Viol* 1992;7:57–69.
10. Cicchetti D, Carlson V. *Child maltreatment.* Cambridge: Cambridge University Press. 1989.
11. Cicchetti D, Rizley R. Developmental perspectives on the etiology, intergenerational transmission and sequelae of child maltreatment. *New Dir Child Maltreat* 1981;11:31–55.
12. Cohn AH, Daro D. Is treatment too late: What ten years of evaluative research tell us. *Child Abuse Negl* 1987;11:433–442.
13. Conte JR. Child sexual abuse: Awareness and backlash. *Future Child* 1994;4:224–232.
14. DePanfilis D. Social isolation of neglectful families: A review of social support assessment and intervention models. *Child Maltreat* 1996:1:37–52; *New Dir Child Maltreat* 1981;11:31–55.

15. Eth S, Pynoos RS. *Post-traumatic stress disorder in children.* Los Angeles, CA: American Psychiatric Association. 1985.

16. Finkelhor D. Current information on the scope and nature of child sexual abuse. *Future Child* 1994;4:31–53.

17. Finkelhor D. The sexual abuse of children: Current research reviewed. *Psychiatr Ann* 1987;17:233–241.

18. Finkelhor D. The trauma of child sexual abuse. *J Interpers Viol* 1988;2:348–366.

19. Friedrich WN. Child victims: Promising techniques and programs in the treatment of child abuse. *Advisor* 1991;4:2.

20. Friedrich WN, Jaworski TM, Berliner L, James B. Sexual abuse treatment practices: A survey. *Advisor* 1994;7:17–24.

21. James B. *Treating traumatized children.* Lexington, MA: Lexington Books. 1989.

22. Kaufman J, Zigler E. The intergenerational transmission of child abuse. In Cicchetti D, Carlson V (eds.), *Child maltreatment,* 129–150. Cambridge: Cambridge University Press. 1989.

23. Melton GB, Flood MF. Research policy and child maltreatment: Developing the scientific foundation for effective protection of children. *Child Abuse Negl* 1994;18:1–28.

24. Nelki JS, Watters J. A group for sexually abused young children: Unravelling the web. *Child Abuse Negl* 1989;13:369–377.

25. Oates RK, Bross DC. What have we learned about treating child physical abuse: A literature review of the last decade. *Child Abuse Negl* 1995;19:463–473.

26. Tufts–New England Medical Center: *Sexually exploited children: Service and research project.* Washington, DC: U.S. Department of Justice (Office of Juvenile Justice and Delinquency Prevention Grant 80-N-AX-001). 1982.

27. Williams LM. Adult memories of childhood abuse: Preliminary findings from a longitudinal study. *Advisor* 1992;5:19–21.

Index

abdominal trauma, 87, 127–129
abuse-focused therapy. *See* cognitive behavioral therapy; treatment; treatment, long-term
abuse histories, 18
  See also documentation of abuse; medical records
adolescent(s)
  dissociative, 24, 25
  sexual offenders, 294–296
  victims of abuse, 19, 26–27
adoption, 304, 310
adult survivors of sexual abuse
  disclosure of abuse by, 67–69
  physical examination of, 73–74
  posttraumatic stress disorder and, 70–71
  psychiatric diagnoses of, 71–72
  psychotherapy and, 72–73
  recovery of memories and, 69–70
  reporting abuse regarding, 74–75
  survivor movement, 75–76
  See also effects of abuse or neglect
affective processing. *See* cognitive behavioral therapy
age of victim
  effect on consequences of abuse, 343–344
  effect on diagnosis, 6, 110, 318–319
aggressive behavior
  in abused children, 16, 95, 120, 137, 146, 273, 350
AIDS, 5–7
alcoholism
  abusive or neglectful parents and, 174, 340
  family assessment and recognition of, 102, 176
  as long-term effect of child abuse, 60, 72
  Munchausen by proxy and, 221
  as risk indicator for parental abuse, 97
  See also substance abuse
American Academy of Pediatrics, 89, 167
  sexual abuse defined by, xv
American Professional Society on the Abuse of Children (APSAC), 203–204, 214

amnesia, selective, 69
  See also memories, of sexual abuse
anal trauma, 10
anger
  in professionals, 48, 50, 85
  as symptom of trauma in children, 15
anger management, 140–141, 143–144
animal abuse, as symptom of trauma in children, 102
anorexia nervosa. *See* eating disorders
anxiety
  management of, 140
  measures for, 139
  as symptom of trauma in children, 15
anxiety disorders, 55, 57, 66, 95
apathy-futility syndrome, 161
asthma, 60, 66
attachment theory, 31, 97–99, 351, 363
  and neglect, 159, 175
attention deficit hyperactivity disorder (ADHD), 16, 24, 101, 119, 121
autonomic arousal, as symptom of trauma, 99
autopsies, 88

battered child syndrome, 81, 304, 329
behavioral methods of treatment for offenders, 297–299
  See also cognitive behavioral therapy
bladder infections, 8, 59
bladder injuries, 128–129
blood transfusions, prohibition of, 187
body image concerns, in victims, 4–5, 67
  See also eating disorders
borderline personality disorder (BPD), 275–276
brain injuries, 86–87, 118–123
breast disease, association with child sexual abuse, 59
bruises, 87–88
bulimia nervosa. *See* eating disorders
burden of proof, 108–109, 252
  See also forensic evidence; legal considerations
burns, 87–88, 124–126

Library of Congress Cataloging-in-Publication Data

Treatment of child abuse : common ground for mental health, medical, and legal
practitioners / edited by Robert M. Reece.
  p. cm.
  Includes bibliographical references and index.
  ISBN 0-8018-6320-1 (alk. paper)
  1. Child abuse—Treatment. 2. Abused children—Rehabilitation. I. Reece,
Robert M.

RJ375.T74 2000
362.76'8'0973—dc21   99-048750